Skin Care Triad: Continence Management, Wound Care, and Therapeutic Positioning

D1451880

Skin Care Triad: Continence Management, Wound Care, and Therapeutic Positioning

Edited by

Jack L. Rook, M.D.
Private practice, Colorado Springs, Colorado

Lyn D. Weiss, M.D.
Clinical Associate Professor of Physical Medicine and Rehabilitation, State University of New York at Stony Brook School of Medicine, Stony Brook; Chairman and Director of Residency Training Program, Department of Physical Medicine and Rehabilitation, Nassau County Medical Center, East Meadow, New York

Deborah D. Hagler, P.T.
Owner and Chief Executive Officer, Cheyenne Mountain Alliance, Inc., Colorado Springs, Colorado

with 7 contributing authors

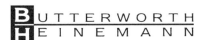

BUTTERWORTH
HEINEMANN

Boston   Oxford   Auckland   Johannesburg   Melbourne   New Delhi

Recognizing the importance of preserving what has been written, Butterworth–Heinemann prints its books on acid-free paper whenever possible.

 Butterworth–Heinemann supports the efforts of American Forests and the Global ReLeaf program in its campaign for the betterment of trees, forests, and our environment.

Library of Congress Cataloging-in-Publication Data
Rook, Jack L.
   Skin care triad : continence management, wound care, and therapeutic positioning / Jack L. Rook, Lyn D. Weiss, Deborah D. Hagler.
      p. cm.
   Includes bibliographical references and index.
   ISBN 0-7506-7035-5
   1. Urinary incontinence. 2. Wounds and injuries. 3. Patients--Positioning. 4. Physical therapy.   I. Weiss, Lyn D. II. Hagler, Deborah D. III. Title.

RC921.I5 R66 2000
616.6'3--dc21

                                                                      99-087183

British Library Cataloguing-in-Publication Data
A catalogue record for this book is available from the British Library.

The publisher offers special discounts on bulk orders of this book.
For information, please contact:
Manager of Special Sales
Butterworth–Heinemann
225 Wildwood Avenue
Woburn, MA 01801-2041
Tel: 781-904-2500
Fax: 781-904-2620

For information on all Butterworth–Heinemann publications available,
contact our World Wide Web home page at: http://www.bh.com

10 9 8 7 6 5 4 3 2 1

Printed in the United States of America

To our children, with our love and gratitude, for helping us keep our perspective on what is truly important

Alaina Rook
Jordan Rook
Ari Weiss
Helene Weiss
Stefan Weiss
Richard Weiss
Jamie Doolittle Hagler
Tiffany Flentje

To our patient and understanding spouses, Jay and Marlene, for their support, humor, encouragement, and understanding of the endless hours we spent on this work

Contents

I Continence Management

Section Editor: Jack L. Rook

II Wound Care

Section Editor: Lyn D. Weiss

III Therapeutic Positioning

Section Editor: Deborah D. Hagler

Contributing Authors

Sergey Bogdan, M.D.
Resident Physician, Department of Physical Medicine and Rehabilitation, Nassau County Medical Center, East Meadow, New York

Anna Dacanay, M.D., O.T.R.
Resident Physician, Department of Physical Medicine and Rehabilitation, Nassau County Medical Center, East Meadow, New York

Mery Elashvili, D.O.
Resident Physician, Department of Physical Medicine and Rehabilitation, Nassau County Medical Center, East Meadow, New York

Deborah D. Hagler, P.T.
Owner and Chief Executive Officer, Cheyenne Mountain Alliance, Inc., Colorado Springs, Colorado

Sara E. Kennedy, O.T.R.
Former Clinical Consultant, Cheyenne Mountain Therapies, Colorado Springs, Colorado

Nashin Manohar, D.O.
Resident Physician, Department of Physical Medicine and Rehabilitation, Nassau County Medical Center, East Meadow, New York

Daniel Mendez, M.D.
Chief Resident, Department of Physical Medicine and Rehabilitation, Nassau County Medical Center, East Meadow, New York

Rajshree Puri, M.D.
Resident Physician, Department of Physical Medicine and Rehabilitation, Nassau County Medical Center, East Meadow, New York

Jack L. Rook, M.D.
Private practice, Colorado Springs, Colorado

Lyn D. Weiss, M.D.
Clinical Associate Professor of Physical Medicine and Rehabilitation, State University of New York at Stony Brook School of Medicine, Stony Brook; Chairman and Director of Residency Training Program, Department of Physical Medicine and Rehabilitation, Nassau County Medical Center, East Meadow, New York

Preface

This text is the first of its kind. It contains comprehensive information on three highly specialized yet strongly interrelated fields of medicine: incontinence, wound care, and positioning. Specifically, the development of skin breakdown and pressure ulcers is often contributed to by improper patient positioning and moist skin caused by urinary incontinence. Optimal treatment of the patient with incontinence requires an awareness on the part of the clinician that moist skin is prone to maceration and breakdown. Optimal treatment of the individual who is elderly, debilitated, or both must incorporate techniques to minimize the sequelae of immobility. This requires a transdisciplinary approach involving nurses, physical and occupational therapists, speech-language pathologists, the patient and his or her family, and the physician. Only through control of incontinence and observance of proper positioning can the debilitated patient be protected against skin breakdown.

Chapters 1–19 are devoted to assessment and treatment of the patient with urinary incontinence. Included is a discussion of the anatomy and neurophysiology of the genitourinary tract (Chapters 1 and 2). Six chapters on assessment procedures for the incontinent patient follow, including the patient history and physical examination (Chapters 3 and 4) and laboratory, urodynamic, and imaging techniques (Chapters 5–7). Chapter 8 describes advanced electrophysiologic techniques used in the assessment of urinary incontinence. Medical complications associated with chronic urinary incontinence are discussed in Chapter 9. Chapters 10–17 each cover the assessment and treatment of a distinct type of urinary incontinence due to either anatomic changes (pelvic floor or sphincter incompetence, enlarged prostate, or extraurethral incontinence), neurologic injury (brain or spinal cord damage), or functional/environmental factors. Chapters 18 and 19 discuss two conditions characterized by prostate enlargement: benign prostatic hypertrophy and prostate cancer. These conditions can be associated with overflow incontinence.

The next section of the text (Chapters 20–26) describes various pressure ulcer types and their management. Included in this section are discussions of basic skin anatomy (Chapter 20), wound classification (Chapter 21), and stages in normal wound healing (Chapter 22). This background information provides a foundation for Chapters 23–25 on the etiology and management of pressure and vascular ulcers. Chapter 26 discusses wound care pain management, a previously neglected but currently evolving field of medicine that is truly in its infancy.

The final section of the book completes the skin care triad concept. Chapter 27, on therapeutic positioning, provides the reader with valuable techniques that can be used by the treatment team to facilitate wound healing and aid in the future prevention of wounds. Wounds may develop due to a whole host of causative factors, including cognitive, functional, environmental, nutritional, neurologic, and anatomic. The vast majority of ulcers are preventable when the caregiver(s) can identify and treat the etiologic factors expediently.

This book has been written to educate those personnel whose jobs involve helping individuals with incontinence and wounds. It is not written for a particular specialty, as currently there is no one group of clinicians who solely address this population of patients. Rather, multiple disciplines can benefit from the information presented here, including physicians, nurses, enterostomal therapists, speech-language pathologists, and physical and occupational therapists. As the field of wound care management grows, subspecialties within each discipline may develop—subspecialties that will require knowledge of salient topics within this text.

J. L. R.
L. D. W.
D. D. H.

Acknowledgments

We thank Sheila Slezak, Secretary, Nassau County Medical Center, East Meadow, New York, for her tireless assistance in the preparation of this manuscript; Dot Smith, for helping to inspire this text and the triad concept; Laurie Rappl, P.T., Span-America Medical Systems, Inc., Greenville, South Carolina, for her knowledge, insight, and tireless efforts to eradicate pressure ulcers; Wayne Rice, P.T., Hot Springs, Arkansas, and Cathy Starkey, P.T., Ft. Walton Beach, Florida, for their pioneering work in pressure ulcer resolution; Kathryn Elizabeth Greenarch Brown for her invaluable assistance with computer-enhanced graphics in Chapters 1–19 and 26; Dick Maxwell, Mary Kircher, and Casey Welch, librarians at Webb Memorial Library, Penrose Hospital, Colorado Springs, Colorado, for their assistance with references; Camie Nemeth; Timothy O. Hall, M.D.; Arlyn Robinson; Karen Oberheim and Leslie Kramer of Butterworth–Heinemann; and Kim Langford of Silverchair Science + Communications.

We also thank our fellow team members and the patients and families who have touched our lives and from whom we have learned. Without them, this book would not have been possible.

Skin Care Triad: Continence Management, Wound Care, and Therapeutic Positioning

I Continence Management

Section Editor: Jack L. Rook

1 Anatomy of the Urinary System

Jack L. Rook

Kidney

The kidneys are a pair of organs located adjacent to spinal levels T12 through L3.[1] Each kidney lies posterior to the peritoneum (retroperitoneum) on the posterior abdominal wall (Figure 1.1). The physiologic function of the kidneys is to remove excess water, salts, and products of protein metabolism from the blood and to maintain its pH. This collection of metabolic waste products removed from the blood, called *urine*, is conveyed to the urinary bladder by ureters.[2]

The fresh adult kidneys are reddish-brown in color and measure approximately 10 cm in length, 5 cm in width, and 2.5 cm in thickness. Each is shaped like a bean, with an extensive convex and smaller concave border. The renal artery enters the kidney through its concavity, known as the *renal hilum*, and the renal vein and ureter exit the organ (Figure 1.2).[1–3]

The cross-sectional anatomy of the kidney helps to explain urine transport. Two distinct sections are noted, the pelvis and the surrounding parenchyma. The renal parenchyma comprises a cortex and medulla that are visible to the unaided eye.[1] The cortex appears as a broad, red-brown, granular layer of tissue that lies immediately beneath the convex border and follows its contours.[3] The renal medulla contains the pyramids, which are conical-shaped structures with bases in the cortex and apices that approach the renal hilus. The renal cortex surrounds the medulla, forming columns and lobules that surround and fill the space between pyramids.[1] In contrast with the dark granular cortex, the cut surface of the medulla is lighter and has a striated appearance. The striations fan out from the apex of the pyramid to its broad base (Figure 1.3).[3]

The macroscopic appearance of the kidney is a reflection of its microscopic organization. The cortex appears granular in appearance secondary to the presence of glomeruli. The linear striations of the medulla are a reflection of the nephron loops and collecting tubules that pass through it.

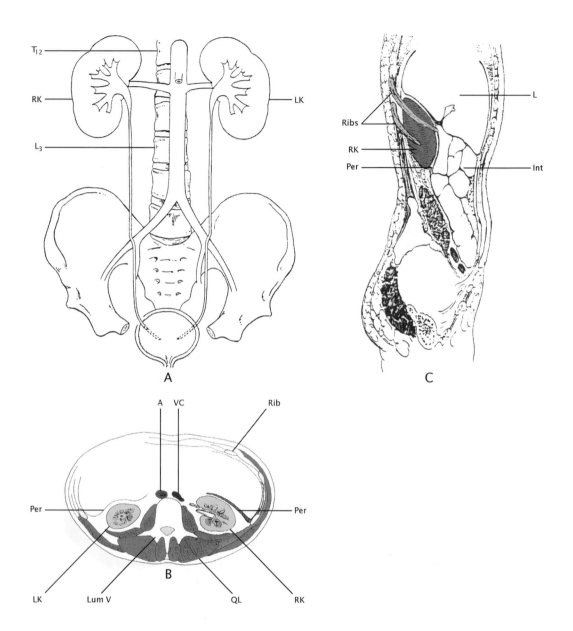

FIGURE 1.1   *Kidney location. (**A**) The kidneys are a pair of organs located adjacent to spinal levels T12 through L3. (**B**) Retroperitoneal location of kidneys (cross-sectional view). (**C**) Retroperitoneal location of kidneys (sagittal view). (T$_{12}$ = T12 vertebra; L$_3$ = L3 vertebra; RK = right kidney; LK = left kidney; Per = peritoneum; L = liver; Int = intestines; A = aorta; VC = vena cava; QL = quadratus lumborum; Lum V = lumbar vertebra.)*

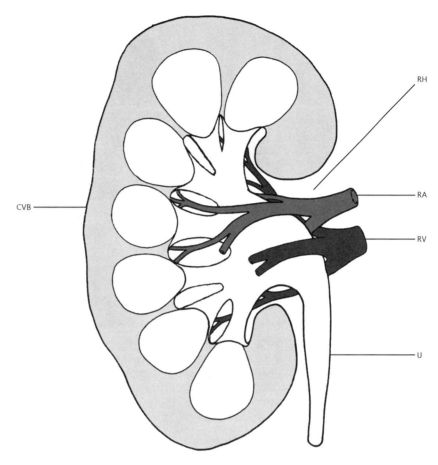

FIGURE 1.2   *The renal artery enters the kidney, and the renal vein and ureter exits through the renal hilum. (CVB = convex border of kidney; RH = renal hilum; RA = renal artery; RV = renal vein; U = ureter.)*

A capsule of dense connective tissue adheres to the renal cortex. The diaphragm, abdominal and quadratus lumborum muscles, as well as the overlying ribs further protect the kidneys. Collectively, these structures form a shock absorber and protective shield that guards each kidney against damage from blunt or penetrating trauma.[1]

Blood Supply of the Kidney

A renal artery, a relatively large vessel arising from the abdominal aorta, supplies each kidney, providing each kidney with large amounts of blood delivered under high pressure. Close to the renal hilus, the renal artery divides into two large branches from which five segmental arteries originate. From each segmental artery, further branches arise that ascend toward the cortex as the interlobar arteries. The interlobar arteries break up into arcuate arteries when they have almost reached

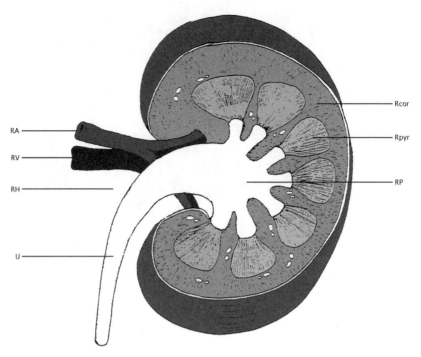

FIGURE 1.3   *The cross-sectional anatomy of the kidney as visible to the unaided eye demonstrates an outer renal cortex (Rcor) surrounding the renal medulla, both of which surround the renal pelvis (RP). The renal medulla constitutes a composite of individual renal pyramids (Rpyr) (conical-shaped structures with bases within the cortex and apices approaching the RP). The renal cortex surrounds the medulla, forming columns and lobules that surround and fill the spaces between the pyramids. (RA = renal artery; RV = renal vein; RH = renal hilum; U = ureter.)*

the corticomedullary border. The arcuate arteries arch over the bases of the medullary pyramids, giving off branches that ascend into the cortex. These smaller vessels run between lobules and are termed *interlobular arteries*. The interlobular arteries give off branches at wide angles on every side. Because these branches immediately enter the substance of surrounding lobules, they are called *intralobular arteries*. The intralobular arteries give rise to the afferent vessels that make up glomeruli (Figure 1.4).[3]

Renal veins are paired with the arteries and empty into the inferior vena cava (Figure 1.5).[1]

Glomerulus

As mammalian organisms became more complex, the blood circulatory system increased in importance in distributing oxygen and food to cells in different parts of the body and in carrying away the cell waste products. This

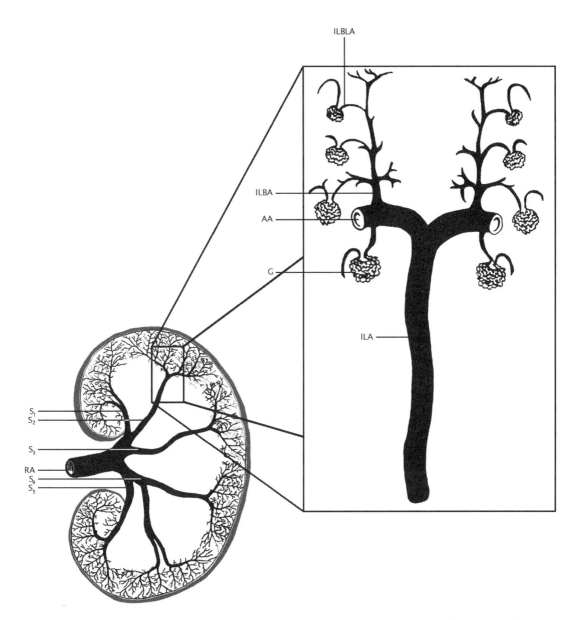

FIGURE 1.4   *The renal arterial system. The renal artery (RA) branches at the renal hilum into five seg-mental arteries (S1–S5). The segmental arteries further branch into interlobar arteries (ILAs), which ascend to the cortex where they further branch as the arcuate arteries (AAs) over the base of the medul-lary pyramid. Smaller arterial vessels that arise from the arcuate arteries and ascend into the cortex are the interlobular arteries (ILBAs), from which the intralobular arteries (ILBLAs) originate. The ILBLAs are the afferent vessels that make up the glomeruli (G).*

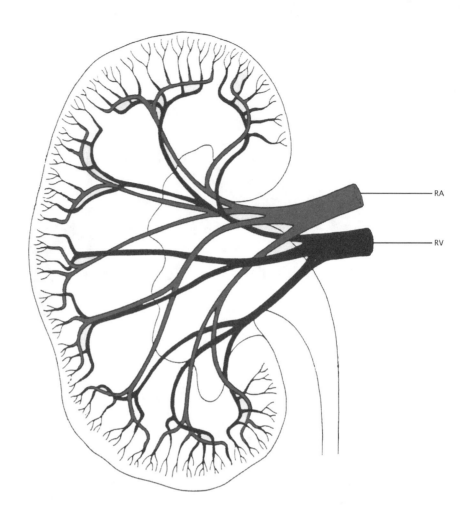

RA

RV

FIGURE 1.5   *The renal vein has branches that pair with the renal arterial system (RA). The renal vein (RV) carries blood, which empties into the inferior vena cava.*

required a mechanism by which waste products could continuously be removed from the blood. In the arrangement that evolved, excretory tubules were segregated and housed within the kidneys. A little cluster of capillaries formed in association with the blind end of each tubule. The human kidneys have millions of such tubules with this arrangement. The thin epithelium at the blind end of each tubule covers the capillaries that push into it. This little capillary cluster that projects into the blind end of each tubule is called a *glomerulus*, and the tissue fluid formed by it is called *glomerular filtrate*. As this filtrate passes along the remainder of the tubule, valuable substances are resorbed, so that the fluid that emerges from its external end as urine (and drains via the ureter into the urinary bladder) has waste products concentrated in it (Figure 1.6).[3]

The glomerular capillaries are designed to produce a tremendous amount of tissue fluid, more so than ordinary capillaries. Hydrostatic pressure remains high (60–70 mm Hg) along the full length of the glomerular capillary.

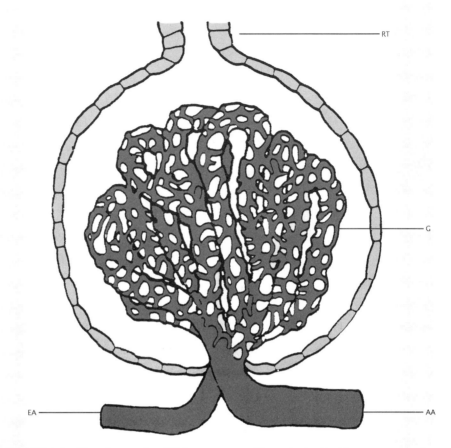

FIGURE 1.6 *The glomerulus (G) is porous capillary cluster that forms an associa-tion with one end of a renal tubule (RT). The afferent arteriole (AA) carries blood to the glomerulus, and the efferent arteriole (EA) carries blood away from it.*

The reason for the high pressure is that each glomerular drains, not into a wide, unobstructed venule, but into an arteriole that offers resistance to the outflow of blood. Because glomerular capillaries are supplied and drained by an arteriole, they actually represent a tuft of capillaries interposed along the course of an arteriole. The arteriole that supplies the glomerular capillaries is termed the *afferent arteriole*, and the arteriole into which the glomerular cap-illaries empty is the *efferent arteriole*. The lumen of the efferent arteriole is narrower than that of the afferent one, creating a situation in which the resis-tance to the exit of blood is enough to maintain a sufficiently high hydrostatic pressure within the glomerular capillary tuft (Figure 1.7).[3]

The endothelium of glomerular capillaries is also specially designed to promote the formation of glomerular filtrate. The cytoplasm of their endo-thelial cells is attenuated and riddled with pores. The pores have a diameter of approximately 1,000 Å. This weak, pore-riddled endothelium responds to blood being pumped into the capillaries under high pressure (60–70 mm Hg) by creating vast amounts of tissue fluid deposited directly into the blind end

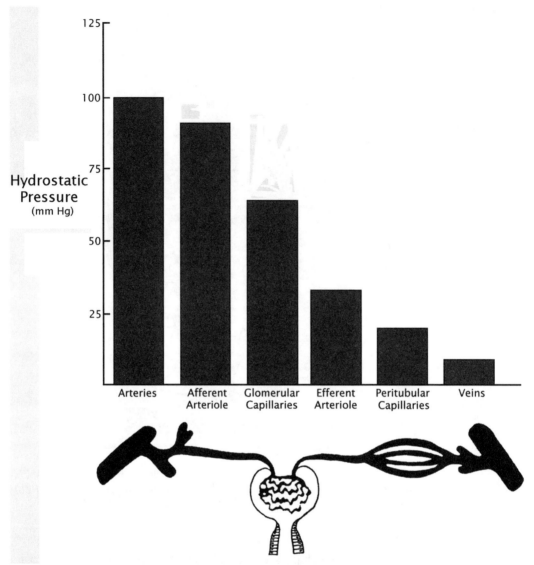

FIGURE 1.7   *The hydrostatic pressure remains high (60–70 mm Hg) along the full length of the glomerular capillary. The lumen of the efferent arteriole is narrower than that of the afferent arteriole, contributing to the high hydrostatic pressure within the glomerular capillary tuft.*

of the nephron. As soon as the tissue fluid passes through the epithelium covering the capillary, it is called *glomerular filtrate.*[3]

The total surface area of the capillaries of a glomerulus has been estimated and measured (there are well over 1 million glomeruli in each human kidney). The estimated total filtration surface of all glomeruli of both kidneys is well over a square meter.

The glomerular capillaries of the two kidneys produce from 170 to 200 liters of tissue fluid each 24 hours. As this fluid moves along the nephrons, almost 99% of it is resorbed through the walls of these tubules and back into the bloodstream.[3]

Nephron

The functional unit of structure of each kidney is the nephron. Each is an excretory tubule with a glomerulus pushed into its blind end. More than a million nephrons are in each human kidney. In a 24-hour period, 1,700 liters of blood pass through the kidneys via the renal arteries. Of these 1,700 liters that pass through glomeruli, 170 liters of tissue fluid (glomerular filtrate) are formed. Thus, every 24 hours, 170 liters of glomerular filtrate are delivered to the tubular portions of nephrons. As this fluid passes along the nephrons, more than 168 liters are resorbed back into the bloodstream so that only approximately 1.5 liters of it emerge into the two ureters each 24 hours to constitute the daily output of urine. Clearly, this is an efficient mechanism for tubular resorption of fluid.[3]

The tubular portion of each nephron exhibits three consecutive segments, which microscopically reveal different structural features, and physiologically perform somewhat different functions. These are termed the *proximal convoluted segment*, the *loop of Henle*, and the *distal convoluted segment*, respectively (Figure 1.8).[3]

Each nephron is so long that it can fit into a kidney only by pursuing a devious course through it. A nephron leads off from the glomerulus in the cortex and pursues a looped and tortuous course in the cortical tissue close to the glomerulus from which it originated. This proximal convoluted tubule then turns down to pursue a fairly straight course to the medulla. This segment of the nephron is termed the *descending limb of the loop of Henle*. The reason for the term *loop* is that the tubule, after descending for various distances into the medulla, loops back and reascends to the cortex. The part that ascends is called the *ascending limb of the loop of Henle*. The segment of the nephron that reenters the cortex is known as the *distal convoluted tubule*. It pursues a mildly tortuous course in the neighboring cortical tissue. It then joins a side branch of one of the many long and straight collecting tubules that extend from the cortex down through the medulla to open through the apex of the pyramid into the renal pelvis (see Figure 1.8).[3]

Collecting System

The collecting tubules comprise a series of drainage ducts into which urine is delivered by distal convoluted tubules. The collecting tubules are not part of the nephrons. They convey urine from nephrons to medullary papillae, where it empties into the calyces of the ureter. Many nephrons drain into each collecting tubule. The collecting tubules form a branched system. The largest ones are known as the *ducts of Bellini* (Figure 1.9).[3]

Renal function requires an obstruction-free, low-pressure transport and storage system from the renal pelvis to the urethral meatus. Disorders of urinary system transport, storage, or expulsive functions endanger urine formation when they lead to obstruction, elevated urinary system pressure, and stasis.[1] With obstruction, urine backs up and the kidney swells, a phenomenon known as *hydronephrosis*. Within the hydronephrotic kidney, no filtration can occur at the glomerular level. Unless

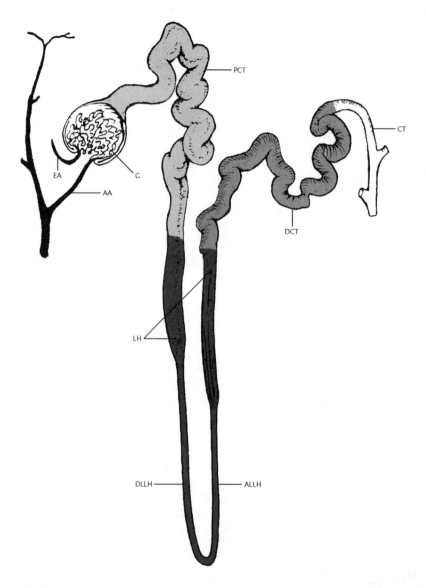

FIGURE 1.8   *The nephron pursues a long and tortuous course through the cortical and medullary renal tissue. The nephron segments include the proximal convoluted tubule (PCT), the loop of Henle (LH), and the distal convoluted tubule (DCT). Fluid generated by the glomerulus (G) travels through the PCT, enters the descending limb of the loop of Henle (DLLH), then passes through the ascending limb of the loop of Henle (ALLH), back into the cortex to join with the DCT that drains into the collecting tubule (CT). (AA = afferent arteriole; EA = efferent arteriole.)*

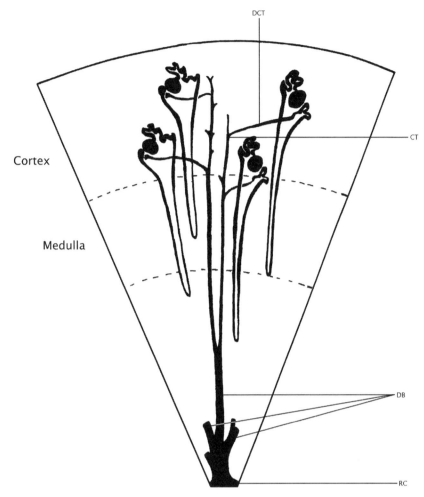

FIGURE 1.9 *The distal convoluted tubules (DCTs) of four nephrons enter into two collecting tubules (CTs) of the renal drainage system. Multiple CTs come together, forming the ducts of Bellini (DB), many of which coalesce and drain into a renal calyx (RC).*

corrected, this will cause a medical emergency, with electrolyte imbalances and potential permanent kidney damage.

Microscopic Appearance of the Kidney

One may ask why the cortex appears granular and the medulla striated on macroscopic inspection. The explanation lies in the microscopic appearance of the kidney. The cortex contains all of the glomeruli and all convoluted parts of the proximal and distal tubules. If a slice is cut through the kidney, the proximal and distal convoluted tubules, being tortuous, are cut in cross and oblique sections. Tubules cut this way, with glomeruli scattered among them, give the cortex a granular appearance when its cut surface is examined by the naked eye.[3] The microscopic appearance (Figure 1.10) delineates the various components that create the granular cortex.

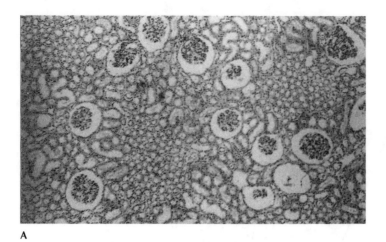
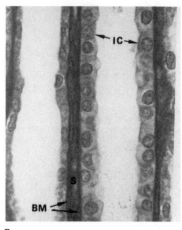

A   B

FIGURE 1.10   *(A) The microscopic appearance of the renal cortex demonstrates glomeruli scattered among cross and oblique sections of proximal and distal convoluted renal tubules. (B) The microscopic appearance of the renal medulla demonstrates a linear cellular arrangement that tends to run a fairly straight course. (BM = basement membrane; Ic = linear cellualr arrangement).*

In the medulla, the loops of Henle and collecting tubules both tend to run a fairly straight course, and the medullary macroscopic cross-sectional appearance is striated.[3] The microscopic appearance of the medulla confirms the linear cellular arrangement (see Figure 1.10).

Renal Pelvis and Ureters

Each kidney drains into the bladder via a renal pelvis and ureter. The renal pelvis is a funnel-shaped structure that originates at the major calyces and tapers into the ureter. The ureter is a continuous tube extending from the renal pelvis, its funnel shaped superior end, to the base of the bladder.[1]

The tube-shaped ureters are muscular ducts that propel urine toward the urinary bladder by peristaltic waves that occur in their walls. Each ureter is approximately 25 cm long and is an expansile, thick-walled, muscular tube with a narrow lumen.[2] The ureter lumen varies in diameter from 0.2 to 1.0 cm. Three areas of the lumen are particularly narrow and susceptible to obstruction by urinary stones, including the ureteropelvic junction, the point where the ureter crosses the iliac arteries, and the ureterovesical junction (Figure 1.11).[1]

Three layers define the microscopic anatomy of the ureters. The innermost layer, an epithelial mucosa consisting of transitional cell epithelium, is resistant to secretion or reabsorption of urine contents. A submucosal lamina propria, containing nerves, vascular elements, and fibroelastic connective tissue, lies just outside the epithelium. The lamina propria is bounded by the muscularis, a layer of smooth muscle.[1] The undistended ureter has a convoluted lumen (Figure 1.12).[4]

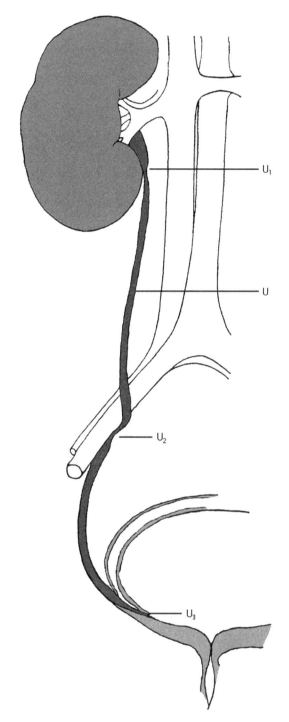

FIGURE 1.11   *Each ureter (U) is particularly narrow and susceptible to obstruction at three sites, including the ureteral pelvic junction (U_1), as the ureter passes over the iliac artery (U_2), and at the ureteral vesical junction (U_3).*

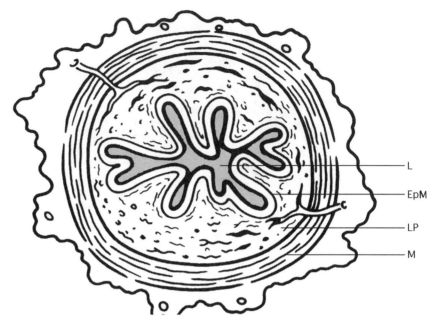

FIGURE 1.12 *Cross-section of a ureter demonstrating three layers, the epithelial mucosa (EpM), the lamina propria (LP), and the muscularis (M), all surrounding a convoluted lumen (L).*

The purpose of the ureteral muscularis is to transport urine from the kidneys to the bladder. Urine does not drain from kidney to bladder because of gravity as at first might be thought. Peristaltic-like waves of contraction sweep down the muscle of the ureter and force urine into the bladder.[3] The muscularis consists of an inner longitudinal and outer circular layer of smooth muscle. The renal pelvis and ureter transport urine from the kidney to the bladder in an antegrade fashion, a process called *efflux*.[1]

The renal pelvis stores only a small amount of urine (15–20 ml) before distension initiates a peristaltic wave, thought to originate from pacemaker cells in the calyces. A single peristaltic wave causes a chain of contraction that forces a bolus of urine through the entire ureteral course to the bladder.[1]

As each ureter enters the bladder wall, it loses its circularly disposed smooth muscle fibers. However, its longitudinal fibers continue through and attach to the wall of the bladder. The contraction of these longitudinally oriented, smooth-muscle fibers helps open the lumen of the ureterovesical segment so as to permit urine to be delivered into the bladder.[3]

The ureters pierce the bladder wall obliquely. The contraction of surrounding bladder detrusor muscle fibers during micturition tends to close the lumen of the ureter as it passes obliquely through the bladder. This, together with valvelike folds of bladder mucosa that

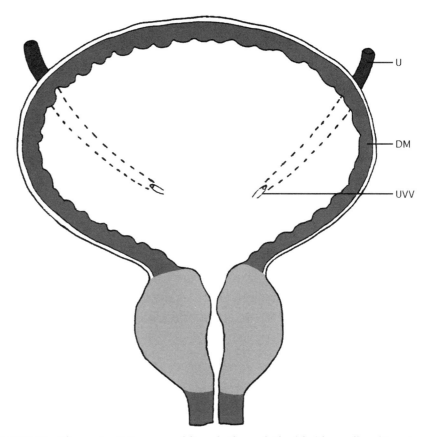

FIGURE 1.13 *The ureter (U) passes obliquely through the bladder wall and terminates at the ureteral vesicle valve (UVV), which opens into the bladder. (DM = detrusor muscle.)*

guard this entrance to the bladder, prevent contractions of the bladder wall from forcing urine back up the ureters in a retrograde fashion (Figure 1.13).[3]

Ureterovesical Junction

The ureterovesical junction represents a transition from the lower portion of the ureter to the adjacent bladder wall. The ureter enters the bladder at the lateral aspect of the trigone muscle. The portion of the ureter that travels through the bladder wall is unique from upper ureteral segments and is called the *intravesical ureter*.[1]

The intravesical ureter is approximately 1.5 cm long, and it terminates at the ureterovesical valve, which opens into the bladder (see Figure 1.13). The intravesical ureter also differs from upper ureteral segments in the arrangement of smooth muscle bundles. Whereas the upper ureteral segments form a complex meshwork of circular and longitudinal muscle layers, the intravesical ureteral muscle bundles are more simply arranged in a longitudinal fashion. These longitudinal muscle bundles span out and terminate in the trigone muscle of the bladder base.[1]

The ureterovesical junction allows urine to pass from the upper urinary tract (kidneys and ureters) to the lower urinary tract (bladder and urethra) and prevents regurgitation of urine in the opposite direction. The antegrade movement of urine from the upper to the lower urinary tract is called *efflux*, and retrograde movement from the bladder to the ureters or kidneys is called *reflux*.[1]

During bladder filling, intravesical pressure remains low and the detrusor muscle relaxed. Thus, pressure produced by peristaltic waves in the ureters propels spurts of urine through the ureterovesical junction into the bladder. In contrast, during micturition, intravesical pressure is elevated for awhile, favoring reflux of urine from the bladder to the upper urinary tract. The ureterovesical junction prevents this unfavorable condition. Immediately before the detrusor muscle contracts, the trigone muscles adjacent to the intravesical ureters contract, functionally closing off its lumen and preventing any urine from moving through the junction. This tone is maintained for approximately 20 seconds after micturition has been completed. Then, the trigone muscles relax, efflux of urine resumes, and the bladder begins to refill with urine.[1]

Urinary Bladder

The urinary bladder is a hollow organ with strong muscular walls located in the pelvis. It is characterized by its distensibility. Its shape, size, and position vary with the amount of urine it contains. An empty bladder lies entirely in the pelvis. As it fills, the bladder dome and upper aspect enter the abdomen, approaching the level of the umbilicus.[1,5]

The bladder is interrupted by three openings: The ureterovesical valves mark the termination of the intravesical ureters; at its most inferior aspect, a single outlet, the bladder neck, connects the bladder to the urethra. The bladder neck and base shape remain fixed, regardless of how much urine the bladder contains. In contrast, the upper parts of the bladder can change shape in response to varying urine volume. The bladder dome enters the abdomen as it fills to 300 ml or more.[1]

The macroscopic appearance of the bladder demonstrates layers of the wall similar to those of the ureter, but the thick muscular coat of the bladder is distinctive. The mucosa in the empty bladder is thrown into numerous folds, which are obliterated when it is distended. Transitional epithelium (urothelium) lines the inner bladder, as in the ureter. However, the bladder epithelium has more cell layers. The vascular submucosa (lamina propria), a thick muscularis layer, and the adventitia lie below the epithelial layer.[4]

The mucous membrane in the empty contracted bladder is thrown into numerous folds or rugae, except in the trigone where the mucous membrane is always smooth because here it is firmly attached to the muscular wall. The openings of the ureters and the urethra are located at the base of the bladder and form the angles of the trigone. The ureters pass

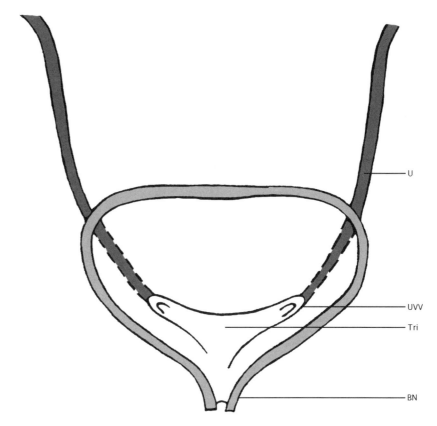

U

UVV

Tri

BN

FIGURE 1.14   *The trigone (Tri) of the bladder extends from the interureteric ridge (between the two ureteral vesical valves [UVVs]) and the bladder neck (BN). The trigone and the BN function as the bladder base, the most fixed aspect of the bladder. (U = ureter.)*

obliquely through the bladder wall, which helps to prevent urine from backing up into the ureter. An increase in intraluminal bladder pressure presses the walls of the ureters together at the ureterovesical junction, preventing reflux and kidney damage. The two orifices of the ureters are connected by the narrow interureteric ridge, the superior margin of the trigone.[5] The trigone and bladder neck function as the bladder base, the most fixed aspect of the bladder, and the rest of the bladder, including the dome, is known as the *bladder body* (Figure 1.14).[6–8]

The lamina propria lies immediately beneath the urothelium. It consists of connective tissue, arteries, veins, lymphatic channels, and nerves. Some of the nerve fibers relay afferent information to the central nervous system about bladder stretch and distension. The smooth muscle bundles of the bladder wall are collectively referred to as the *detrusor muscle*. The adventitia layer of the bladder is composed of connective tissue.[1]

The microscopic anatomy of the bladder is also characterized by these four layers, the urothelium, the vascular submucosa, the smooth muscle bundles of the detrusor, and the protective adventitia (Figure 1.15). The

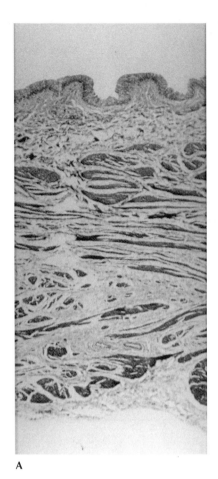
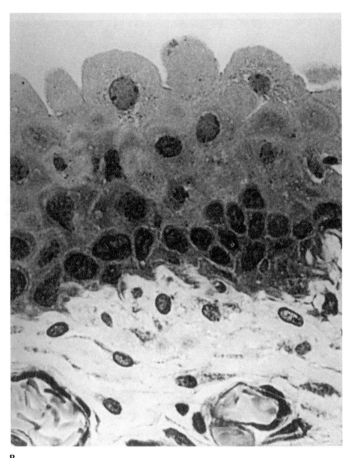

A   B

FIGURE 1.15   **(A)** *The microscopic anatomy of the bladder is characterized by four layers, the urothelium, the vascular submucosa, the smooth muscle bundles of the detrusor, and the outer adventitia.* **(B)** *The urothelium is made up of transitional epithelial cells that are six to eight cells deep in the empty bladder.*

urothelium is made up of transitional epithelial cells that are six to eight cells deep in the empty organ. As the bladder fills, the urothelium increases its surface area to accommodate the increasing volume of urine by stretching to only two to three cells thick. The urothelium is remarkable for its impermeability to reabsorption of water or solutes, a characteristic necessary to prevent reaccumulation of urinary waste products within the systemic circulation before micturition.[1]

The muscularis is composed of a thick coat of muscle fibers arranged in anastomosing bundles, between which is loose connective tissue.[4] The wall of the bladder is composed chiefly of these smooth muscle fibers collectively called the *detrusor muscle*. The detrusor consists of three layers, external and internal layers of longitudinal fibers and a middle layer of circular fibers.[5]

The trigone musculature continues into the circumferential smooth muscle of the proximal urethra.

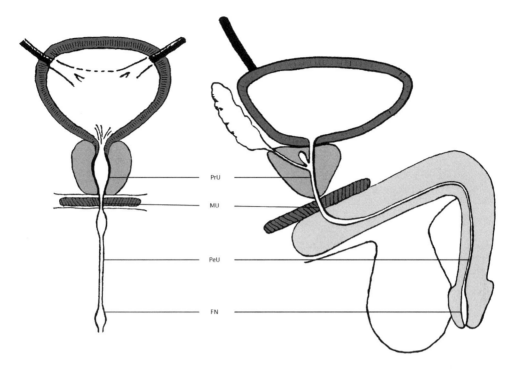

FIGURE 1.16 *The male urethra is divided into three segments, the prostatic urethra (PrU), the membranous urethra (MU), and the penile urethra (PeU). The PrU extends through the prostate, the MU pierces the pelvic diaphragm, and the PeU travels through the penis to its termination at the fossa navicularis (FN).*

Urethra

The urethra extends from the bladder neck to an external meatus. It has a sphincter mechanism that serves the dual purpose of preventing leakage between episodes of micturition and serving as a nonobstructive conduit during urination.[1]

Male Urethra

The urethra in the male, a channel 15–20 cm long, conveys urine from the urinary bladder to the external urethral orifice (meatus) located at the tip of the glans penis. For descriptive purposes, the male urethra is divided into three segments (prostatic urethra, membranous urethra, and penile urethra).[5] After exiting the bladder at the bladder neck, the proximal prostatic urethra extends approximately 3 cm through the prostate. Just below the prostate, the membranous urethra pierces the pelvic floor muscles (pelvic diaphragm, urogenital diaphragm). The distal most penile urethra travels from the membranous segment, through the penis, to its termination at the fossa navicularis (a dilatated chamber that lies near the corona of the glans penis) (Figure 1.16).[1]

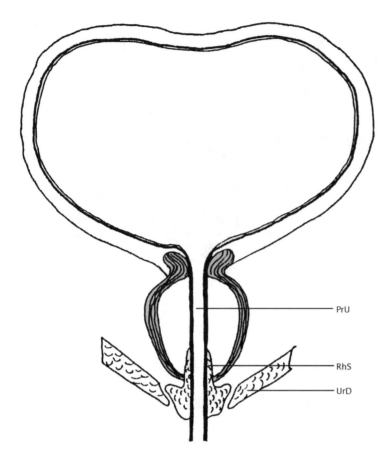

PrU

RhS

UrD

FIGURE 1.17   *The external voluntary sphincter mechanism is made up of a rhabdosphincter (RhS) (which consists of smooth muscle fibers of the prostatic urethra [PrU] that merge with periurethral striated muscle fibers) and the urogenital diaphragm (UrD).*

The prostatic urethra begins at the internal sphincter, at the apex of the trigone. It descends through the prostate, and ends at the superior layer of fascia overlying the urogenital diaphragm.[5] The prostatic urethra contains both smooth and striated muscle. The smooth muscle comes from the bladder trigone and extends down through the proximal portion of the prostatic urethra. Within the prostate, the smooth muscle merges with specialized C-shaped periurethral striated muscle fibers (rhabdosphincter), which in conjunction with the urogenital diaphragm makes up the external voluntary sphincter mechanism (Figure 1.17).[6, 9]

Due to the close relationship of the prostate to the prostatic urethra, enlargement (hypertrophy) of the gland may obstruct the urethra. Such an obstruction can be relieved by a transurethral resection of the prostate.[5]

The second part of the male urethra, the membranous urethra, is the shortest and narrowest portion (approximately 1 cm long) of the urethral segments. It descends from the apex of the prostate to the bulb of the penis and traverses the muscle of the urogenital diaphragm. Its narrowness results from the surrounding sphincter musculature, which also makes the membranous urethra the least distendible part of the channel.[5]

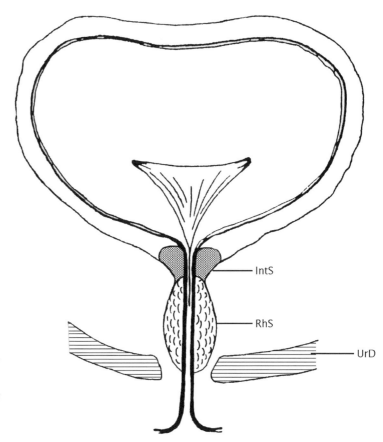

FIGURE 1.18   *At the base of the bladder is the internal urethral sphincter (IntS) made up of smooth involuntary muscle bundles. The voluntary sphincter mechanism consists of specialized striated muscle fibers, the rhabdosphincter (RhS), and the pelvic floor urogenital diaphragm (UrD).*

The third part of the male urethra, the penile urethra, is the longest urethral segment (approximately 15 cm). It begins where the urethra passes into the corpus spongiosum of the penis and ends at the external urethral orifice. Its lumen is approximately 5 mm in most places, but is expanded in the bulb of the penis to form the fossa navicularis.[5]

Female Urethra

Compared with the male system, the female urethra traces a relatively short, straight course from the bladder neck to the external meatus. It is made up of a single segment that corresponds to the prostatic and membranous parts of the male urethra.[1,5]

The female urethra is a short (2–6 cm) muscular tube lined by mucous membrane.[5] At the base of the bladder is the internal urethral sphincter, which contains smooth (involuntary) muscle bundles. Its middle third is lined by specialized, C-shaped striated muscle fibers (rhabdosphincter) that, along with the periurethral pelvic floor striated muscles (urogenital diaphragm), form the external voluntary sphincter mechanism (Figure 1.18).[1, 6]

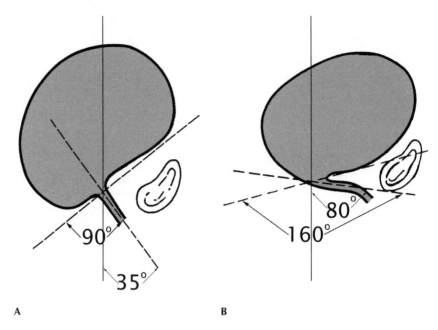

FIGURE 1.19 **(A)** The normal urethral vesicle angle is 90 degrees and the normal vertical urethral angle 30–35 degrees. The presence of normal angles indicates a well-supported bladder and urethra. **(B)** Increases in the vertical urethral angle to more than 35 degrees and an increase in the urethral vesicle angle to more than 100 degrees may indicate loss of urethral support, increased urethral mobility, and poor pelvic support, all of which may be associated with incontinence.

The female urethra is shorter and less complex than that of the male. Urethral resistance depends more on proper orientation of the bladder neck and a competent internal sphincter, and less on the external sphincter. The ovarian hormone, estrogen, modulates the integrity of pelvic floor muscles in women. In premenopausal women, estrogen helps maintain the tone of these structures by stimulating estrogen receptors in the pelvic floor musculature.[6,10]

Anatomic features that help promote continence in women include a normal angle from the urethra to the bladder neck (urethrovesical angle: normal is 90 degrees); a normal vertical urethral angle (30–35 degrees); and a normal urethral length. The presence of normal angles indicates a well-supported bladder and urethra. Increases in the vertical urethral angle to more than 35 degrees may indicate loss of urethral support with increased urethral mobility. Increases in the urethrovesical angle to more than 100 degrees may indicate poor funneling of the bladder neck. Such abnormalities suggest poor pelvic support and may be associated with incontinence (Figure 1.19).[6]

Pelvic Floor Muscles

The pelvic floor muscles, the two levator ani muscles and two coccygeus muscles, form the funnel-shaped pelvic diaphragm (Figure 1.20).[5] The pelvic floor muscles extend from the anterior to the posterior aspects of the bony pelvis, forming a sling that supports the pelvic contents.

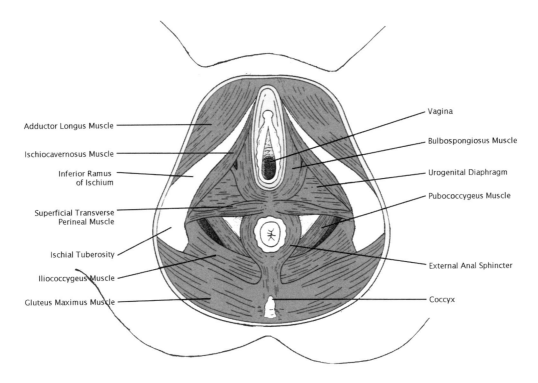

Adductor Longus Muscle

Ischiocavernosus Muscle

Inferior Ramus
of Ischium

Superficial Transverse
Perineal Muscle

Ischial Tuberosity

Iliococcygeus Muscle

Gluteus Maximus Muscle

Vagina

Bulbospongiosus Muscle

Urogenital Diaphragm

Pubococcygeus Muscle

External Anal Sphincter

Coccyx

FIGURE 1.20   *The pelvic floor muscles (pelvic diaphragm) extend from the anterior to the posterior aspects of the bony pelvis, forming a sling that supports the pelvic contents. The urethra, vagina, and anal canal perforate the pelvic diaphragm.*

The pelvic diaphragm is the fibromuscular floor of the confluent abdominopelvic cavity that supports the contents of the pelvis (urethrovesical unit, rectum, and reproductive organs).[1,5] The pelvic diaphragm is perforated by the urethra and the anal canal in the male and by the urethra, the vagina, and the anal canal in the female.[5] The pelvic floor periurethral muscles contribute to the urethral external sphincter mechanism.[1] These muscles are striated and under control of the somatic (voluntary) nervous system.

To help maintain continence, the muscular pelvic diaphragm supports the pelvic viscera and resists the downward thrust accompanying increases in intra-abdominal pressure. In contrast, during micturition the two levator ani muscles contract, and along with the anterior abdominal muscles assist in compressing the abdominal and pelvic contents. This action is an important part of micturition.[5]

References

1. Gray M. Color Atlas of Genitourinary Anatomy and Physiology. In M Gray (ed), Genitourinary Disorders. St. Louis: Mosby, 1992;1–19.
2. Moore KL. The Abdomen. In KL Moore (ed), Clinically Oriented Anatomy. Baltimore: Williams & Wilkins, 1980;121–292.

3. Ham AW. The Urinary System. In AW Ham (ed), Histology. Philadelphia: JB Lippincott, 1974;744–781.
4. Di Fiore MSH. Excretory System. In MSH Di Fiore (ed), Atlas of Human Histology. Philadelphia: Lea & Febiger, 1979;172–181.
5. Moore KL. The Perineum and Pelvis. In KL Moore (ed), Clinically Oriented Anatomy. Baltimore: Williams & Wilkins, 1980;293–418.
6. Wheeler JS, Peters MJ. Anatomy and Physiology of Voiding. In DB Doughty (ed), Urinary and Fecal Incontinence—Nursing Management. St. Louis: Mosby, 1991;1–22.
7. Elbadawi A. Neuromorphologic basis of vesicourethral function. I. Histochemistry, ultrastructure, and function of the intrinsic nerves of the bladder and urethra. J Neurourol Urodyn 1982;1:3.
8. Elbadawi A, Schenk EA. Dual innervation of the mammalian urinary bladder: a histochemical study of the distribution of cholinergic and adrenergic nerves. Am J Anat 1966;119:405.
9. Clegg EJ. The musculature of the human prostatic urethra. J Anat 1959;91:345.
10. Tapp AJS, Cardozo LD. The post-menopausal bladder. Br J Hosp Med 1986;35:20.

2   The Neurophysiology of Micturition

Jack L. Rook

The bladder functions as a filling and storage compartment for urine. At controlled intervals, the bladder also expels its contents through the process of micturition. In adults, voluntary control of micturition via normal functioning of the urethrovesical unit is called *urinary continence*. Urinary continence relies on three mechanisms: an anatomically intact urinary system; integration of neural impulses between regions in the brain, spinal cord, and peripheral nervous system; and a competent urethral sphincter mechanism.[1] This chapter is a discussion of the second mechanism, the neurophysiology of micturition.

Maintaining continence requires neural modulation between the brain, spinal cord, and peripheral nervous system. An ascending system exists that transmits information about bladder distension to the central nervous system. Sensory receptors in the bladder wall respond to distension, sending impulses through peripheral nerves to the dorsal horn of the spinal cord, stimulating an ascending system that travels to the brain. At the pontine level are synapses with third-order cells, which relay information about bladder distention to cortical brain centers in the frontal cortex (Figure 2.1).

A descending system also exists that starts in the frontal cortex and travels to the pons, spinal cord, and, ultimately, to the bladder (Figure 2.2). Information from the pontine micturition center travels to two spinal cord regions: the thoracolumbar spinal cord (origin of the sympathetic nervous system [SNS]); and the sacral spinal cord between segments S1 and S4 (origin of the sacral parasympathetic and somatic nervous system).

The sympathetic and parasympathetic nervous systems are components of the autonomic nervous system (ANS). The ANS differs from the somatic nervous system in that it plays a major role in bladder functioning. The SNS modulates bladder filling, while the parasympathetic nervous system (PNS) modulates bladder emptying, both involuntary

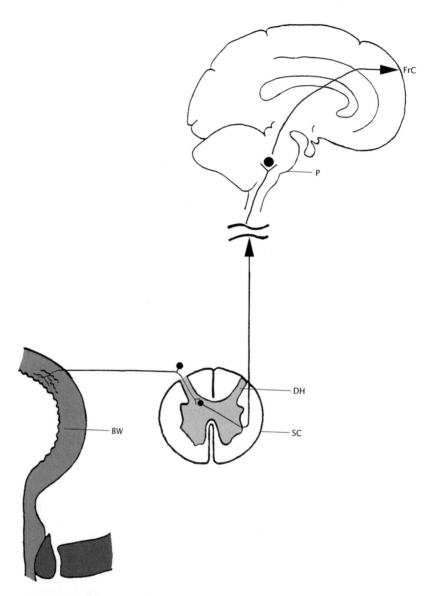

FIGURE 2.1 *The ascending system transmits information about bladder distention to the central nervous system. Sensory receptors in the bladder wall (BW) send impulses through peripheral nerves into the dorsal horn (DH) of the spinal cord (SC). A second-order sensory neuron travels from the spinal cord to the brain, stimulating third-order cells in the pons (P) that relay the information about bladder distention to cortical brain centers in the frontal cortex (FrC).*

phenomena. In contrast, the somatic nervous system modulates voluntary control of the external sphincter.[1,2]

The net effect of the cortical influence on the process of micturition is to suppress detrusor contraction until the individual wishes to urinate. It does this through inhibitory synapses with the pontine micturition center. In a continent adult, the pons initiates voiding only when "permis-

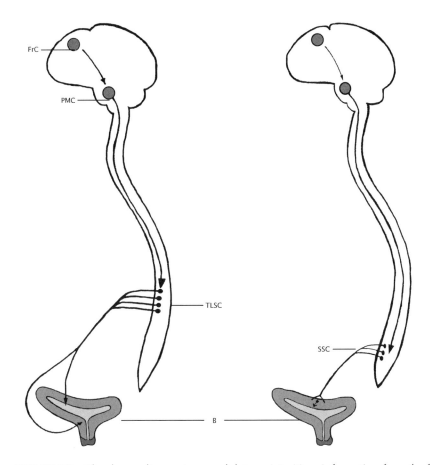

FIGURE 2.2   *The descending system modulates micturition. Information from the frontal cortex (FrC) travels to the pontine micturition center (PMC) carrying information about inhibition or initiation of micturition. Pathways from the PMC then travel to two spinal cord regions, the thoracolumbar spinal cord (TLSC) and the sacral spinal cord (SSC). Information from these spinal cord regions then travels via peripheral nerves to the urinary bladder (B).*

sion" has been given by higher brain centers. The response is a contraction of the bladder and coordinated relaxation of pelvic floor muscles, allowing efficient emptying.[1]

Neurologic Modulation of the Bladder and Sphincters (Urethrovesical Unit)

Afferent or Ascending Sensory Pathways

Sensory information concerning bladder filling and increasing bladder tension is relayed to the spinal cord and brain via somatic afferent

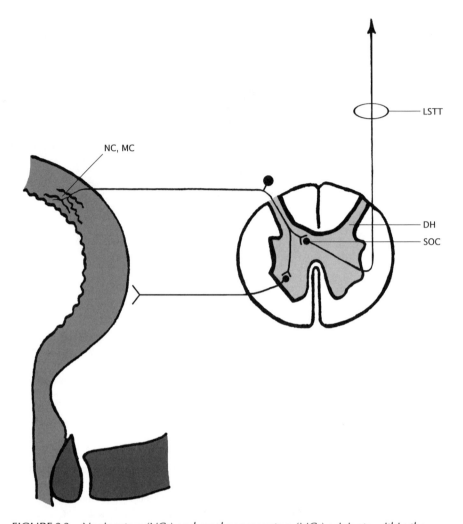

FIGURE 2.3 *Nociceptors (NCs) and mechanoreceptors (MCs) originate within the bladder wall. Their fibers travel via the autonomic and pudendal nerves into the dorsal horn (DH) of the spinal cord where synapses occur with second-order pain transmission cells (SOCs). The axons from the second-order cells cross the spinal cord to the lateral spinothalamic tract (LSTT), and the afferent information ascends toward the brain.*

nerve pathways. Pain and mechanical receptors (nociceptors and mechanoreceptors) originate within the bladder wall. Information about stretching of the bladder wall and mucosal pain is mediated via afferent nerve pathways that emanate from these receptors. As the bladder fills, impulses concerning distension and eventually pain travel via the pelvic, hypogastric, and pudendal nerves into the dorsal horn of the spinal cord. There, they set off local reflexes to maintain bladder tone. Synapses occur with second-order cells whose axons cross the spinal cord to the lateral spinothalamic tract where these fibers ascend to the brain (Figure 2.3).

More activity exists within second-order spinal cord transmission cells as the bladder further distends. Third-order cells within the pons transmit this information to cortical centers that produce sensation and ultimately help to modulate voluntary control of the bladder.[1,3,4]

Descending Pathways That Influence Bladder Activity

Two distinct descending pathways exist, which begin in the cortex of the brain that have an influence on bladder activity; the autonomic (corticoreticular and reticulospinal) tracts and the corticospinal tract. The corticoreticular and reticulospinal tracts control bladder activity through an effect on the sympathetic and parasympathetic nerve centers within the spinal cord. On the other hand, the corticospinal tract follows an uninterrupted course from the motor cortex to the sacral spinal cord alpha and gamma motor neurons. This pathway controls the voluntary, striated external sphincter (Figure 2.4).[2,5]

A detrusor motor area is located in the frontal cerebral cortex. The thalamus, hypothalamus, basal ganglia, and, possibly, the limbic system also influence bladder function. All of these brain regions have synaptic connections with the brain stem's pontine micturition center.[1]

The pontine micturition center plays an important role in controlling the detrusor reflex. Two regions (nuclei) within the pons directly modulate the act of micturition. One nuclear center instigates the detrusor reflex, while the other nucleus coordinates pelvic floor relaxation with the bladder contraction.[1,6,7]

The pontine micturition center is controlled by the frontal cortex, which can either facilitate or inhibit pontine activity. Hence, impulses to inhibit detrusor contraction are transmitted from the frontal cortex to the pons via the corticoreticular tract. The pontine impulses then travel along the reticulospinal tract to the sympathetic thoracolumbar outflow, effectively inhibiting detrusor contraction (see Figure 2.4).[2] In infants, the pontine micturition center acts without input from higher centers in the brain. Thus, the infantile pons responds directly to afferent input from stretch receptors in the bladder, producing a reflex voiding response coordinated to filling with urine, without cortical inhibitory control.[1]

Reticular formation refers to a matrix of nuclei in the core of the brain stem. The pontine micturition center (part of the reticular formation) receives a large input from the frontal cortex via corticoreticular fibers. The pontine reticular formation gives rise to a major projection of fibers that go to the spinal cord. These are uncrossed pontine reticulospinal tract fibers. This tract conveys information from higher levels to the preganglionic sympathetic and parasympathetic neurons to influence bladder function and sphincter muscle control of the urinary tract (see Figure 2.4).[5]

Autonomic sympathetic nerve pathways originate at the thoracolumbar cord (T11 to L2), and travel to the bladder neck and proximal urethra. SNS activity supports urine storage by stimulating sphincter muscle fibers in the bladder neck and proximal urethra to contract. Autonomic parasympathetic nerve pathways originate at the sacral

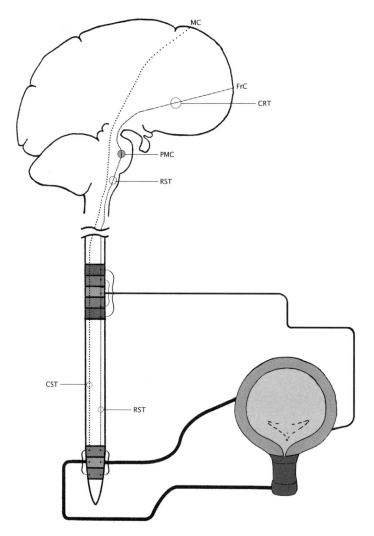

FIGURE 2.4 *Two distinct descending pathways begin in the cortex of the brain and influence bladder activity. An autonomic pathway travels via the cortical reticular (CRT) and reticulospinal (RST) tracts from the frontal cortex (FrC) to the pontine micturition center (PMC), and then to sympathetic and parasympathetic nerve centers within the spinal cord. The cortical spinal tract (CST) follows an uninterrupted course from the motor cortex (MC) to alpha and gamma motor neurons in the sacral spinal cord.*

cord (S2 through S4). Parasympathetic fibers travel to the bladder wall and support emptying of the bladder by stimulating detrusor contraction (Figure 2.5).[1,2]

Somatic (voluntary) efferent nerve pathways originate in the motor cortex. These upper motor neuron fibers travel via the corticospinal tract to the pudendal nucleus in the sacral spinal cord (bypassing the pons). Local fibers originate at the sacral cord (S2 through S4) pudendal nucleus. These lower motor neuron fibers originate from the pudendal nucleus

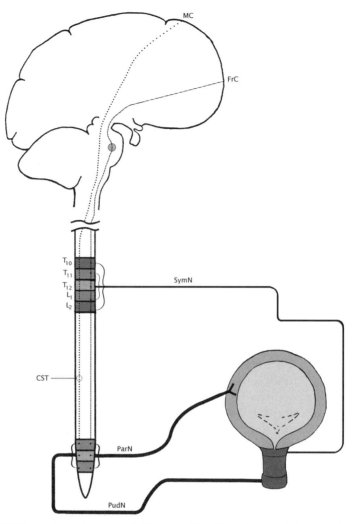

FIGURE 2.5 *Autonomic sympathetic nerve (SymN) pathways originate at the thora-columbar spinal cord (T10–L2) and travel to the bladder neck and proximal urethra. Autonomic parasympathetic nerves (ParN) originate at the sacral cord (S2–S4) and travel to the bladder wall, stimulating detrusor contraction. Upper motor neuron fibers travel from the motor cortex (MC), through the cortical spinal tract (CST) to the pudendal nucleus in the sacral cord (S2–S4). Lower motor neuron fibers originate from the puden-dal nucleus and travel through the pudendal nerve (PudN) to muscles of the pelvic floor and external sphincter. (FrC = frontal cortex.)*

and travel through the pudendal nerve to muscles of the pelvic floor and striated external sphincter (see Figure 2.5).[2,5]

The upper motor neurons that originate in the cortex travel via the corticospinal tract also termed the *pyramidal tract*. The corticospinal tract passes through the posterior limb of the internal capsule, then breaks up into bundles, and finally recollects as a discrete bundle known as the *pyramid of the medulla*. Within each pyramid, most of the corticospinal tract fibers cross (decussate) to the opposite side.

This region is referred to as the *level of pyramidal tract decussation*. Approximately 90% of the fibers cross at this level and descend through the spinal cord as the lateral corticospinal tract. With respect to the urethrovesical unit, the lateral corticospinal tract has fibers that pass to the sacral portion of the spinal cord, synapsing on alpha and gamma lower motor neurons, which together make up the pudendal nerve. These motor neurons innervate striated muscles of the pelvic floor (under voluntary control) (see Figure 2.5).[5,8]

In summary, the external sphincter and other perineal muscles are composed of striated muscle innervated by motor fibers traveling within the pudendal nerve. Skeletal muscle activity results from the net influence of alpha and gamma motor neurons that originate within the ventral horn of the spinal cord. Collectively, these neurons are referred to as *lower motor neurons*. Their cell bodies reside within the central nervous system, and their axons make synaptic contact with striated muscles through myoneural junctions (motor endplates).[5]

Autonomic Nervous System

The ANS, although a part of the peripheral nervous system, is the functional division that innervates smooth and cardiac muscle, and glands of the body. It consists of motor fibers only. Individuals do not have control of their ANS. It functions at a subconscious level. For example, this system controls heart rate, blood pressure, opening and closing of the pupil, peristalsis within the gastrointestinal tract, bowel functioning, bladder functioning, and sexual functioning. The ANS regulates the activity of smooth and cardiac muscles and glands and integrates these activities with one another and with somatic motor function.[8]

Local reflex stimuli and integrative influences from the brain stem and hypothalamus govern autonomic neurons. The spinal cord acts as a mediator of messages from higher nervous centers in the brain and pons.[8]

Unlike the somatic motor system, the autonomic system reaches its effector organs by a two-neuron chain, the pre- and postganglionic neurons. The preganglionic neuron originates within the intermediolateral gray column of the respective spinal cord segment. The postganglionic neuron is located in an outlying ganglion and innervates the end organ.[8]

Both parasympathetic and sympathetic systems contain two neurons between the spinal cord and periphery. The first synapse for both systems is cholinergic (transmitting the neurotransmitter acetylcholine). For the sympathetic system, this synapse is either in the paravertebral chain of sympathetic ganglia or farther away in the prevertebral ganglion plexuses (Figure 2.6). The initial parasympathetic synapse typically lies close to or within the innervated viscera (Figure 2.7).[9]

The preganglionic fibers of the ANS have their cell bodies of origin in two regions of the spinal cord. The sympathetic division of the ANS consists of fibers that arise in the intermediolateral gray column of the lower thoracic and upper lumbar (thoracolumbar) segments of the spinal cord. The parasympathetic outflow fibers arise from intermediolateral cell bodies in the gray matter of sacral segments two

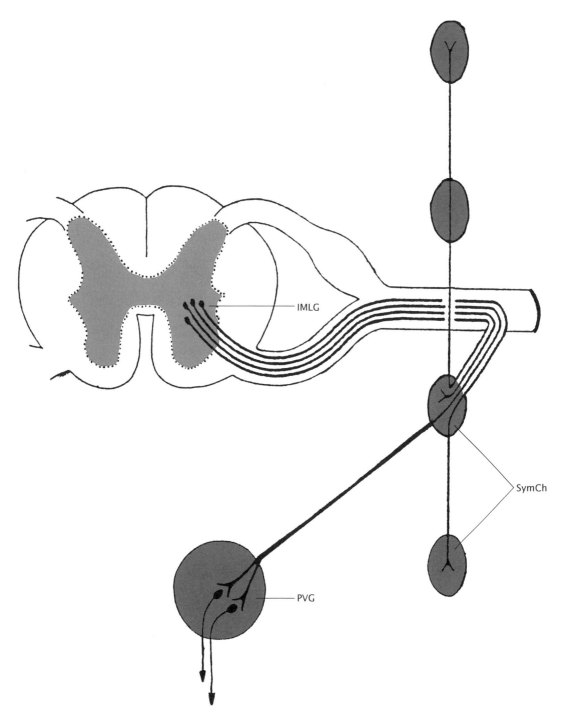

FIGURE 2.6   *The autonomic nervous system reaches its effector organs by a two-neuron chain. The preganglionic neuron originates within the intermediolateral gray (IMLG). For the sympathetic system, the preganglionic neuron fiber synapses either in the paravertebral chain of sympathetic ganglion (SymCh) or farther away in the prevertebral ganglion plexus (PVG).*

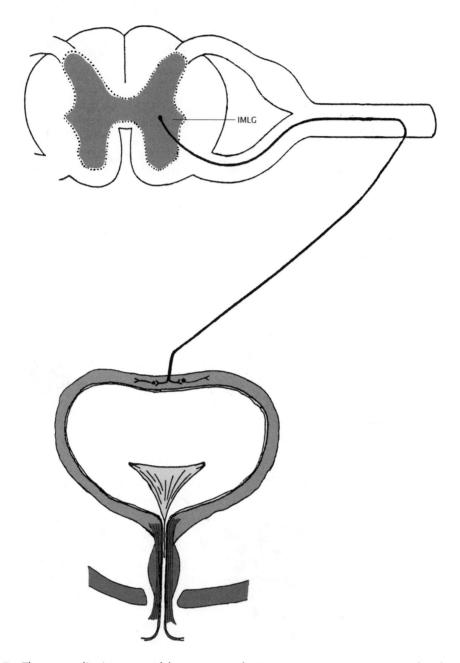

FIGURE 2.7   The preganglionic neuron of the parasympathetic nervous system originates within the inter-mediolateral gray (IMLG) portion of the sacral spinal cord. The preganglionic nerve fibers of the parasympa-thetic system synapse with postganglionic cells that are close to or within the innervated viscera, in this case the bladder wall.

through four. The sympathetic and parasympathetic divisions of the ANS are differentiated not only on their site of origin, but also on the basis of the neurotransmitters released at the terminals of the post-ganglionic fibers. It was noted in the preceding paragraph that the first synapse for the both systems was cholinergic. The terminals of the parasympathetic postganglionic fibers also liberate acetylcholine and thus are classified as cholinergic. The terminals of the sympathetic postganglionic fibers release norepinephrine and thus are classified as adrenergic.[8]

Many organs receive fibers from both the sympathetic and parasympathetic systems. When dual innervation occurs, the fibers frequently have opposing effects. For example, parasympathetic fibers to the bladder cause bladder evacuation, while sympathetic fibers have the opposite effect, promoting storage.[8]

Therefore, efferent nerve supply of the urinary bladder includes both the sympathetic and parasympathetic outflow. The sympathetic fibers travel along the superior hypogastric plexus to the bladder and bladder outlet, and parasympathetic fibers travel through the pelvic splanchnic nerve to these same structures. The somatic fibers (not part of the ANS) travel via the pudendal nerve (sacral cord segments two through four) to the external sphincter and pelvic floor (Figure 2.8).[10]

Sympathetic Nervous System

The myelinated preganglionic fibers of the SNS originate in the intermediolateral gray column of the thoracolumbar cord. They leave the spinal cord with the motor fibers of the ventral roots, but soon separate from the spinal nerves to form the white rami communicantes that enter the chain ganglia of the sympathetic trunks. The trunks are paired, ganglionated chains of nerve cell bodies and fibers that extend along either side of the vertebral column from the base of the skull to the coccyx (Figure 2.9). Some of the fibers of the white rami synapse with postganglionic neurons in the sympathetic trunk ganglion nearest their point of entrance. Other preganglionic fibers pass up or down the chain to end in a paravertebral ganglia higher or lower than the level of entrance. A third group of preganglionic fibers passes through the paravertebral ganglion into a thoracic or lumbar splanchnic nerve, terminating in an abdominal or pelvic prevertebral ganglion. It is this third group of sympathetic fibers that travels to the bladder. (Figure 2.10).[8]

Therefore, the sympathetic supply to the bladder originates in cells of the intermediolateral gray column from cord segments T10 to L2. Their axons pass through the sympathetic trunk to reach the inferior mesenteric ganglion. Postganglionic fibers then travel through the hypogastric and vesical plexuses to the wall of the bladder (see Figure 2.10).[8]

In summary, the origin of the SNS with respect to the bladder is in the intermediolateral gray region of the thoracolumbar spinal cord. Myelinated axons from this region exit through ventral roots and pass through the sympathetic trunk, traveling through lumbar splanchnic nerves to the inferior

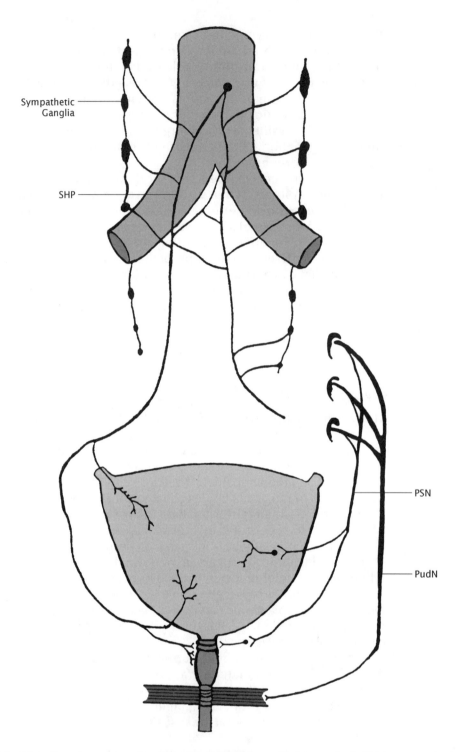

FIGURE 2.8   *The afferent nerve supply of the urinary bladder and sphincter includes the sympathetic and parasympathetic outflow, and the somatic fibers. The sympathetic fibers travel along the superior hypogastric plexus (SHP) to the bladder and bladder outlet. The parasympathetic fibers travel through the pelvic splanchnic nerve (PSN) to these same structures. The preganglionic parasympathetic fibers synapse with short postganglionic fibers located near the innervated structure. The somatic lower motor neuron fibers originate in the sacral spinal cord and travel via the pudendal nerve (PudN) to the external sphincter and pelvic floor.*

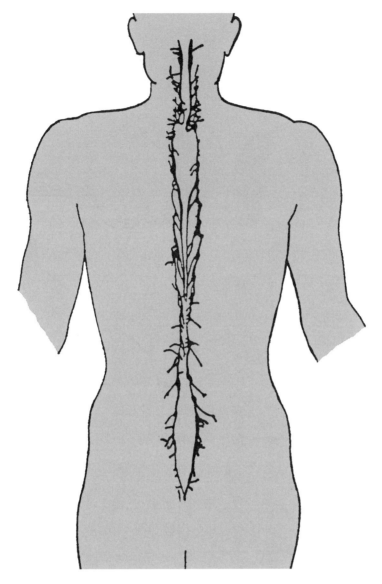

FIGURE 2.9   *The sympathetic trunks are paired ganglionic chains of nerve cell bodies and fibers that extend along either side of the vertebral column from the base of the skull to the coccyx.*

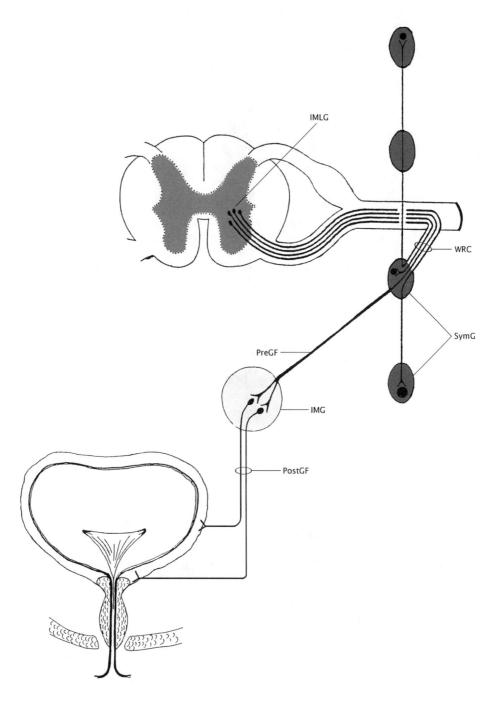

FIGURE 2.10   *The myelinated preganglionic fibers (PreGF) of the sympathetic nervous system originate in the intermediolateral gray (IMLG) of the thoracolumbar spinal cord. Their fibers branch off of the motor nerve root via the white rami communicantes (WRCs), and pass through the sympathetic ganglion chain (SymG) to synapse with postganglionic neurons in the inferior mesenteric ganglion (IMG). The postganglionic sympathetic fibers (PostGF) travel through the hypogastric and vesical plexuses to the wall of the bladder.*

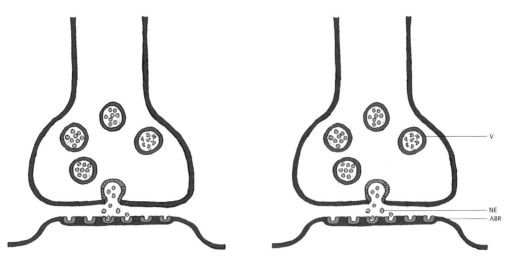

FIGURE 2.11   *The sympathetic nerve terminal contains vesicals (V) of the sympathetic neurotransmitter, norepinephrine (NE). Two types of receptors on the bladder respond to norepinephrine, alpha and beta receptors (ABRs).*

mesenteric ganglion. Here, the myelinated preganglionic sympathetic fibers synapse with a postganglionic neuron in the inferior mesenteric ganglion. The neurotransmitter released is acetylcholine. The postganglionic sympathetic nerve fibers travel through the hypogastric and vesical plexuses to the muscular layers of the bladder where they release norepinephrine. The effect of SNS activity is bladder storage due to relaxation of detrusor muscle and contraction of the involuntary sphincter.[1,8,9]

At the termination of each sympathetic nerve fiber within the bladder is the nerve ending, the boldest portion of the nerve, within which are vesicals of the neurotransmitter norepinephrine. Norepinephrine released from sympathetic nerve endings travels to receptors on bladder musculature. Two types of receptors exist that respond to norepinephrine, alpha and beta receptors. Beta receptors found on the detrusor muscle respond to norepinephrine by causing relaxation, thus favoring filling and storage. Alpha receptors at the bladder neck, proximal urethra, and rhabdosphincter respond to norepinephrine by contracting, thus increasing the sphincter closure tension and further promoting the filling and storage functions of the urethrovesical unit. The overall effect of the SNS is storage of urine (Figure 2.11).[1]

Parasympathetic Nervous System

The sacral portion of the spinal cord (conus medullaris) contains the sacral micturition center. Motor control of the urinary bladder results from parasympathetic activity. The preganglionic fibers of parasympathetic nerves that travel to the bladder have their cell bodies in the intermediolateral gray matter of sacral cord segments 2, 3, and 4. Their fibers enter the pelvic splanchnic nerves, pass through the vesical plexus, and terminate on ganglia located in the wall of the bladder, bladder neck, and

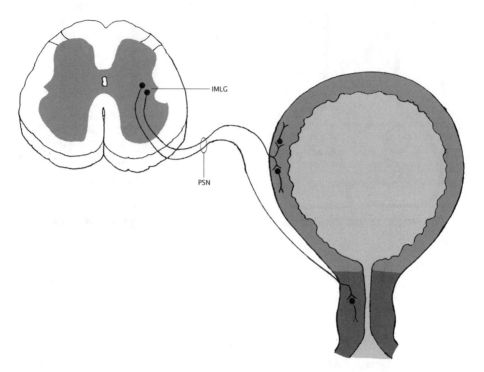

FIGURE 2.12   *The parasympathetic nerves that travel to the bladder have their cell bodies in the inter-mediolateral gray matter (IMLG) of the sacral cord segments two, three, and four. Their fibers pass through the pelvic splanchnic nerves (PSN) and synapse with postganglionic nerve ganglia located in the wall of the bladder, bladder neck, and rhabdosphincter. The postganglionic fibers are quite short.*

rhabdosphincter. Short postganglionic fibers go to detrusor and involuntary sphincter muscles (Figure 2.12).[2,8]

The PNS is concerned with emptying the bladder. Stimulation of the PNS contracts the detrusor, opens the neck of the bladder into the urethra, and empties the bladder. The preganglionic synapse is cholinergic. The postganglionic neuron lies within the wall of the bladder, and the postganglionic parasympathetic fibers are very short. The postganglionic neurotransmitter is also acetylcholine. Cholinergic (muscarinic) receptors in the bladder wall and rhabdosphincter respond by causing contraction of detrusor muscle and relaxation of the sphincter mechanism, respectively, promoting micturition (see Figure 2.12).[1]

In summary, parasympathetic signals arise from nerve cell bodies at sacral levels 2 through 4. These signals promote voiding, causing detrusor contraction and sphincter relaxation.

Overall Neural Control of Micturition

To properly evaluate voiding dysfunction, one must understand the normal cycle of micturition. The cycle begins when the bladder receives urine through the ureters. As the bladder slowly fills, pressure inside the bladder remains low (due to the presence of transitional epithelium, which allows the bladder to distend greatly without an increase in pressure). When the detrusor muscle reaches a certain threshold of distension, sensory nerve endings, including mechanoreceptors and nociceptors in the bladder wall, are stimulated, transmitting the sensation of fullness to the spinal cord through the pelvic nerves.[2] The first-order afferent sensory fibers synapse within the dorsal horn of the spinal cord onto second-order cells that travel across the spinal cord and up toward the brain via the spinothalamic tract. Third-order cells emanating from the thalamus go to the cerebral cortex, relaying the information about bladder distension (see Figures 2.1 and 2.3).[1,2]

The micturition threshold is the point during bladder filling when the individual feels the urge to void (usually at a volume of 300–400 ml in adults). At this point, a continent individual waits for the appropriate time to initiate the voiding reflex. Until that person can reach an appropriate place to void, his or her cortical functioning inhibits the pontine micturition center via fibers of the corticoreticular tract. Activity of the SNS promoting involuntary bladder filling and continence is unopposed. Fibers that travel via the corticospinal tract directly to the sacral spinal cord stimulate alpha motor neurons (that make up the pudendal nerve), traveling to the external sphincter to aid the individual in voluntarily promoting continence (see Figure 2.5).[1,2,5,11,12]

As the individual waits to void, increased activity within corticospinal and pudendal nerve fibers results in voluntary contraction of the external sphincter.[2] At the same time, reticulospinal tract fibers that originate in the pons stimulate the thoracolumbar SNS, and sympathetic outflow increases. Continence is maintained because of detrusor relaxation and internal sphincter smooth muscle contraction. This occurs because of noradrenergic stimulation of alpha receptors on the internal sphincter and beta receptors on the detrusor muscle.[1,8]

At an appropriate time and place, micturition ensues. The cortex releases its inhibitory control over the pontine micturition center, and parasympathetic input to the bladder predominates. Activity in the reticulospinal fibers, which travel to the PNS, increases. This in effect turns on the motor center for bladder contraction, located in the sacral spinal cord. Increased activity within the PNS causes contraction of the bladder and relaxation of the internal sphincter. Corticospinal (voluntary) fibers decrease their stimulation of alpha and gamma motor neurons within the sacral cord, promoting relaxation of the external sphincter. This sequence of events is known as the *micturition reflex*.[1,2,8,11,12]

In summary, bladder distension causes afferent sensory information to travel through the dorsal horn of the spinal cord and ultimately to the brain, reaching the cortex. Until the person reaches an appropriate social destination to initiate voiding, the cortex creates an inhibitory effect on the pontine micturition center. Unopposed activity of the SNS promotes continence through bladder relaxation and contraction of the internal sphincter. In addition, voluntary contraction of the external sphincter occurs. At the appropriate time and place, the frontal cortex releases its inhibitory effect on the pons, and the pons mediates a synchronized relaxation of the bladder outlet with contraction of the detrusor muscle, the micturition reflex. This strong reflex response empties the bladder completely and automatically. When the bladder is empty, the detrusor contraction stops, the sphincter closes, and filling and storage resume.[1,2,8]

Effect of Neurologic Lesions on Micturition

Knowing that the brain and pons coordinate the function of the bladder and the urethral sphincters, the clinician can understand the patterns of bladder function associated with certain neurologic lesions.

Cortical lesions, particularly located in the frontal cerebral cortex, cause a loss of cortical inhibition to the pons. This results in uninhibited detrusor activity. However, coordination between the bladder and the sphincters continues in such a patient because the pontine/sacral axis has been preserved. This pattern of uninhibited reflexive detrusor activity causes the symptoms of frequency, urgency, and incontinence that are seen in cortical stroke patients. An uninhibited bladder occurs with frontal cerebrovascular accidents, dementia, and in patients who have normal-pressure hydrocephalus.

A lesion below the pontine level, but above the sacral spinal cord (e.g., an upper motor neuron spinal cord injury), results in a loss of coordinated bladder sphincter activity because the pontine/sacral axis has been disrupted. This common finding (bladder sphincter dyssynergia) in patients with upper motor neuron spinal cord injuries and multiple sclerosis, if not treated, can lead to diseases of the upper urinary tract such as pyelonephritis, hydronephrosis, stone disease, and renal insufficiency.

The lower motor neuron bladder occurs with lesions of the sacral spinal cord or its nerve roots (cauda equina). Here, there is loss of parasympathetic and somatic input to the bladder and sphincter. This results in a flaccid bladder and overflow incontinence. Lower motor neuron lesions occur with spinal cord cauda equina injuries, with severe lumbar spinal stenosis, and in patients who have autonomic or peripheral neuropathy, or both.

Normal Cystometry and Electromyography

The normal voiding pattern can be recorded easily by basic simultaneous cystometry and electromyography. The cystometrogram (CMG) measures bladder function and the electromyogram (EMG) records the activity of pelvic floor and sphincter muscles. The normal voiding pattern recorded by the CMG shows a low bladder pressure at low bladder volumes. As the bladder fills to a volume of 300–400 ml, the patient feels a sensation of fullness and then urgency. The EMG reveals increasing muscle activity in the pelvic floor when the patient first feels the urge to void. At the micturition threshold, the

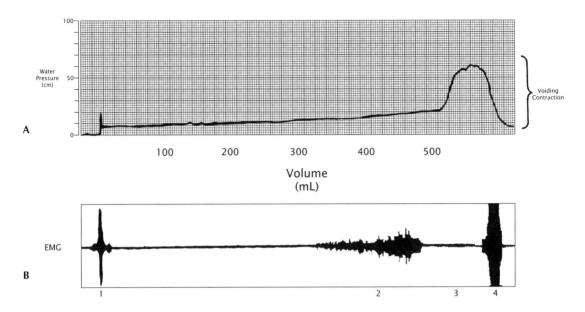

FIGURE 2.13   *(A) The normal voiding pattern recorded by the cystometrogram shows a low bladder pressure at low bladder volumes. As the bladder fills to a volume of 300–400 ml, the patient experiences a sensation of fullness. A rapid increase in bladder pressure indicates bladder contraction. (B) The electromyogram is silent during bladder contraction, indicating appropriate sphincter relaxation.*

EMG is silent and the CMG shows a rapid change in bladder pressure, which indicates a bladder contraction with appropriate sphincter relaxation. This is the normal voluntary voiding pattern as measured by the CMG and EMG (Figure 2.13).

Further elaboration on the equipment used, how it works, and various patterns of disease activity are provided in Chapter 6.

References

1. Gray M. Color Atlas of Genitourinary Anatomy and Physiology. In M Gray (ed), Genitourinary Disorders. St. Louis: Mosby, 1992;1–19.
2. Blaivas JG, Oliver L. Pathophysiology of Urinary Incontinence. In DB Doughty (ed), Urinary and Fecal Incontinence—Nursing Management. St. Louis: Mosby, 1991;23–46.
3. DeGroat WC, Kawatani M. Neurologic control of the urinary bladder. J Neurourol Urodyn 1985;4:285.
4. Maggi CA, Meli A. Review: the role of neuropeptides in the regulation of the micturition reflex. J Auton Pharmacol 1986;6:133.
5. Gilman S, Winans SS. The Descending Pathways. In S Gilman, SS Winans (eds), Manter & Gatz's Essentials of Clinical Neuroanatomy and Neurophysiology (6th ed). Philadelphia: FA Davis, 1982;25–32.

6. Griffiths D, Holstege G, Dalm E, de Wall H. Control and coordination of bladder and urethral function in the brain stem of the cat. Neurol Urodyn 1990;9:63.
7. Holstege G, Griffiths DJ, DeWall H, Dalm E. Anatomic and physiologic observations on supraspinal control of bladder and urethral sphincter muscle contractions in the cat. J Comp Neurol 1986;250:449.
8. Gilman S, Winans SS. The Autonomic Nervous System. In S Gilman, SS Winans (eds), Manter & Gatz's Essentials of Clinical Neuroanatomy and Neurophysiology (6th ed). Philadelphia: FA Davis, 1982;149–156.
9. Goldberg S. Autonomic System and Hypothalamus. In S Goldberg (ed), Clinical Neuroanatomy Made Ridiculously Simple. Miami: Med-Master, 1987;60–66.
10. Moore KL. The Perineum and Pelvis. In KL Moore (ed), Clinically Oriented Anatomy. Baltimore: Williams & Wilkins, 1980;293–418.
11. Elbadawi A, Schenk EA. Dual innervation of the mammalian urinary bladder: a histochemical study of the distribution of cholinergic and adrenergic nerves. Am J Anat 1966;119:405.
12. Gosling J. The structure of the bladder and urethra in relation to function. Urol Clin North Am 1979;6:31.

3   Assessment: Patient History

Jack L. Rook

A thorough history is the first component of a complete assessment of the patient with incontinence. Ideally, the history is obtained by oral interview of the patient. However, some elderly or cognitively impaired patients may be unable to provide an adequate history. In such a case, the history may need to come from the caretaker, family member, or nurse most familiar with the patient.

The patient work up should start with a "chief complaint" followed by some brief "identifying information" about the patient (age, pertinent diagnosis, and duration of the bladder control problem), before proceeding with the history of present illness. Consider the following example:

> Chief complaint: Urinary dribbling after voiding and a feeling of incomplete bladder emptying.
>
> Identifying information: 68-year-old man with a history of benign prostatic hypertrophy (BPH) who has been having urinary dribbling over the past 2 years.

After this introduction, the interviewer moves to a structured series of questions to elicit data concerning voiding patterns, urologic history related to incontinence, overall neurologic and general medical condition, surgical history, and current medications.[1]

History of Present Illness

Bladder Voiding Patterns

Begin the history portion of the interview by finding out about the individual's problematic voiding pattern. If the patient is able to void spontaneously, then information should be obtained about diurnal frequency, nocturia, hesitancy to void, urgency to void, and force of urinary stream.[2]

To determine diurnal frequency, the interviewer should ask the individual to describe a typical time interval between trips to the bathroom. The normal pattern is to urinate no more than every 2 hours during waking hours.[1]

The interviewer then assesses nocturnal patterns of urination (nocturia) by asking the person how many times he or she awakens from sleep by the desire to void. One episode of nocturia each night is considered normal, and elderly individuals may awaken as often as twice each night without associated voiding dysfunction. Excessive urinary frequency (diurnal or nocturnal, or both) indicates sensory urgency disorder (cystitis, urinary infection), bladder instability (uninhibited neurogenic bladder), or urinary retention (BPH, lower motor neuron bladder).[1] Urgency describes an acute onset of the need to urinate. The patient with urge incontinence often describes episodes of precipitous urination and "inability to reach a toilet in time."

Urinary hesitancy refers to a delay in the initiation of voiding, which normally commences within 15 seconds. Patients with hesitancy often wait considerably longer to initiate voiding.

Characteristics of Urinary Stream

Next, the force and character of the urinary stream are assessed. The patient is asked to describe the stream, and the interviewer attempts to classify it as normal, explosive, intermittent, or poor.

The normal urinary stream should begin within 15 seconds of an attempt to initiate voiding and then be expressed continuously until the person feels that his or her bladder is completely emptied. The individual should not have to strain to maintain the stream and should be able to interrupt micturition on command. A normal urinary stream indicates effective bladder emptying but does not rule out the possibility of abnormalities in bladder filling and storage.[1]

The female patient with an explosive stream typically describes it as particularly forceful and brief, occurring without straining, with an inability to interrupt the stream on command. The explosive stream is often associated with stress incontinence resulting from reduced outlet resistance.[1]

The patient with an intermittent or poor urinary stream pattern often states that the stream stops before they feel "finished" with micturition, and that the force of the stream is decreased. He or she must strain to increase its force or wait several minutes before completing micturition. Urinary hesitancy often is associated with poor urinary stream. A feeling of incomplete bladder emptying, poor urinary stream, and a prolonged postvoid dribble typically occurs in men with prostatic obstruction. Poor urinary flow may also be caused by inadequate detrusor contractility (lower motor neuron bladder).[1]

Containment Devices

Some individuals who spontaneously void also wear a urine containment device, such as a pad or diaper, to cope with their incontinence. Such patients should be questioned as to the type of product worn and how often it is changed. This information gives some indication of the severity and frequency of incontinence. Individuals with severe urinary leakage must use a diaper either to contain leakage between spontaneous voiding or to contain all urinary output. The interviewer should determine how long the patient has used pads or diapers to manage leakage and what elimination patterns led to their use.[1]

Condom catheters are frequently used among male spinal cord injured–patients. These devices may also help men with incompetent bladder outlets after prostatic operations for BPH or cancer of the prostate.

Intermittent Catheterization

Some patients manage urinary elimination by intermittent catheterization. The interviewer should determine the prescribed versus the actual schedule of catheterization.[1]

Indwelling Catheter

Some people manage their bladder with an indwelling catheter. The interviewer should attempt to determine why a catheter was first used and for how long it has been worn. When considering a bladder management program for the patient with an indwelling catheter, one must determine whether the person is willing to remove the catheter and try another program, such as intermittent catheterization, or whether he or she simply wishes to keep the catheter and prevent leakage around the tube.[1] Other important inquiries of the patient with a chronic indwelling catheter should include the frequency of any prior urinary tract infections, the presence of bladder calculi (which frequently develop in patients with indwelling catheters and can increase the frequency of urinary infections), the use of maintenance antibiotic medications, and antibiotic allergies (particularly to sulfa drugs, which are commonly used to treat urinary infections).

Patterns of Incontinence

Once patterns of urinary elimination and the bladder management program have been determined, the patient is asked to describe his or her patterns of incontinence.

Stress Incontinence

Stress incontinence occurs when physical exertion produces urinary leakage. The degree of stress incontinence ranges from mild to severe. The patient is asked whether leakage occurs with coughing, sneezing, or heavy lifting. Leakage that occurs only with physical exertion is a symptom of mild to moderate stress incontinence. Patients with severe stress incontinence report leakage that occurs whenever they assume an upright position or engage in any form of physical exertion, no matter how slight. Stress incontinence is distinguished from urge incontinence by the fact that leakage is not associated with a sense of urgency to urinate.[1]

Instability Incontinence

Instability incontinence is classically defined as "contraction of the bladder without its owner's permission that results in urinary leakage." In other words, involuntary detrusor contractions cause the leakage. Subtypes of instability incontinence include uninhibited bladder incontinence, urge incontinence, and reflex incontinence.[1,3]

Uninhibited Urinary Bladder Incontinence

Uninhibited urinary bladder incontinence occurs in patients with central nervous system cortical injury (stroke, Alzheimer's dementia, normal-pressure hydrocephalus [NPH]). These patients urinate at varying times and with varying degrees of bladder fullness. Uninhibited bladder incontinence occurs due to interference with the normal cortical inhibitory influence on the pontine micturition center.

Urge Incontinence

Urge incontinence is the symptom produced when bladder instability occurs in an individual who has intact sensory function of the lower urinary tract. Bladder instability may occur as a result of urinary infection, cystitis due to medications or chemotherapy, or an inflammatory condition of the bladder wall. The patient often describes episodes of precipitous urination and an inability to reach a toilet in time.[1]

Reflex Incontinence

Reflex incontinence is the pattern produced when bladder instability occurs in an individual who does not have normal sensory function of the lower urinary tract. The most common cause of reflex incontinence is a lesion or disease of the spinal cord above sacral levels (upper motor neuron lesion) that produces an unstable bladder with loss of pelvic floor and bladder sensation. The patient with reflex incontinence may state that the bladder empties itself at unpredictable times. Some patients can stimulate micturition by stroking the suprapubic area or inner thigh or by pulling pubic hair. However, they are unable to voluntarily initiate or inhibit voiding. Despite the absent or diminished sensations of filling, these patients are often able to describe atypical warnings of impending micturition, such as tingling in the legs or abdomen. Some spinal cord–injured patients are not aware that they are voiding until they perceive urine leaking onto their skin.[1,4]

Continuous Incontinence

Continuous incontinence refers to constant urinary leakage. It occurs due to sphincter incompetence or when congenital or acquired anatomic defects cause urine to bypass the normal sphincter mechanism. Some patients have both normal spontaneous voiding and continuous dribbling not associated with urgency or physical exertion.[1]

Causes of continuous incontinence include sphincter trauma, urinary fistula, and ectopic ureter. With sphincter trauma, the outflow tract may be converted into an open conduit after surgical trauma from prostatectomy or other bladder outlet procedures. In such cases, continuous-dribbling incontinence results, and the bladder possesses no storage potential. This is generally easily identified by the patient's history of recent urologic surgery and postoperative continuous incompetence.

Urinary fistula more commonly occur in women. Vesicovaginal fistula, the most common variety, may result from obstetric surgical trauma, radiation therapy, or malignancy. Urinary loss is usually continuous.

Incontinence due to an ectopic ureter is uncommon and occurs exclusively in females. In incontinent cases, the ectopic ureter opens beyond the urinary sphincter, most commonly into the distal urethra. In this variety of incontinence, the patient has a normal voiding pattern, but has continuous urine leakage between voiding. Characteristically, there is more significant leakage on arising in the mornings, when the dilatated ectopic system empties, as the upright position is assumed.[5]

Functional Incontinence

The term *functional incontinence* refers to urinary leakage caused by environmental or functional factors. Cognitive deficits or lack of motivation produced by organic brain syndrome or mental health disorders may contribute to functional incontinence. The patient with functional incontinence frequently has cognitive or communication deficits that render the patient an unreliable historian. In such cases, family members or caretakers should supplement the patient's history.

Functional incontinence is not always associated with a pathologic condition of the urinary system or voiding mechanism. However, any type of incontinence can be exacerbated by functional factors. Examples of functional factors that lead to incontinence include impaired mobility and environmental obstructions.[1]

An environmental assessment is important for any patient suspected of having a functional component to their incontinence. Careful questioning of the patient or caregiver about the home environment must be done.

Bathroom assessment of lighting and flooring are important. Lighting in the bathroom should be adequate, and a night-light is recommended for patients with nocturia. The floor should not be particularly slick or cluttered with objects that may cause a fall. Rugs that slide easily on the floor should not be used. The patient should have adequate access to the bathroom. The doorframe should be wide enough to provide access for individuals who use assistive devices such as a cane, crutches, walker, or wheelchair. Toilet height and its accessibility for transfers from a wheelchair should be assessed if indicated. The distance of the bathroom from key locations in the home (sleeping, eating, and living areas) should be determined. Ideally, the toilet should be close to where the individual spends most of his or her time.

The clinician should question the patient about environmental obstacles that impede access to the bathroom, such as dimly lit passageways, slick floors, loose rugs, or stairs. Limitations to this line of questioning exist, and, ultimately, a physical inspection of the home environment may be necessary.[1]

Overflow Incontinence

Overflow incontinence occurs when symptoms of dribbling or leakage are caused by an inability to effectively and completely empty the bladder. This condition occurs with urinary retention due to outlet obstruction (as in prostatic enlargement), as well as due to poor detrusor contraction. The person with overflow incontinence commonly reports urinary frequency, nocturia, and dribbling with leakage. Often, the patient is aware of incomplete bladder emptying and feels only partial relief after voiding. With long-term urinary retention, however, patients damage sensory fibers within the detrusor muscle, and the detrusor fibers stretch and become incompetent. Long-term obstructed patients may deny feelings of incomplete bladder emptying due to loss of sensation of bladder filling and larger bladder capacity.[1,6]

Fluid Intake

After the pattern of urinary elimination is assessed, the interviewer determines the pattern of daily fluid intake. The individual should be asked to describe the types and amounts of fluids he or she consumes during a typical day. Specifically, the patient is asked to estimate the volume of water, clear juices, citrus juices, and caffeinated beverages consumed.[1]

Review of Systems

Assessment of urinary incontinence should include evaluation of the patient's neurologic and urologic function and the medical and surgical history.

Neurologic Disorders

Disorders of the central (brain and spinal cord) and peripheral nervous system often contribute to urinary system dysfunction.

Common brain disorders that might contribute to voiding dysfunction include cerebrovascular accident (CVA), tumor, NPH, multiple sclerosis (MS), parkinsonism, and Alzheimer's disease.[7,8]

When evaluating the patient who has had a CVA, he or she should be questioned about the location and extent of the stroke. The two most common anatomic types of CVA include strokes involving the carotid circulation and strokes involving the vertebrobasilar or posterior circulation. The internal carotid arteries branch to become the anterior and middle cerebral arteries. These arteries supply major portions of the cerebral hemispheres. On the other hand, the vertebrobasilar system supplies the brain stem and the cerebellum (Figure 3.1). Damage involving these different circulations produces a variety of distinct symptomatology. The most common symptoms described in carotid circulation ischemia include hemiparesis, hemisensory loss, monocular blindness, facial numbness, lower facial weakness, aphasia, headache, dysarthria, and visual field loss (Table 3.1). Common signs and symptoms of vertebrobasilar ischemia include ataxia, hemisensory loss, vertigo, hemiparesis, dysarthria, dysphagia, syncope or lightheadedness, headache, deafness or tinnitus, and diplopia.[4,5]

The carotid artery circulation supplies the anterior and middle cerebral arteries. The anterior cerebral artery provides blood to the motor cortex

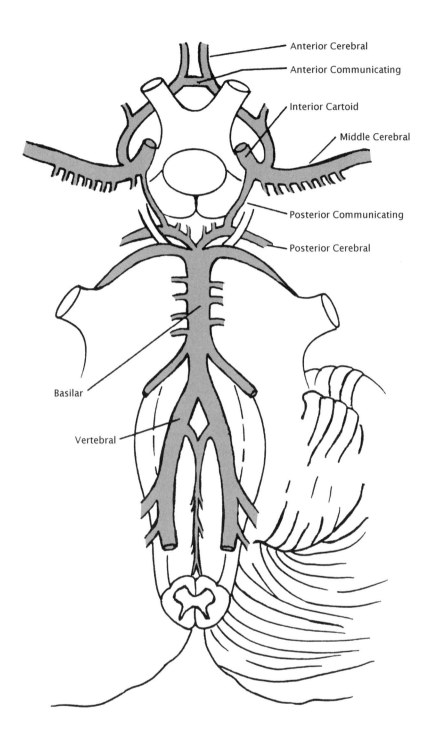

Anterior Cerebral

Anterior Communicating

Interior Cartoid

Middle Cerebral

Posterior Communicating

Posterior Cerebral

Basilar

Vertebral

FIGURE 3.1 *Arterial arrangement at the base of the brain: The internal carotid arteries branch to become the anterior and middle cerebral arteries. These arteries supply major portions of the cerebral hemispheres. The posterior vertebral basilar system supplies the brain stem and cerebellum. It begins as the two vertebral arteries, which merge to form the basilar artery that courses over the brain stem. This further branches to become the posterior cerebral arteries. The anterior and posterior circulations are connected through anterior and posterior communicating arteries. This region is known as the* circle of Willis.

TABLE 3.1 Most common symptoms of carotid circulation ischemia

Symptom	Frequency (%)
Hemiparesis	65
Hemisensory loss	60
Monocular blindness	35
Facial numbness	30
Lower facial weakness	25
Aphasia	20
Headache	20
Dysarthria	15
Visual field loss	15

supplying the leg and to the frontal cortex. Ischemia or infarction within an anterior cerebral artery distribution would produce a lower extremity hemiparesis, which could impair mobility and lead to functional incontinence. In addition, involvement of the frontal cortex, a critical center with regards to inhibition of the pontine micturition center, could result in an uninhibited neurogenic bladder. Involvement of the middle cerebral artery could cause hemiparesis, visual field loss, and major cognitive and language deficits, all of which may impair safe mobility and contribute to functional incontinence (Figure 3.2).

Patients with vertebrobasilar circulation strokes could have ataxia and balance difficulties that make safe ambulation to the bathroom difficult.[8]

Likewise, brain tumors can involve different areas of the brain, producing a variety of clinical syndromes. The type of tumor should be discussed with the patient to determine whether it is benign and treatable or

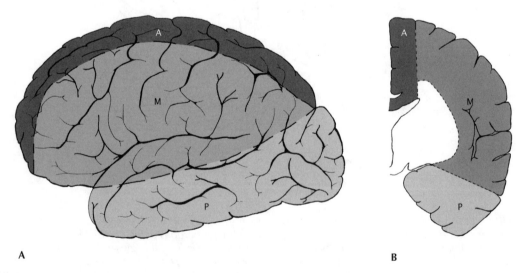

A   B

FIGURE 3.2   *Cerebral regions supplied by the anterior (A), middle (M), and posterior (P) cerebral arteries.* **(A)** *Left lateral view.* **(B)** *Cross-sectional view.*

whether it is malignant, in which case prognosis should be evaluated. The location of the tumor is important as involvement of certain regions could lead to specific deficits as mentioned in the previous stroke discussion. The most recent computed tomography scan or magnetic resonance imaging scan should be reviewed to determine extent of involvement. Previous treatment with chemotherapy should be assessed, as certain chemotherapeutic agents can cause interstitial cystitis or even a peripheral neuropathic process that could affect bladder functioning.

Some patients develop NPH. Typically, these patients present with a triad of symptomatology, including a slowly progressive gait disorder, cognitive impairment, and urinary incontinence. This is an important triad to identify, as NPH is a treatable condition. Workup would include a computed tomography or magnetic resonance imaging scan, which demonstrate dilatated ventricles and compressed sulci and gyri within the brain. If the patient is found to have NPH, prompt treatment, including insertion of a ventriculoperitoneal shunt by a neurosurgeon, should be pursued to alleviate the condition.[9]

MS is a neurologic disorder characterized by damage to white matter pathways throughout the central nervous system (brain and spinal cord). The symptomatology of an MS patient depends on the location of the lesion(s). Neurologic dysfunction results from partial, complete, or intermittent block of nerve conduction through demyelinated areas. Signs and symptoms depend on the location of the lesions: Lesions of the optic nerves result in optic neuritis. In the cerebrum, cognitive and behavioral changes can occur; in the spinal cord, weakness, spasticity, numbness, bowel, bladder, and sexual dysfunction can occur; in the brain stem, vertigo, nystagmus, internuclear ophthalmoplegia, dysarthria, and dysphagia can occur; and with lesions in the cerebellum or basal ganglia, ataxia and tremor can occur.[10]

MS patients with cognitive impairment may develop problems with functional incontinence. Those with high spinal cord white matter lesions or upper extremity tremor may not be able to perform intermittent catheterization. Those with suprasacral spinal cord lesions have an upper motor neuron bladder characterized by detrusor sphincter dyssynergia. There may be varying degrees of paralysis or spasticity, or both, leading to mobility problems in these patients. Patients with difficulty swallowing (dysphagia) could have inadequate oral intake with increased incidence of urinary tract infections.

Bladder dysfunction occurs in just about every patient with MS. In the early stages of MS, urodynamic studies have demonstrated almost any combination of increased or decreased detrusor, bladder neck, and external sphincter tone. In general, however, the end-stage bladder is one of detrusor sphincter dyssynergia in which the spastic detrusor muscle contracts against a closed outlet. This can produce reflux with upper urinary tract damage.[10]

Patients with Parkinson's disease have problems related to mobility and upper extremity tremors, and 10–15% of these patients develop cognitive dysfunction due to the development of Alzheimer's disease. The incidence of dementia increases to 65% in parkinsonian patients older than 80 years of age. These symptoms could contribute to functional incontinence.[11,12]

Alzheimer's disease is the most common and most important degenerative disease of the brain. Severe degrees of diffuse cerebral atrophy evolving over a few years, associated with dementia, are the hallmark of Alzheimer's disease. A gradual development of forgetfulness is the major symptom. Once the memory disorder has become pronounced, other failures in cerebral function become increasingly apparent. Visual spatial orientation also becomes defective. The patient may become lost even within his or her own home. Late in the disease, patients develop difficulty in locomotion. Weakness, rigidity, and tremor may appear in a parkinsonian fashion. Ultimately, the patient loses the ability to stand and walk, and he or she has to be fed and bathed. The patient sinks into a state of relative akinesia and mutism. Bowel and bladder incontinence occurs due to mobility issues as well as loss of inhibitory control over the urine micturition center.

No evidence exists that any of the proposed forms of medical therapy for Alzheimer's dementia has any salutary effect whatsoever. Patients function best when there is little change in their environment. They need structured and orderly surroundings, scheduled daily activities, and posting of signs in the home indicating the locations of household objects. The Alzheimer patient's caretaker should be questioned about extent of disease and cognitive impairment, severity and management of incontinence, patient mobility, and home environment.[11]

Traumatic spinal cord injury (SCI) represents 70% of all spinal cord paralysis. The majority of victims are male and 80% of the victims are younger than age 40 years. Atraumatic causes of SCI represent the other 30% of spinal paralysis. Common atraumatic causes of SCI include atherosclerosis of the spinal arteries, viral and bacterial diseases (Guillain-Barré, viral transverse myelitis, osteomyelitis, and epidural abscess), degenerative diseases (spinal muscular atrophy, amyotrophic lateral sclerosis, MS), tumor (primary tumors such as meningioma or astrocytoma, and secondary tumors such as lung, prostate, breast, thyroid, kidney, and lymphoma), spinal arthritis with spinal stenosis, and radiation myelopathy, which may occur in cancer patients. The term *spinal cord injury* refers to damage of any of the neural elements within the spinal cord, including the cord itself and the cauda equina (lumbar, sacral, and coccygeal nerve roots) (Figure 3.3). An upper motor neuron injury implies a lesion above the level of the cauda equina and conus medullaris. A lower motor neuron lesion implies injury below the conus.

For complete accuracy, sensory and motor levels on both sides of the body must be identified. Recognition of critical levels allows predictions of obtainable functional goals; the lower the level of SCI, the greater functional potential.

1. Lesions above C4 require continuous respiratory support, with mechanical ventilation or phrenic nerve stimulation.
2. The C5 quadriplegic patient is dependent for all activities of daily living, although with training and special equipment, certain functional upper extremity activities can be accomplished.
3. The C6 quadriplegic patient is partially independent for self-care and completely independent for many hand functions by the use of hand

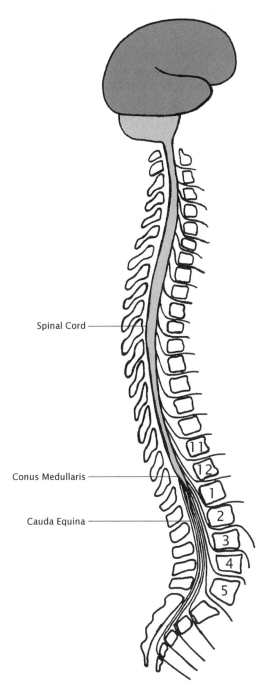

Spinal Cord

Conus Medullaris

Cauda Equina

FIGURE 3.3   *The neural elements of the spinal cord include the spinal cord itself and its termination, which occurs at around the T12–L1 vertebral bodies known as the* conus medullaris *and the* cauda equina *(lumbar, sacral, and coccygeal nerve roots).*

cuffs into which a pen, fork, or toothbrush can be inserted. With tenodesis splints, grasping can be accomplished.

4. The majority of patients with C7 quadriplegia should be completely independent for activities of daily living in a wheelchair-accessible environment.

5. Lesions below the thoracic level result in paraplegia. It is possible for most patients with paraplegia to ambulate with crutches and orthoses, although, generally, only those with lumbar lesions and some pelvic and lower extremity control will ever ambulate functionally.[13,14]

With respect to spinal level and ability to manage bladder dysfunction, those patients with lesions above C6 are completely dependent for bladder management. They are not able to catheterize themselves due to lack of hand intrinsic muscle control. They are not able to transfer themselves due to weak triceps muscles. They require assistance with bed mobility. Patients with C7 lesions are able to transfer themselves to and from the commode due to the strong triceps muscles that are innervated by the C6 and C7 nerve roots. These patients may be able to catheterize themselves, as they do have their finger flexors and in conjunction with special equipment, they should be able to obtain a fairly good grip with any utensils used. Patients with lesions at the C8 or T1 level should be independent with bowel and bladder functioning if adequately instructed. They have hand intrinsic musculature for straight catheterization and strong triceps for transfers.

Questions concerning the current bladder management program should be asked of the SCI patient (indwelling, straight, or condom catheterization). Some patients with upper motor neuron lesions frequently can initiate urination at will by scratching their abdomen or pulling pubic hairs. This can be discussed with the patient. The SCI patient should be asked about medications used to treat his or her bladder dysfunction (oxybutynin [Ditropan], bethanechol chloride [Urecholine], alpha blockers), any surgical procedures performed to prevent detrusor sphincter dyssynergia (sphincterotomy), and the results of prior urodynamic studies (upper motor neuron bladder, detrusor sphincter dyssynergia).

The upper motor neuron SCI patient may have body spasticity associated with a reflexive bladder. Severe spasticity can interfere with transfers and mobility. This could lead to functional incontinence in patients who might be better able to mobilize and transfer themselves if their spasticity were well controlled. The SCI patient should be questioned about his or her ability to mobilize and transfer. This should be compared to the overall spinal neurologic level to determine if the patient is optimally using his or her abilities.

SCI patients with chronic indwelling catheters are particularly prone to urinary tract infections. The patient should be questioned as to how often the catheter is changed, the frequency of infections, the development of urinary stones (commonly associated with frequent bladder infections), and the use of medications for treatment or prophylaxis of infections.

Other potential complications that can occur in the SCI patient with bladder dysfunction should be sought. A severe and potentially lethal one is autonomic dysreflexia. Autonomic dysreflexia is a syndrome associated with the sudden onset of hypertension, headache, bradycardia, sweating, piloerection (goose bumps), facial flushing, dilated pupils, nasal stuffiness, and blurry vision. It occurs with lesions above T5 or T6 and results from increased reflex activity in the sympathetic nervous system precipitated by noxious stimuli below the level of injury. This could include bladder distention, bladder stones, or decubiti. Basically, any noxious input below the injured spinal cord level could trigger autonomic dysreflexia. Therefore, proper bladder evacuation is critical in high paraplegic and quadriplegic patients to prevent this potentially lethal complication.[13,14] Likewise, skin breakdown, which could occur with bowel or bladder incontinence, must be optimally treated. SCI patients should be questioned as to their need for a caretaker.

SCI patients with sacral or cauda equina injuries (which could occur due to lumbar spinal stenosis in elderly patients), typically have a lower motor neuron bladder with a poorly contracting detrusor muscle. These patients need to initiate either intermittent catheterization, straining techniques such as Credé's maneuver, or condom catheterization. Questions should be asked about the individual's voiding program. Last, questions about skin breakdown are appropriate for the lower motor neuron SCI patients who tend to have severe muscle wasting below the level of their lesion. Patients with upper motor neuron lesions develop spasticity, which helps maintain muscle tone. It is the lower motor neuron patients who, although they are more mobile, are prone to development of decubiti due to the prominence of bony structures after extreme muscle atrophy.

Peripheral and Autonomic Neuropathy

Patients with chronic nerve damage resulting from a diffuse polyneuropathy may have involvement of the autonomic nervous system (which controls visceral organs, including the bowel and bladder). Questions should be asked to possibly elicit a history of underlying neuropathy. The symptoms of extremity numbness, tingling, or burning paresthesias, and difficulty walking are all consistent with a polyneuropathy diagnosis. A previous history of alcoholism, diabetes, or heavy metal exposure can contribute to the development of a diffuse polyneuropathy. There may be concomitant problems in other systems indicative of autonomic neuropathy such as cardiac conduction defects, gastrointestinal motility problems, and sexual dysfunction. Previous electrodiagnostic (electromyelogram or nerve conduction velocity) studies or a nerve biopsy may have confirmed the diagnosis of chronic neuropathy. The development of muscle atrophy (usually from the knees down bilaterally) and foot drop suggests advanced disease.

Urologic History

The patient should be questioned about his or her urologic history. Painful, burning urination (dysuria) could represent a current urinary tract infection. Previous urinary tract infections, how often they occur, and whether they are associated with fever or blood within the urine should be delineated. Fever often indicates upper tract involvement, particularly if flank pain is associated with it.

Some patients have congenital urologic disorders, which result in vesicoureteral reflux. This should be evaluated, as chronic vesicoureteral reflux can ultimately lead to upper tract damage and chronic renal failure.

Any history of urinary calculi (bladder or kidney stones) should be evaluated, including the number (one or multiple) of previous episodes of colic and the type of stones that have previously been identified. This can give clues as to the underlying metabolic abnormality that leads to their development. Patients should be questioned as to whether prior stones were treated by lithotripsy, surgery, endoscopic retrieval, or whether they were allowed to pass spontaneously.

A number of systemic disorders could lead to the production of kidney stones. For example, metabolic disorders that result in high serum calcium levels (hypercalcemia) can lead to the development of calcium stones within the urinary system. Some patients with hyperthyroidism also develop this problem. Adolescents are more prone to hypercalcemia if they need to be immobilized, due to their rapid bone growth during adolescence. Any patient suddenly immobilized after SCI is subject to this electrolyte abnormality. Excessive dietary calcium or vitamin D intake can lead to high urine calcium levels and the development of stones. Therefore, questions about diet, calcium, and vitamin intake are appropriate when presented with a patient with urinary stone disease.

Patients who have a history of gouty arthritis have high uric acid levels. Uric acid stones are common in this population. Last, there are a number of enzyme disorders that can lead to the development of oxalate stones. Crohn's disease is also associated with a higher than normal incidence of oxalate stones.

If the patient has a history of urinary system tumor, the type of tumor and prior or current treatment (chemotherapy, radiation therapy, and surgery) should be discussed. If the patient previously had blood in the urine (hematuria), the cause of this problem, amount of bleeding (microscopic hematuria versus gross hematuria), and prior treatment for this problem should be outlined.

The patient should be questioned about any prior inflammatory bladder problems. Possible causes include urinary tract infection, interstitial cystitis, bladder tumors, radiation cystitis, and/or chemotherapy-induced cystitis. The presence of urinary infections and inflammatory bladder lesions could lead to urgency incontinence.[2]

The patient should be questioned as to whether he or she has renal dysfunction. Patients with chronic upper tract problems due to stones, vesicoureteral reflex, or chronic infection, could develop chronic renal failure. If so, the patient should be questioned as to the severity of his or her renal dysfunction, the results of recent laboratory data, and whether prior renal ultrasound demonstrated small kidneys (indicative of chronic renal failure), or large kidneys (which could indicate hydronephrosis, a subacute and possibly reversible process due to obstruction).

Medications Affecting Continence and Detrusor Contractility

A number of medications that reduce detrusor contractility exist, including antispasmodics, anticholinergics, antipsychotics, antidepressants, antiparkinsonian agents, opioids, and recreational drugs. These medications could contribute to urinary retention and overflow incontinence.

Medications that increase detrusor contractility include the cholinergic agents bethanechol chloride and bethanechol. Cholinergic medications may prove helpful for patients with lower motor neuron bladder due to cauda equina SCI, polyneuropathy, or neuropathy.

Medications that reduce sphincter resistance include alpha-blocking drugs and skeletal muscle relaxants. These medications may help improve voiding in patients with upper motor neuron SCI and detrusor sphincter dyssynergia, and in men with BPH (a disorder associated with urinary retention, overflow incontinence, and urge instability).

Medications that increase sphincter resistance include the alpha sympathomimetics. These drugs may improve continence in women with mild stress incontinence and in men with incontinence after prostatectomy (Table 3.2).[2]

Surgical History

Any genital or urinary procedures, abdominal or pelvic surgery, neurosurgical procedures, and spinal orthopedic procedures should be investigated. In women, the number of vaginal deliveries may lend insight into potential causes of stress incontinence. With respect to prior spinal orthopedic or neurosurgical procedures, patients with a history of surgery for treatment of low back pain or spinal stenosis may have had previous nerve root damage that could result in bladder dysfunction.

Voiding Diary

A voiding diary can provide valuable adjunctive information to complement the history portion of the patient assessment. The voiding diary can provide information about a patient's patterns of urinary elimination. It can be used as part of the initial assessment of incontinence and may be used again to evaluate the effectiveness of an instituted bladder management program. The diary should document both diurnal and nocturnal voiding patterns and episodes of incontinence. Most patients, their caretakers, or their nurses can easily keep an accurate and complete record. The diary should be placed near the bathroom or bedside commode to facilitate prompt documentation. Keeping a diary for a short time, perhaps 2–3 days, can provide a solid baseline of information.[1]

The simplest voiding diary documents only patterns of urinary elimination. It contains three columns for the recording of time, voiding, and leakage. The patient places a check or an X in the respective column each time he or she voids, or discovers urine leakage.[1]

In a more sophisticated diary, the recorder documents the actual volume of urine voided. For as long as the diary is being kept, the patient voids only

TABLE 3.2 Medications that can affect urinary continence

Medications that reduce detrusor contractility	Antiparkinsonian agents
Antispasmodics and anticholinergics	Anticholinergic agents
Gastrointestinal agents	Akineton (biperiden HCl)
Bentyl (dicyclomine HCl)	Artane (trihexiphenidyl HCl)
Donnatal	Benadryl (diphenhydramine HCl)
Levsin (hyoscyamine sulfate)	Cogentin (benztropine mesylate)
Pro-Banthine (probantheline bromide)	Kemadrin (procyclidine HCl)
Robinul (glycopyrrolate)	Levbid (hyoscyamine sulfate)
Urinary tract agents	Levsin (hyoscyamine sulfate)
Cystospaz (hyoscyamine)	Opioid analgesics (see Chapter 24 for list of
Ditropan (oxybutinin chloride)	opioids)
Levsin (hyoscyamine sulfate)	Recreational drugs/cannabis
Urised	Medications increasing detrusor contractility
Urispas (flavoxate HCl)	Cholinergic agents
Antipsychotics	Urecholine (bethanechol chloride)
Phenothiazine and combinations	Medications reducing sphincter resistance
Compazine (prochlorperazine)	Alpha-blocking agents
Etrafon (perphenazine and amitriptyline HCl)	Cardura (doxazosin mesylate)
Serentil (mesoridazine besylate)	Dibenzyline (phenoxybenzamine HCl)
Stelazine (trifluoperazine)	Hytrin (terazosin HCl)
Thorazine (chlorpromazine HCl)	Minipress (prazosin HCl)
Trilafon (perphenazine)	Skeletal muscle relaxants
Antidepressants	Baclofen
Tricyclic antidepressants	Dantrium (dantrolene sodium)
Asendin (amoxapine)	Flexeril (cyclobenzaprine HCl)
Elavil (amitriptyline HCl)	Norflex (orphenadrine citrate)
Etrafon (perphenazine and amitriptyline HCl)	Parafon Forte (chlorzoxazone)
Limbitrol (chlordiazepoxide and amitriptyline	Robaxin (methocarbamol)
HCl)	Skelaxin (metaxalone)
Norpramin (desipramin HCl)	Soma (carisoprodol)
Pamelor (nortriptyline HCl)	Valium (diazepam)
Sinequan (doxepin HCl)	Medications increasing sphincter resistance
Tofranil (imipramine pamoate)	Alpha sympathomimetics
Triavil (perphenazine and amitriptyline HCl)	Decongestants
Vivactil (protriptyline HCl)	Appetite suppressants

into a graduated collection device. The time and volume of voided urine are recorded. Because it is difficult to estimate the volume of leakage, incontinence is recorded only as a checkmark. Correlating the occurrence of wetness with events of daily living and recording the amount of fluid consumed throughout the day provides additional information.[1]

The voiding diary provides information about patients' patterns of urinary elimination. Normal voiding intervals are at least 2 hours long and should be no longer than 4–6 hours except during sleep. Variance from these norms suggests urinary frequency, infrequent voiding pattern, or incontinence.[1]

Urinary incontinence is assessed by counting the number of times the person recorded leakage and by correlating the occurrence of wetness with events of daily living. The patient with stress incontinence may have documented that leakage occurs during periods of activity and exercise. The patient with bladder instability and urge incontinence may record leakage associated with increased fluid consumption. Patients with over-

TABLE 3.3   Patient history

Chief complaint	Normal-pressure hydrocephalus
Identifying information	Multiple sclerosis
History of present illness	Parkinson's disease
Bladder voiding patterns	Alzheimer's disease
Diurnal frequency	Spinal cord injury
Nocturia	Level of injury
Hesitancy	Current bladder management program
Urgency	Upper motor neuron versus lower motor neuron
Characteristics of urinary stream	bladder
Normal	Complications of bladder dysfunction (spasticity,
Explosive	autonomic, dysreflexia, incontinence,
Intermittent	decubiti)
Poor	Peripheral or autonomic neuropathy
Containment devices	Urologic history
Diaper	Previous urinary tract infection
Pad	Congenital urologic disorders
Condom catheter	Urinary calculi
Intermittent catheterization	Hyperuricemia (gout)
Indwelling catheter	Hypercalcemia (hyperparathyroidism)
Patterns of incontinence	Hyperoxaluria (Crohn's disease)
Stress	Urinary system tumor
Instability	Hematuria
Urge	Inflammatory bladder problems
Reflex	Renal dysfunction
Continuous	Medications affecting continence and detrusor
Functional	contractility (see Table 3.2)
Environmental assessment	Surgical history
Bathroom	Genitourinary
Lighting	Abdominal/pelvic
Flooring	Spinal orthopedic/neurosurgical procedures
Distance from bedroom to bathroom	Number of vaginal deliveries
Fluid intake	Voiding diary
Review of systems	Fluid intake
Neurologic disorders	
Cerebrovascular accident	
Brain tumor	

flow incontinence due to urinary retention often document particularly frequent urination and leakage during the sleeping hours. Patients with extraurethral incontinence record that the frequency or magnitude of leakage is unaffected by changes in position or activity levels.[1]

Fluid Intake

Assessment of fluid consumption helps correlate patterns of fluid intake with patterns of urination and incontinence. This process often provides clues as to the cause of incontinence and may offer solutions to some bladder management problems. For example, the person with frequent nocturia may not realize that he or she consumes a large amount of fluid just before bedtime. The solution to this problem would be to refrain from nighttime fluid consumption.[1]

Table 3.3 summarizes the comprehensive history for the incontinent patient.

References

1. Gray M. Assessment of Patients with Urinary Incontinence. In DB Doughty (ed), Urinary and Fecal Incontinence: Nursing Management. St. Louis: Mosby, 1991;47–94.
2. Gray M. Assessment. In Gray M (ed), Genitourinary Disorders. St. Louis: Mosby, 1992;20–31.
3. Alfaro R. Applying Nursing Diagnosis and Nursing Process: A Step-By-Step Guide (2d ed). Philadelphia: JB Lippincott, l990.
4. Gray ML, Dougherty MC. Urinary incontinence: Pathophysiology and treatment. J Enterost Ther 1987;14:152.
5. Webster GD. Urinary Incontinence. In MI Resnick, RA Older (eds), Diagnoses of Genitourinary Disease. New York: Thieme-Stratton, 1982;517–534.
6. Gray ML. Urinary Retention. In JM Thompson (ed), Mosby's Manual of Clinical Nursing (2d ed). St. Louis: Mosby–Year Book, 1989.
7. Garrison SJ, Rolak LA, Dodaro RR, O'Callaghan AJ. Rehabilitation of the Stroke Patient. In DeLisa JA (ed), Rehabilitation Medicine: Principles and Practice. Philadelphia: JB Lippincott, 1988;565–584.
8. Adams RD, Victor M, Ropper AH. Cerebral Vascular Diseases. In RD Adams, M Victor, AH Ropper (eds), Principles of Neurology (6th ed). New York: McGraw-Hill, 1997;777–873.
9. Adams RD, Victor M, Ropper AH. Disturbances of Cerebrospinal Fluid and Its Circulation, Including Hydrocephalus and Meningeal Reactions. In RD Adams, M Victor, AH Ropper (eds), Principles of Neurology (6th ed). New York: McGraw-Hill, 1997;623–641.
10. Cobble ND, Wangaard C, Kraft GH, Burks JS. Rehabilitation of the Patient with Multiple Sclerosis. In JA DeLisa (ed), Rehabilitation Medicine: Principles and Practice. Philadelphia: JB Lippincott, 1988;612–634.
11. Adams RD, Victor M, Ropper AH. Degenerative Diseases of the Nervous System. In RD Adams, M Victor, AH Ropper (eds), Principles of Neurology (6th ed). New York: McGraw–Hill, 1997;1046–1107.
12. Mayeux R, Chen J, Mirabello E, et al. An estimate of the incidence of dementia in idiopathic Parkinson's disease. Neurology 1990;40:1513.
13. Stover SL, Donovan WH, Freed MM, et al. Rehabilitation in Spinal Cord Disorders (2d ed). Chicago: American Academy of Physical Medicine and Rehabilitation, 1985.
14. Staas WE, Formal CS, Gershkoff AM, et al. Rehabilitation of the Spinal Cord Injured Patient. In JA DeLisa (ed), Rehabilitation Medicine: Principles and Practice. Philadelphia: JB Lippincott, 1988;635–659.

4   Assessment: Physical Examination of the Genitourinary System

Jack L. Rook

After completion of the history, the clinician begins a systematic physical examination designed to elucidate specific findings pertinent to the assessment and management of the patient with incontinence. Because of the sensitive nature of the genitourinary system evaluation, both the history and physical examination should be performed in an environment that ensures patient confidentiality and privacy. In general, a clinician should be chaperoned whenever examining the genitourinary system.[1,2]

The overall order of the physical examination should include a general survey with evaluation of vital signs, followed by examination of the abdomen, male or female genitalia, rectum, and a neurologic examination.

General Survey

During the general survey, the examiner should observe the patient's apparent state of health, signs of distress, skin color, weight, fine motor activity, gait, personal hygiene, mood, speech, and state of awareness. A limited mental status evaluation can be done during the history portion of the evaluation.[1,3]

The patient's cognition can be evaluated throughout the historical interview and physical examination, including an assessment of orientation, alertness, and his or her ability to recall, store, and synthesize the skills needed to perform self-care functions.[1] The patient's motivation and interest in altering behaviors to cope with his or her incontinence are also assessed. Assessment of a patient's cognitive status and motivational level is critical to establishment of an effective bladder management program.[2]

Next, vital signs should be checked (pulse, respiratory rate, blood pressure, and temperature). Abnormal vital signs may be a reflection of compromised renal function. Elevated blood pressure may be renal vascular in origin (stenosis of the renal artery is a common cause of hypertension).

Patients with chronic renal failure and uremia have a characteristic ammonia-like breath odor that the examiner should become familiar with.

Note the color of the skin, its vascularity, any lesions, edema, and the condition of the nails. With chronic renal failure, skin integrity may be altered, with easy bruising and slow wound healing. Chronic anemia may be noted as pallor accompanied by pale conjunctiva, general weakness, and decreased physical endurance. The hair may appear thin and brittle, the nails cracked, and there will be weight loss and muscle wasting detected as a result of protein wasting.[1,3]

Next evaluate mobility, transfer skills, and dexterity. Gait is initially assessed as the patient walks into the examination room. Assess how well the patient ambulates and the use of assistive devices (walker, cane, or wheelchair). Note ability to transfer onto the examination table.

Observe and assess the patient's motor skills and dexterity as he or she removes clothing and undergarments in preparation for examination of the genitalia. The examiner notices the type of clothing the patient wears, the condition of the clothing, and the skill and speed with which the patient manipulates zippers, buttons, belts, shoelaces, or hook and loop material.[2]

After the patient has disrobed, evaluate the back. Check for costovertebral angle tenderness. After examining the back, evaluate the lower extremities for obvious signs of muscular asymmetry or general atrophy that may indicate neurologic abnormality.[2,3]

An abdominal examination, genital and rectal examination, and a screening neurologic examination follow the general survey.

Abdominal Examination

For descriptive purposes, the abdomen is divided into four quadrants by imaginary lines crossing at the umbilicus: right upper, right lower, left upper, and left lower quadrants (Figure 4.1).

Several structures may reveal themselves to the palpating hand, including the liver edge, portions of the large bowel, the pulsating aorta and iliac arteries, and the lower pole of the right kidney (the left kidney is rarely palpable).[4]

The kidneys are posterior organs, protected above by the ribs and posteriorly by the back muscles. The costovertebral angles formed by the lower border of the rib cage and vertebral column are clinically useful landmarks (Figure 4.2).[5]

Essential conditions for a good abdominal examination include good lighting, full exposure of the abdomen, and a relaxed patient. To achieve relaxation, the patient should have an empty bladder; he or she should lie comfortably in a supine position (with a pillow for his or her head and perhaps under the knees) with arms kept at his or her sides or folded across the chest. The clinician should have warm hands, a warm stethoscope, and short fingernails; the patient may require distraction with conversation or questions during the abdominal examination, and tender areas should be examined last.[4]

From the patient's right side proceed in an orderly fashion with inspection, auscultation, percussion, and palpation.

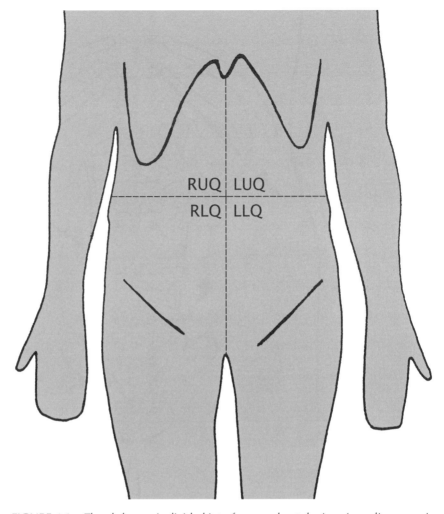

FIGURE 4.1   *The abdomen is divided into four quadrants by imaginary lines crossing at the umbilicus: right upper quadrant (RUQ), right lower quadrant (RLQ), left upper quadrant (LUQ), and left lower quadrant (LLQ).*

Inspection

From the right side of the bed, inspect the abdominal skin, noting the presence, size, and location of surgical scars. They indicate surgical procedures that may have involved the urinary system and adjacent structures.[1]

Evaluate the contour of the abdomen and check for symmetry, local bulges, and masses. A centrally located suprapubic bulge may indicate a distended bladder or pregnant uterus. A visible mass of the upper abdominal quadrants may indicate the presence of a renal tumor or an obstructed hydronephrotic kidney.[1,5]

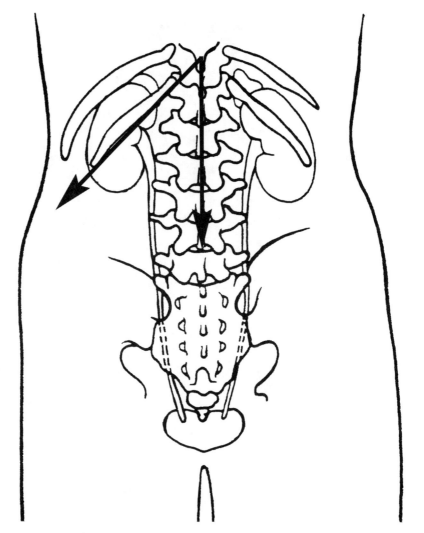

FIGURE 4.2   *The costovertebral angle* (arrows) *is formed by the lower border of the rib cage and the spinous processes of the vertebral column.*

Auscultation

Auscultation before percussion and palpation is recommended, as the latter maneuvers may alter the frequency of bowel sounds. Listen in all four quadrants, noting the frequency and character of bowel sounds. Normally, there are clicks and gurgles occurring at a frequency of 5 to 34 per minute. Evaluating the presence of bowel sounds is important immediately after urologic surgery.[1,5]

Bowel sounds may be increased due to diarrhea or an early intestinal obstruction. Bowel sounds may be decreased or absent after urologic surgery. Before deciding bowel sounds are absent, sit down and listen for 2 minutes or even longer.[5]

Percussion

Percuss the abdomen lightly in all four quadrants to assess the general distribution of tympany and dullness. Tympany usually predominates. Normally, a bladder holding 150 ml of fluid or less remains below the pubic symphysis so that percussion reveals tympany in the suprapubic area. In contrast, suprapubic dullness predominates with a distended bladder.[1,5]

Light Palpation

Light palpation is helpful in identifying muscular resistance, abdominal tenderness, and some superficial organs and masses. A large tender abdominal or pelvic mass, urinary system infection, or distended bladder may produce resistance on light palpation of the abdomen and suprapubic area.[1,5]

Deep Palpation

Deeper palpation is required to delineate abdominal organs and masses. The clinician uses the palmar surfaces of the fingers to feel in all four quadrants. Any masses are noted, including their location, size, shape, consistency, pulsations, mobility, and magnitude of tenderness provoked by palpation. If tenderness is present, test for rebound tenderness by firmly and slowly pressing in, then quickly withdrawing the fingers. *Rebound tenderness* refers to any pain elicited during the withdrawal maneuver. Rebound tenderness suggests peritoneal inflammation.[1,5]

The kidneys are then assessed for tenderness and masses. To evaluate the right kidney, place the examiner's supporting, left hand behind the patient's right loin, between the rib cage and iliac crest. The right hand is placed behind the right costal margin with fingertips pointing to the left. The hands are then pressed firmly together. Because of the posterior location of the kidneys, palpation should be deep. As the patient takes a deep breath, the examiner tries to feel the lower pole of the right kidney come between his or her fingers during exhalation. If the kidney is palpable, the clinician attempts to describe its size, contour, and tenderness (Figure 4.3).[5]

The left kidney can also be evaluated from the patient's right side. The examiner supports the patient's left loin with his or her left hand while the right hand palpates the anterior abdominal wall (Figure 4.4A). Capturing the left kidney between the examiner's hands is more easily done from the patient's left, however, with the left hand behind the patient and right hand in front (Figure 4.4B). A normal left kidney is rarely palpable.[5]

Causes of kidney enlargement include hydronephrosis, neoplasm, and polycystic disease.[5]

Kidney tenderness is usually assessed during examination of the back. The examiner's left palm is placed over each costovertebral angle. The left hand is then struck with the ulnar surface of the right fist. Normally, the patient should perceive a jar or thud. Costovertebral angle pain or tenderness during this maneuver suggests kidney infection.[5]

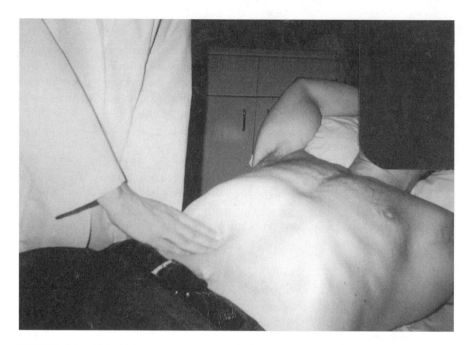

FIGURE 4.3 *Right kidney examination with the examiner standing to the right of the patient.*

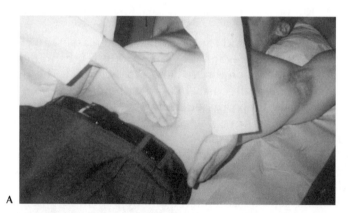

A

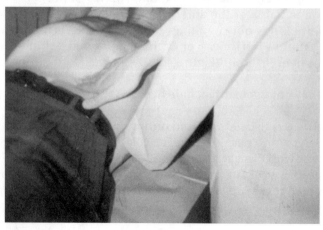

B

FIGURE 4.4 *(A) The left kidney can also be evaluated from the patient's right side. (B) However, capturing the left kidney between the examiner's hands is more easily done from the patient's left, with the left hand behind the patient, and the right hand in front.*

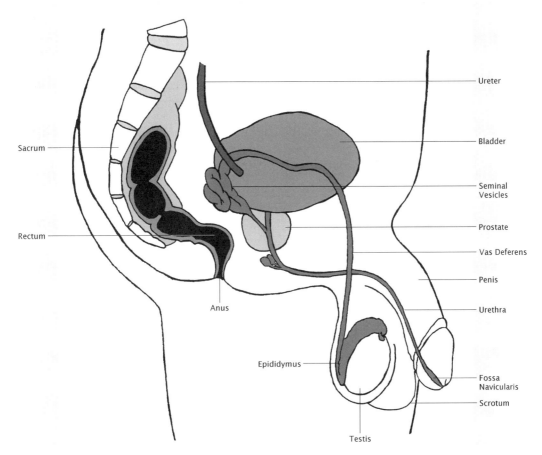

FIGURE 4.5   *The male genitalia, prostate, bladder, anus, and rectum.*

Labels in figure: Sacrum, Rectum, Anus, Epididymus, Testis, Ureter, Bladder, Seminal Vesicles, Prostate, Vas Deferens, Penis, Urethra, Fossa Navicularis, Scrotum

Male Genitalia

Examination of the male genitalia should include a general inspection followed by evaluation of the penis, scrotum, anus, and rectum. The anatomy of the male genitalia, prostate, anus, and rectum can be reviewed in Figure 4.5.

General Examination

The perineal skin should be checked for integrity. Men with significant urinary leakage may have rashes and ulcerations related to urinary leakage.[1]

When inspecting the penis, the prepuce or foreskin should be retracted if it is present. This step is essential for detection of chancre and carcinoma. A syphilitic chancre presents as an oval or round, dark red, painless erosion or ulcer with an indurated base, usually associated with nontender enlarged inguinal lymph nodes. Carcinoma of the penis may present as an indurated nodule or ulcer that is usually nontender. It occurs almost exclusively in men who are not circumcised in childhood, and the prepuce may mask it. Any persistent penile sore must be considered suspicious.[4]

To evaluate the urethral meatus, the glans penis is pressed between thumb and forefinger. The mucosa of the fossa navicularis (terminal portion of the urethra) should readily separate, exposing pink, moist tissue. Discharge should be absent. Scarring or inability to expose distal mucosa may indicate stenosis with coexisting voiding dysfunction.[1]

In Peyronie's disease the patient has a palpable nontender hard plaque just beneath the skin, usually along the dorsum of the penis. He complains of crooked, painful erections.[4]

Palpation

Next, the shaft of the penis is palpated between thumb, index, and middle fingers. Gloves should be used. Any abnormality should be assessed, noting tenderness, induration, size, and contour. Last, the scrotal skin is inspected for any nodules, inflammation, or ulcers. The scrotum should be lifted up to inspect its posterior surface as well, observing its contour and its contents, noting any evidence of swelling.[4]

Anus and Rectum: Male Examination

Anatomy

The gastrointestinal tract terminates in a short segment, the anal canal. It is normally held in a closed position by action of the voluntary external and involuntary internal sphincters, the latter an extension of the muscular smooth muscle coat of the rectal wall.

Above the anal and rectal junction, the rectum balloons out and turns posteriorly. In the male, the prostate gland is palpable anteriorly as a rounded prominence approximately 2.5 cm in length (see Figure 4.5). A shallow median sulcus or groove separates its two lateral lobes.[6]

Male Rectal Examination

Many examiners prefer to do a male rectal examination on an ambulatory patient while he is standing, with hips flexed and upper body resting across the examination table. For the nonambulatory patient, however, the lateral position is necessary, and some examiners prefer to use it routinely. The patient is asked to lie on his left side with his right hip and knee somewhat flexed and his buttocks close to the edge of the examination table near the examiner. The examiner's right hand is gloved and the index finger lubricated. The left hand then spreads the buttocks apart and the sacral, coccygeal, and perianal areas are inspected for inflammation, rashes, or excoriations. The patient is then asked to strain down, which relaxes the sphincter. As the sphincter relaxes, the lubricated and gloved index fingertip is gently inserted into the anal canal, in a direction pointing toward the umbilicus. This examination causes the patient to feel as if he is moving his bowels. The patient should be told of this affect before the procedure is performed.

The examiner notes the tone of the anal sphincter. Sphincter tightness occurs with anxiety, whereas laxity results from neurologic disease, particularly involving the spinal lumbosacral nerve roots.

The examining hand is then turned so that the index finger can examine the anterior rectal surface. The lateral lobes, median sulcus, size, shape, and consistency, and any nodularity or tenderness of the prostate should be noted.

The normal prostate gland is palpated through the anterior rectal wall as a rounded, heart-shaped structure approximately 2.5 cm in length that projects less than 1 cm into the rectal lumen. The median sulcus should be felt between the two lateral lobes. Only the posterior surface of the prostate is palpable.

With benign prostatic hypertrophy, a common condition in men over 50 years of age, the prostate presents as a firm but elastic, smooth, and symmetrical enlargement of the gland. The hypertrophic prostate may bulge more than 1 cm into the rectal lumen, and the hypertrophied tissue tends to obliterate the median sulcus.

In contrast to the enlarged, elastic tissue of benign prostatic hypertrophy, a hard irregular nodule, glandular asymmetry, and variation of its consistency might suggest the diagnosis of prostate carcinoma. With advanced disease, the carcinoma grows in size, obliterates the median sulcus, and may extend beyond the confines of the gland, producing a fixed, hard, irregular mass.

The acutely inflamed prostate gland of prostatitis is swollen, tender, and often asymmetric.[6]

Palpation of the prostate may cause emission of fluid into the urethra. Any secretions obtained during digital examination should be cultured to test for bacterial infection of the gland.[1]

After palpating the prostate, the examiner completes the rectal examination by assessing the bulbocavernosus response. With the index finger still in the rectum, the examiner gently squeezes the glans penis. A positive response (anal wink) occurs when the sphincter contracts around the examiner's finger. The anal wink indicates that neurologic pathways between the sacral roots and the pelvic floor muscles are intact. Persistent anal relaxation (a negative bulbocavernosus response) may indicate denervation. Last, the examiner asks the patient to contract the anal sphincter around the index finger, assessing volitional control of the pelvic floor muscles (which are mediated by the corticospinal tracts).[2]

Female Genitalia

Anatomy

The anatomy of the external female genitalia includes the vulva, the mons pubis (a hair-covered fat pad overlying the symphysis pubis), the labia majora (rounded folds of adipose tissue), the labia minora (thinner pinkish folds that

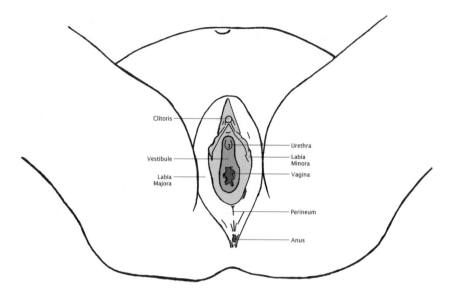

FIGURE 4.6   *The anatomy of the external female genitalia, the introitus, perineum, and anus.*

extend anteriorly to form the prepuce), and the clitoris (Figure 4.6). The *vestibule* refers to the fossa between the labia minora; in its posterior portion lie the vaginal opening or introitus, and the urethral orifice opens into the vestibule between the clitoris and vagina. The term *perineum* refers to the pelvic floor tissues between the introitus and anus.[7]

The vagina, a hollow tube extending upward and posteriorly between urethra and rectum, terminates in the cup-shaped fornix. Almost at right angles to it sits the uterus, a pear-shaped fibromuscular organ. Its cervix protrudes into the vagina. A round or slitlike depression, the external os of the cervix, marks the opening of the uterine cavity. From each side of the uterus extends a fallopian tube. Each tube has a fringed funnel-shaped end that curves toward an ovary. Each ovary is an almond-shaped structure averaging approximately 3.5 × 2.0 × 1.5 cm in size (Figure 4.7).[7]

Technique of Examination

The patient should be lying in the lithotomy position, thighs flexed and abducted, feet resting in stirrups, and buttocks extending slightly beyond the edge of the examination table. Relaxation is essential for an adequate examination. To achieve relaxation, the patient should have a chance to empty her bladder, following which she should lie as comfortably as possible with her head supported by a pillow, draped appropriately, with arms at her sides or folded across her chest. The clinician should explain in advance each step in the examination, avoiding any sudden or unexpected movements, have warm hands and a warm speculum, and should monitor the examination when possible by watching the patient's face.

Equipment within reach should include a good light, a vaginal specu-

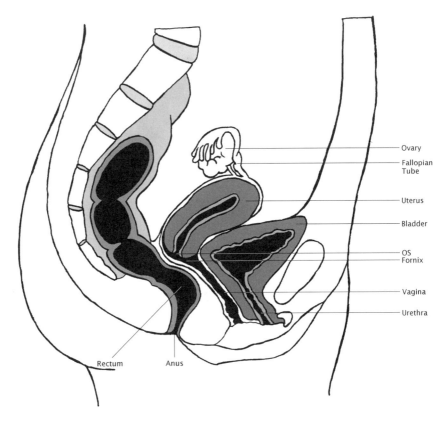

FIGURE 4.7   *The vagina, a hollow tube extending upward and posteriorly between the urethra and rectum, terminates in the cup-shaped fornix. At right angles to it sits the uterus, whose cervix protrudes into the vagina. A round or slitlike depression, the external os of the cervix, marks the opening of the uterine cavity. From each side of the uterus extends a fallopian tube, with its fringed, funnel-shaped end curving toward an ovary.*

lum of appropriate size, and materials for bacteriologic cultures and Papanicolaou (Pap) smears. Gloves should be worn. A female assistant customarily attends male examiners.

The clinician should be seated comfortably when inspecting the patient's external genitalia (mons pubis, labia) and perineum. With a gloved hand, the labia majora are separated for inspection of the labia minora, clitoris, urethral orifice, and the vaginal opening or introitus. Any inflammation, ulceration, discharges, swelling, or nodules are noted and palpated. An ulcerated raised, red vulvar lesion in an elderly woman may indicate vulvar carcinoma.[7]

The skin of the perineum is inspected for rashes or lesions. Women with significant urinary incontinence may have altered skin integrity as a result of ammonia contact dermatitis from chronic exposure to urine.[1] When leakage is continuous or frequent, a red maculopapular rash with satellite lesions (consistent with fungal infection) is commonly found.[2]

The well-estrogenized vaginal vault is pink and moist and nontender to

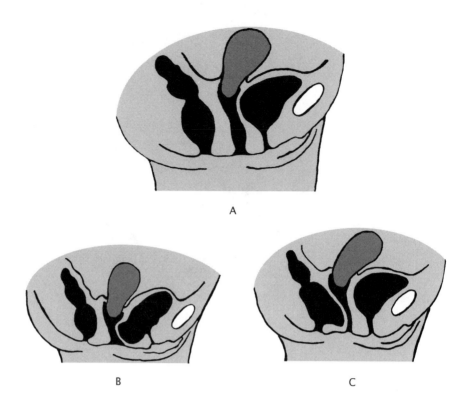

A

B   C

FIGURE 4.8   *(A) Schematic representation of normal uterine, bladder, and rectal support. (B) A cystocele is present when the anterior wall of the vagina, together with the bladder above it, bulges into the vagina. (C) A rectocele is formed by the anterior and downward bulging of the posterior wall together with the rectum behind it into the vagina.*

the touch. The estrogen-deficient vaginal mucosa may be pale, dry, and tender to the touch.[1,2]

Next, support of the vaginal outlet is assessed. With the labia separated by the middle and index fingers, the patient strains down. Any bulging of the vaginal walls is noted during straining. A cystocele is present when the anterior wall of the vagina, together with the bladder above it, bulges into the vagina and, when severe, out of the introitus. A rectocele is formed by the anterior and downward bulging of the posterior wall together with the rectum behind it (Figure 4.8).[7]

Prolapse of the uterus also results from weakness of the supporting structures of the pelvic floor. It is often associated with a cystocele or a rectocele, or both. The prolapsed uterus becomes retroverted and descends down the vaginal canal. In first-degree prolapse, the cervix is still well within the vagina. In second degree, it is at the introitus. In third-degree prolapse, the cervix and vagina are outside the introitus (Figure 4.9).[7]

Next, circumvaginal (pelvic floor) muscle strength is evaluated by asking the woman to squeeze the examining finger. Intact circumvaginal

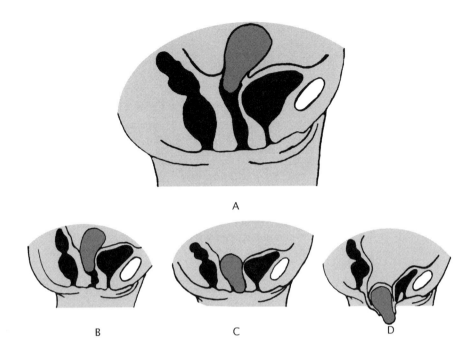

FIGURE 4.9 *(A)* *Schematic representation of normal uterine support.* *(B)* *In first-degree prolapse, the cervix is still well within the vagina.* *(C)* *In second-degree prolapse, the cervix is at the introitus.* *(D)* *In third-degree prolapse, the cervix and vagina are outside the introitus.*

muscles should squeeze against the finger in an anteroposterior manner, pulling it up toward the cervix.[1]

Speculum Examination

The clinician proceeds with speculum insertion while the patient is still straining down. With two fingers just inside the introitus, and gentle downward pressure on the perineum, the other hand introduces a closed warm and lubricated speculum at a downward 45-degree angle. The blades should be held obliquely with pressure exerted toward the posterior vaginal wall to avoid the more sensitive anterior vaginal wall.

After the speculum has entered the vagina, its blades are rotated to a horizontal position, maintaining the pressure posteriorly. The blades are opened after full insertion and maneuvered so that the cervix comes into full view (Figure 4.10).[7]

Next, the cervix is inspected, including its os, color (covered by smooth pink epithelium), position (normally located in the midline), and any ulcerations, nodules, masses, bleeding, or discharge.[7] Normally, cervical discharge is odorless, clear, and varies in consistency from viscus to clear and thin. Discharge from bacterial or fungal infection is malodorous and yellow, gray, or green.[1]

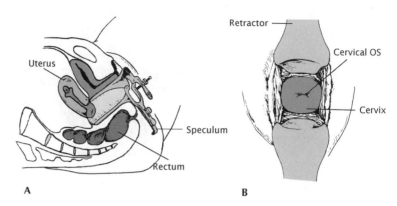

A   B

FIGURE 4.10 *(A) After the speculum has entered the vagina, its blades are rotated to a horizontal position, maintaining the pressure posteriorly. (B) The blades are opened after full insertion and maneuvered so that the cervix comes into full view.*

The cervix should be located in the midline. Any deviation to the left or right may indicate a mass, adhesions, or pregnancy.[1] The normal nulliparous cervical os is small and either round or oval. After childbirth, the cervical os presents as a slitlike appearance. Carcinoma of the cervix presents as a hard, granular lesion, which bleeds easily, proceeding later to an extensive irregular growth.[7]

To obtain cervical samples for Pap smear or cytology, the speculum blades are secured in an open position by tightening the thumbscrew.

Withdraw the speculum slowly, maintaining it in its open position. As the speculum is withdrawn, inspect the cervix for evidence of forward migration, indicating uterine prolapse. During withdrawal, inspect the vaginal mucosa, noting its color, inflammation, discharge, ulcers, or masses. Close the blades as the speculum emerges from the introitus, avoiding excessive stretching of the mucosa.[7]

Next, a single blade of the speculum is inserted to inspect for signs of pelvic descent. First, with the blade oriented posteriorly and the patient bearing down, any herniation of the bladder into the vaginal vault is noted. Next, the blade is oriented anteriorly toward the bladder. As the patient bears down, the clinician again observes for herniation, this time of the rectum into the vaginal space. Herniation of the anterior vaginal wall is a cystocele, and posterior wall herniation is called a *rectocele*. Last, observe the urethra for leakage associated with the physical stress of coughing or bearing down (stress urinary incontinence).[1]

Bimanual Examination

A bimanual examination follows inspection with the speculum. With a glove removed from one hand, the lubricated index and middle fingers of the gloved examining hand are gently and gradually inserted into the vaginal vault, allowing adequate time for the patient to relax her circumvaginal muscles.[1] The examiner's thumb should be abducted, with ring and little fingers flexed into the palm, and pressure exerted posteriorly. Any nodularity, masses, or tenderness within the vaginal wall is noted, including the region of the urethra and bladder anteriorly. Next, the cervix is gently palpated circumferentially, then gently moved from side to side, noting its mobility. A normal cervix moves 1–2 cm without causing discomfort. A tender, fixed cervix may indicate pelvic inflammatory disease, ectopic pregnancy, or pelvic mass.[1,7]

Next, the ungloved hand is placed on the patient's abdomen approximately midway between the umbilicus and symphysis pubis, and downward pressure is exerted toward the pelvic hand. The uterus should be identified, noting its size, shape, consistency, mobility, tenderness, and any masses. Uterine enlargement suggests pregnancy or benign or malignant tumors.[7]

With the abdominal hand pressing downward in the right lower quadrant and pelvic hand in the right lateral fornix, the right ovary and any adnexal masses are identified. Three to 5 years after menopause, the ovaries have usually atrophied and are no longer palpable. A palpable ovary in a postmenopausal woman may suggest an ovarian tumor. A normal ovary is somewhat tender. Repeat the procedure on the left side.[7]

Female Rectal Examination

A digital rectal examination completes the female genital evaluation and further assists in evaluating the integrity of the pelvic floor musculature. The rectum is usually examined after the female genitalia, while the patient is still in the lithotomy position.[1,6] The lubricated, gloved index finger is gently inserted into the rectum, and the tone of the anal sphincter is assessed during insertion. The finger is left in place while the bulbocavernosus reflex (BCR) is performed. The other hand is used to tap the clitoris or, when an indwelling catheter is in place, to place gentle traction against the bladder neck. A positive BCR occurs when tapping of the clitoris or traction on an indwelling catheter produces tightening of the anal sphincter around the examiner's finger. This response indicates grossly intact neurologic pathways between the pelvic floor muscles and the sacral nerve roots. A negative BCR associated with abnormal anal sphincter tone may indicate denervation. Before removing the finger, the examiner asks the patient to tighten the anal sphincter, a maneuver allowing assessment of volitional control of the pelvic floor muscles (mediated by the corticospinal tracts).[2]

Precautionary Measures during Pelvic Examination

When performing either a pelvic or rectal examination, the examiner should never contaminate the tube of lubricant by touching it with his or her gloved hand after touching the patient. The lubricant should always be dropped onto the gloved fingers; if accidentally contaminated, the lubricant's tube should discarded. An alternate is to use individual packets of lubricant.

A risk of spreading infection between vagina and rectum exists. Gonorrhea may infect the rectum as well as female genitalia. Therefore, it is recommended that gloves be changed between vaginal and rectal examination to avoid spreading infection.[7]

Neurologic Examination

Survey of Mental Status and Speech

During the course of the interview and examination, the clinician can make many observations relevant to the patient's mental status. This information may be sufficient for many patients; however, the presence of neurologic disease or the suspicion of emotional or intellectual dysfunction indicates further evaluation of cognitive functions including orientation, attention and concentration.

By skillful questioning, the patient's orientation to time (the time of the day, the day of the week, month, date, year, and duration of hospitalization), place (of his or her residence, hospital, city, state), and person (his or her own name, the names of relatives and professional personnel) can often be determined in the context of the interview. For example, the patient can be asked about specific dates or times, his or her address, and names of family members.

Assessment tools for attention span and concentration include digit span, serial counting, memory, and abstract reasoning. To assess digit span, a series of digits of varying length is read to the patient at a rate of approximately one per second, and the patient is asked to repeat them. Poor performance of digit span is characteristic of organic brain disease or dementia.

Serial sevens or serial threes are assessed by instructing the patient to, "starting from 100, subtract seven, and keep subtracting seven." The effort required and the speed and accuracy of responses are evaluated. Normally, a person can complete serial sevens in 1.5 minutes, with fewer than four errors. If the patient cannot do serial sevens, he or she should be asked to try serial threes or to count backward. Still easier tests are counting forward or reciting the alphabet. Poor performance suggests organic brain disease.

Most questions relevant to memory can be asked in the context of the interview, including inquiries that test both remote memory (birthdays and anniversaries) and recent memory (events of the day). Poor recent memory occurs in organic brain disease.

The capacity to reason abstractly is tested by asking patients the meaning of proverbs such as "a stitch in time saves nine" or "don't count your chickens before they're hatched." Patients with organic brain disorders may often give concrete responses or interpretations.[8]

Motor System

A screening procedure for the motor system is an evaluation of gait. As the patient walks across the examination room or down a hallway, his or her posture, balance, arm swing and leg movements are observed. Normally, balance is easy, arms swing at the sides, and when turning, the face and head lead the rest of the body.[9]

Spastic hemiparesis causes an abnormality of gait. The patient ambulates with one arm flexed close to the side and immobile. The leg is circled stiffly outward and forward (circumducted), often with dragging of the toe. This gait pattern is associated with unilateral upper motor neuron disease such as a stroke.

A sensory ataxia occurs with loss of position sense in the legs. The gait is unsteady and wide based with the feet far apart, and with each step lifted high and brought down with a slap. The patient watches the ground to guide his or her steps and cannot stand steadily with feet together when eyes are closed (positive Romberg's test). To perform the Romberg's test, the patient is asked to stand with feet together and without support from his or her arms. Ability to maintain an upright posture first with eyes open, then with eyes closed is noted. Normally, only minimal swaying occurs. If a patient has ataxia from cerebellar disease (cerebellar ataxia), he or she may have difficulty standing with his or her feet together with eyes open or closed. When the patient is ataxic because of decreased position sense (sensory ataxia), vision can compensate for the sensory loss and he or she can stand fairly well with eyes open. With eyes closed, however, balance decompensates. This phenomenon constitutes the positive Romberg's sign. Sensory ataxia occurs with advanced polyneuropathy.

A parkinsonian gait is associated with the basal ganglia defects of Parkinson's disease. During gait, posture is stooped, hips and knees slightly flexed, arm swings are decreased, and steps are short and often shuffling. The parkinsonian patient turns around stiffly.[9]

Next, testing patient grip and "drift sign" can screen upper extremity motor function. After assessing grip strength, the patient is asked to close his or her eyes and for 20–30 seconds to hold his or her arms straight in front of him or her, with palms up. Watch how well he or she maintains this position. Tendency of one forearm to pronate or downward drift of an arm with flexion at the elbow suggests a hemiparesis.[9]

Next, lower extremity manual muscle testing is performed.

- To test flexion at the hip, the patient attempts to raise his or her leg against the examiner's hands placed on the patient's thighs.
- To test abduction at the hip, the patient is asked to spread his or her legs against the examiner's hands, which are placed firmly on the bed outside the patient's knees.
- For adduction testing, the patient attempts to bring his or her legs together while the examiner places hands firmly on the bed between the patient's knees.
- To test flexion at the knee, the patient tries to keep his or her knees bent as the examiner tries to straighten the respective leg.
- Asking the patient to straighten a flexed knee against resistance assesses knee extension.
- Ankle plantar and dorsi flexion is assessed by asking the patient to push down and pull up against the examiner's hand.[9]

Symmetric proximal muscle weakness suggests myopathy, and symmetric distal weakness suggests neuropathy or polyradiculopathy due to spinal stenosis. Unilateral weakness in a particular muscle group suggests radiculopathy.

Sensory System

The patient is asked to close his or her eyes for sensation testing. Sensation is assessed in the most important dermatomes relative to an evaluation of the urinary system, including the lumbar and sacral nerve root dermatomes. The patient's ability to perceive a particular stimulus is compared in symmetric areas on each side of the body. Distal and proximal areas of the extremities are assessed when testing pain, temperature, and touch. Vibration and position sense testing is initiated distally, and, if normal, proximal testing can be omitted. Any area of sensory loss should have its boundaries mapped out. For sensory testing, the following stimuli can be used. For pain assessment, a safety pin is used, with its sharp and blunt end used as stimuli, and the patient is asked whether it feels sharp or dull. For light touch, the examiner's fingertip or a fine wisp of cotton is used, and the patient responds whenever his or her skin is touched. For vibration testing, a relatively low-pitch tuning fork (128 cycles per second) is tapped on the heel of the examiner's hand and placed firmly over the distal interphalangeal joint of the patient's big toe. The patient is asked whether he or she feels pressure or vibration and when the vibration stops (after the examiner touches the ends of the tuning fork). For position testing, the patient's big toe is grasped by its sides between the examiner's thumb and index finger; avoiding friction against the other toes, it is moved, and the patient attempts to identify whether the toe is moving up or down.[9]

Reflexes

To elicit deep tendon reflexes, the patient should relax. The muscle to be tested is mildly stretched, and its tendon is then struck briskly, producing a sudden additional tendon stretch. The patient's limbs should be symmetrically positioned and the sides compared. If the patient's reflexes are symmetrically diminished or absent, reinforcement techniques are used. This involves isometric contraction of other muscles that may increase reflex activity. For example, if arm reflexes are diminished or absent, asking the patient to lock his or her fingers together and pull one hand against the other can reinforce them.

Reflexes are graded on a 0 to 4+ scale: 4+ indicates very brisk, hyperactive reflexes often associated with clonus (rhythmic oscillations between flexion and extension); 3+ reflexes are brisker than average but not necessarily indicative of disease; 2+ reflexes are average or normal; 1+ reflexes are somewhat diminished or low normal; 0 reflexes indicate no response. If 1+ or 0 reflexes are obtained, reinforcement techniques should be attempted. Hyperactive reflexes (3+, 4+) suggest upper motor neuron disease, and hypoactive reflexes (0, 1+) suggest lower motor neuron disease or polyneuropathy.

Reflexes that should be assessed include the biceps (C5, C6), triceps (C7, C8), brachioradialis (C5, C6), knee (L2, L3, L4), and ankle reflexes (S1 and S2 nerve roots). The ankle reflex is performed with the leg somewhat flexed at the knee and the foot dorsiflexed at the ankle. The examiner then strikes the Achilles' tendon and watches for a planter flexion response at the ankle.

The plantar response (Babinski's reflex) tests the L4 through S2 nerve roots. With a moderately sharp object, such as a key, the examiner lightly strokes the lateral aspect of the sole from the heel to the ball of the foot, curving medially across the ball. The toes normally flex. Dorsiflexion of the great toe with fanning of the other toes indicates upper motor neuron disease (Babinski's response).

If the reflexes are hyperactive, the examiner tests for ankle clonus. With the knee supported in a partly flexed position, the examiner uses his or her other hand to sharply dorsiflex the foot and maintain it in dorsiflexion. Rhythmic oscillations between dorsiflexion and plantar flexion (clonus) indicate upper motor neuron disease. No clonus is the norm.[9]

References

1. Gray M. Assessment. In M Gray (ed), Genitourinary Disorders. St. Louis: Mosby, 1992;20–31.
2. Gray M. Assessment of Patients with Urinary Incontinence. In DB Doughty (ed), Urinary and Fecal Incontinence: Nursing Management. St. Louis: Mosby, 1991;47–94.
3. Bates B. The Physical Examination of the Adult: an Overview. In B Bates (ed), A Guide to Physical Examination (2d ed). Philadelphia: JB Lippincott, 1979;31–34.
4. Bates B. Male Genitalia and Hernias. In B Bates (ed), A Guide to Physical Examination (2d ed). Philadelphia: JB Lippincott, 1979;221–229.
5. Bates B. The Abdomen. In B Bates (ed), A Guide to Physical Examination (2d ed). Philadelphia: JB Lippincott, 1979;200–220.
6. Bates B. Anus and Rectum. In B Bates (ed), A Guide to Physical Examination (2d ed). Philadelphia: JB Lippincott, 1979;249–256.
7. Bates B. Female Genitalia. In B Bates (ed), A Guide to Physical Examination (2d ed). Philadelphia: JB Lippincott, 1979;230–248.
8. Bates B. Mental Status. In B Bates (ed), A Guide to Physical Examination (2d ed). Philadelphia: JB Lippincott, 1979;359–366.
9. Bates B. The Nervous System. In B Bates (ed), A Guide to Physical Examination (2d ed). Philadelphia: JB Lippincott, 1979;311–358.

5   Imaging of the Urinary Tract

Jack L. Rook

Radiography

Introduction

Radiography (roentgenography) is the oldest method of urologic imaging, having been used to demonstrate radiopaque urinary calculi shortly after the discovery of x-rays by Wilhelm Roentgen in 1895. Since then, it has continued to be useful diagnostically in every branch of medicine. More recently developed imaging techniques, such as radionuclide scanning, ultrasonography, computed tomography (CT), and magnetic resonance imaging (MRI), are complementing, and, in some instances, replacing long-established uroradiographic techniques.[1]

X-rays are electromagnetic waves with wavelengths that are only 1/10,000 the length of visible light rays. Because of this short wavelength, x-rays can penetrate dense substances to produce images or shadows that can then be recorded on photographic film placed behind the subject. The basic principle of radiography rests with the fact that differences in density between various body structures produce images of varying light or dark intensity on the x-ray film. Dense structures appear white, air-filled areas are black, and various tones of gray represent varying degrees of tissue density through which the x-ray beams have passed. A radiopaque contrast medium is frequently used to help distinguish separate structures, thus making x-rays easier to interpret. Roentgenography is safe when properly used by trained personnel.[1,2]

Although newer techniques are replacing radiography for diagnosis of some urologic problems, radiography remains the backbone of urologic practice. It is often the first and single most effective examination. The most commonly used uroradiologic studies are plain abdominal films, intravenous urograms, cystourethrograms, urethrograms, and angiograms.[1] This chapter discusses these uroradiologic studies.

Use of Contrast Media

Diagnosis of certain pathologic conditions requires that visualization of details be highlighted by the presence of contrast media in the area. Such radiographic contrast media include various iodine-containing liquids. Water-soluble iodine preparations can be administered by several routes. Intravascular contrast is especially useful in urographic and angiographic x-ray studies. Adverse reactions can occur particularly with intravenous urographic contrast media. Whereas most reactions are minor (e.g., nausea, vomiting, hives, rash, or flushing), and require no specific treatment other than reassurance, cardiopulmonary and anaphylactic reactions can occur with little or no warning and can be life-threatening or fatal. Various reports describe the incidence of death due to intravascular injection of contrast media to range anywhere from 1 per 10,000 to 1 per 70,000.[1,2] However, there are no reliable methods for pretesting patients for possible adverse reactions. Thus, the risks and benefits of using intravascular, iodine-based, urographic contrast media should be carefully evaluated beforehand with each patient.[1]

Treatment for adverse reactions involves the use of antihistamines, epinephrine, vascular volume expanders, cardiopulmonary drugs, and any other treatment procedure deemed necessary by the nature and severity of the reaction. The radiographer must always be alert to the possibility of a reaction, and emergency equipment should be readily available. Death from an allergic reaction can occur if severe symptoms go untreated. Staff in attendance must be qualified to administer cardiopulmonary resuscitation, should it be necessary.[1,2]

Advantages and Disadvantages

Radiography produces excellent anatomic images of almost any body part. Costs of equipment and examinations are considerably less than those of most other imaging systems. Space requirements for radiographic equipment are not excessive, and because there are many specialists exclusively trained in radiography, its use is not confined to large medical centers.[1]

The major disadvantage of radiographic imaging is its fundamental basis in ionizing radiation. Exposure of the human body to x-rays carries certain risks. Exposing reproductive organs to radiation may cause genetic alterations (mutations) in the exposed person's offspring. Somatic mutations (those that occur in body tissue other than reproductive cells) may also occur in tissue receiving excessive or repeated doses of radiation. For example, radiation can be the cause of cancer that develops many years after exposure.[1,2]

During the first trimester of pregnancy, the fetus is especially at risk for genetic alterations. Precautions must be taken to prevent or minimize radiation exposure to the pregnant uterus.[2]

The dangers of radiation exposure arise from the absorption of relatively large amounts of radiation over a short time and from cumulative effects of smaller amounts received over longer times. Moreover, the cumulative effects of radiation may not become evident for several years.[2]

Plain Film of the Abdomen

Background

A plain film of the abdomen, frequently called a *kidney-ureter-bladder* (KUB) film, is the simplest uroradiologic study and the first performed in any radiographic examination of the urinary tract. It is done before intravenous pyelography or other renal studies.

A KUB x-ray is an anteroposterior film study of the kidneys, ureters, and bony pelvis that does not require the use of contrast media. It is done to aid the diagnosis of intra-abdominal diseases, such as nephrolithiasis or soft-tissue masses. KUB films may provide information on the size, shape, and position of the liver, spleen, and kidneys; may demonstrate bony abnormalities; and may give information about the state of the kidneys and extrarenal urinary tract.[1–3]

Because kidney outlines can usually be seen on plain abdominal films, the size, number, shape, and position of the kidneys can be determined. The size of normal kidneys varies widely between individuals. The kidney length is a convenient radiographic measurement. The average adult kidney is approximately 12–14 cm long, and the left kidney is ordinarily slightly longer than the right one. As a rule of thumb, the normal adult kidney is approximately 3.5 times the height of the second lumbar vertebra.[1]

Procedure

The patient, wearing a hospital gown, lies flat on the x-ray table, and all metallic objects are removed from the abdominal area. A second film may be taken with the patient standing or sitting. The patient must remain still during the study. Bowel preparation using cathartics and enemas is required when a KUB is obtained before an intravenous pyelogram. No preparation is used when a KUB is done as a single study or before a cystogram, voiding cystourethrogram, or video urodynamic testing.[2,3]

Clinical Implications

Normally, the renal shadows noted on a KUB allow a rough determination of renal size and location. The ureters are not normally clearly defined, although the urinary bladder can often be identified by the shadows it casts, especially in the presence of concentrated (high-specific gravity) urine.

Abnormal results may reveal calcium deposits, tumors, stones, and abnormalities of kidney size, shape (i.e., "horseshoe-shaped" kidneys), and position.

Calculi may be visualized within the renal pelvis, ureters, bladder, or prostate (Figure 5.1). The KUB may not detect every urinary stone, particularly if the calculi are small, obscured by bowel contents, or radiolucent.[1–3]

The KUB also is used to detect bowel gas patterns that may be abnormal in the presence of large abdominal, pelvic, or renal mass. Large tumors and masses (ovarian or uterine) may also displace normal bowel configurations. Calcifications are occasionally seen with kidney cancer, or they may suggest primary disease elsewhere (e.g., the occasional patient with nephrocalcinosis whose underlying primary disease is hyperparathyroidism).

The KUB also provides an anteroposterior view of the spine. Evaluation of anatomic defects of the bony spinal column may indicate neuropathic

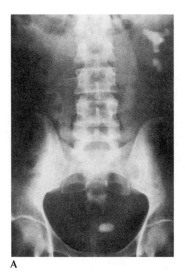
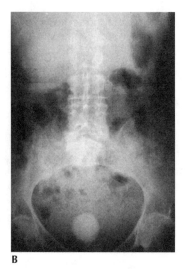
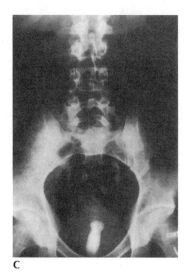

A   B   C

FIGURE 5.1   *Plain x-ray films showing: (**A**) stag horn calculus in the left kidney; (**B**) bladder calculus; and (**C**) prostatic calculus. (Reprinted with permission from P Abrams, RCL Feneley, DA Gillatt, et al. [eds]. Case Presentations in Urology. Oxford, UK: Butterworth–Heinemann, 1993;79, 86, 89.)*

bladder dysfunction caused by dysraphism or advanced degeneration of the lower spine.[1–3]

Intravenous Urography and Pyelography

Background

Intravenous urography (IVU) is among the most frequently ordered tests in cases of suspected renal disease or urinary tract dysfunction. An IVU is indicated during the initial investigation of any suspected urologic problem, especially to diagnose kidney and ureter lesions and impaired renal function.[2] Excretory urograms are simple to perform, are well tolerated by most patients, and can usually demonstrate a wide variety of urinary tract lesions. Occasionally, however, retrograde urography (see Retrograde Urogram) may be required if the patient has a history of significant adverse reaction to intravascular contrast media.[1]

The term *intravenous urogram* is preferred to *intravenous pyelogram* (IVP) because urogram implies visualization of the entire urinary tract, whereas *pyelogram* refers specifically to visualization of the kidneys. When performing an IVU, radiopaque iodine contrast agent concentrates in the urine shortly after injection. As this occurs, a series of x-ray films are made at predetermined intervals. Information about urine transport from the renal pelvis to the bladder is evaluated by means of these sequential x-rays.[2]

IVU films show kidney size, shape, and structure; ureters; bladder; and the degree to which the bladder can empty. Renal function is evaluated by noting the intervals from injection of the contrast material to its first appearance in each kidney and the excretion time of the radiopaque iodine by each kidney. Kidney disease, ureteral or bladder stones, and tumors can be detected with IVU. X-rays of the partly filled bladder provide a limited cystogram, and the patient's ability to empty the bladder is assessed through a postvoiding x-ray.[2,3]

Procedure

The radiographer must observe iodine contrast test precautions. Contraindications to performing this test include allergy to intravenous iodine contrast material, cutaneous iodine-based cleansing solution, or shellfish (which have a high iodine content). Other absolute contraindications include combined renal and hepatic disease, oliguria, or renal failure.[2,3]

The patient should abstain from all food, liquid, and medication (if possible) for 12 hours before examination. Usually, the patient takes a laxative the evening before the examination and receives an enema the next morning. Adequate bowel preparation helps minimize visual obscurity caused by fecal material and bowel gas in the abdomen.[2,3]

To begin the study, a preliminary x-ray film is taken with the patient in a supine position to assure the bowel is empty and kidney location can be visualized. Next, the intravenous contrast material is injected. Initially, a small amount of contrast is injected, and the patient is monitored carefully for urticaria, rhonchi, or shortness of breath. If there is no allergic reaction, the intravenous infusion can continue. The amount of iodine commonly used in patients with normal renal function is approximately 300 mg/kg of body weight.[1,2] During and after the intravenous contrast injection, the patient is assessed for untoward signs of an allergic reaction, such as respiratory difficulty, diaphoresis, numbness, palpitations, shock, respiratory distress, precipitous hypotension, fainting, convulsions, urticaria, or cardiopulmonary arrest. Emergency drugs, equipment, and supplies should be readily available, along with personnel equipped to handle such a situation.

After injection of the contrast material, at least three x-ray films are taken at predetermined intervals. After these films are taken, the patient voids before the final film is taken to determine the ability of the bladder to empty.[2]

Acute renal failure is a rare but serious postprocedural complication. Adequate fluid intake should be encouraged, and ideally the patient should be observed for adequacy of urinary output (at least 30 ml per hour) after an IVU.[3]

Clinical Implications

The normal IVU demonstrates the proper size, shape, and position of the kidneys, ureters, and bladder. Normal kidneys are approximately three and one-half vertebral bodies in length.

With normal renal function, the kidney outline appears on x-ray film 2–5 minutes after injection of contrast material. At this time, threadlike strands of contrast material begin to appear in the calyces. When the second film is taken 5–7 minutes after contrast injection, the entire renal pelvis should be visualized. Subsequent films show the ureters and

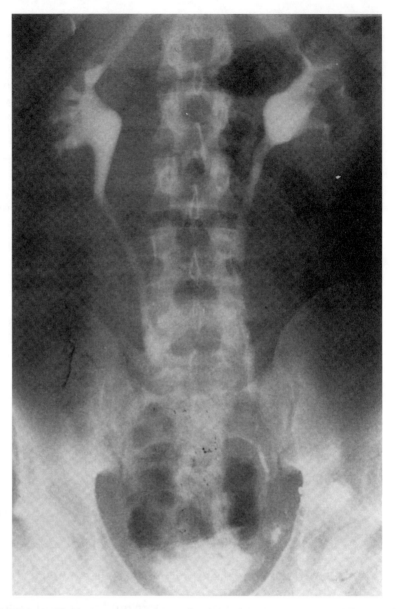

FIGURE 5.2 *The intravenous urogram after 5–7 minutes post–contrast injection demonstrates the entire renal pelvis, ureters, and bladder as contrast material makes it way into the lower urinary tract. (Reprinted with permission from N Cetti, RS Kirby [eds]. Trauma to the Genitourinary Tract. Oxford, UK: Butterworth–Heinemann, 1997;33.)*

bladder as the contrast material makes its way into the lower urinary tract (Figure 5.2). Last, no evidence of residual urine should be found on the postvoid film.[2]

Abnormal IVU findings may reveal altered size, form, and position of the kidneys, ureters, and bladder. Only one kidney, or an enlarged kidney or kidneys (hydronephrosis, or polycystic disease) may be visualized (Figure 5.3).[2]

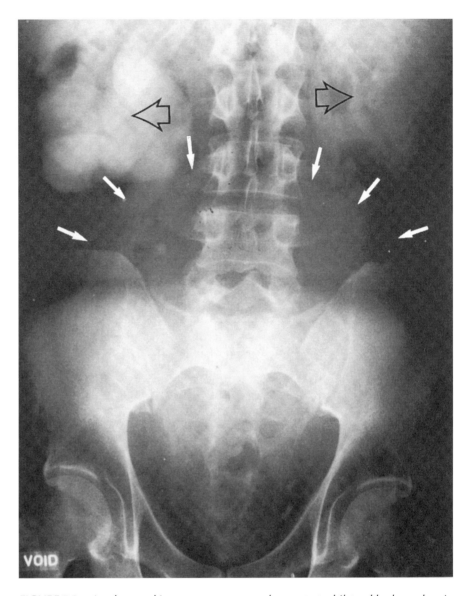

FIGURE 5.3   *An abnormal intravenous urogram demonstrates bilateral hydronephrosis (open arrowheads) and a vastly distended bladder up to the level of the umbilicus (dome of bladder delineated by white arrows). (Reprinted with permission from MB Chancellor, JG Blaivas [eds]. Practical Neuro-Urology: Genitourinary Complications in Neurologic Disease. Boston: Butterworth–Heinemann, 1995;242.)*

Renal or ureteral calculi (stones) (Figure 5.4), cystic disease (Figure 5.5), or tumor (Figure 5.6) may be identified. Renal injury subsequent to trauma may manifest as extravasation of contrast material. Prostate enlargement in the male may be seen during the cystogram phase of the IVU.[2]

A time delay in radiopaque contrast visualization is indicative of renal dysfunction. No contrast visualization may indicate poor renal function. Evidence of renal failure in the presence of normal-sized kidneys suggests

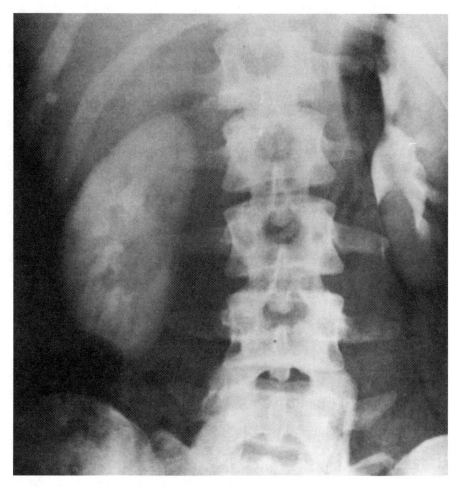

FIGURE 5.4   *Intravenous urogram in acute ureteric obstruction by a stone. Note dense right nephrogram with delayed opacification of dilatated calyces. (Reprinted with permission from NJ O'Higgins, GD Chisholm, RCN Williamson [eds]. Surgical Management [2d ed]. Oxford, UK: Butterworth–Heinemann, 1991;684.)*

an acute rather than chronic disease process. Delayed contrast visualization in the presence of irregular scarring of the renal outlines suggests chronic pyelonephritis.[2]

Retrograde Urogram

Background
Retrograde urography is a moderately invasive procedure. It requires cystoscopy and placement of catheters in the ureters through which a radiopaque, contrast medium is introduced into the ureters or renal collecting structures. Radiograms of the abdomen are then taken. The study, which requires local or general anesthesia, and which is technically more difficult than an excretory urogram, must be performed by a urologist.[1]

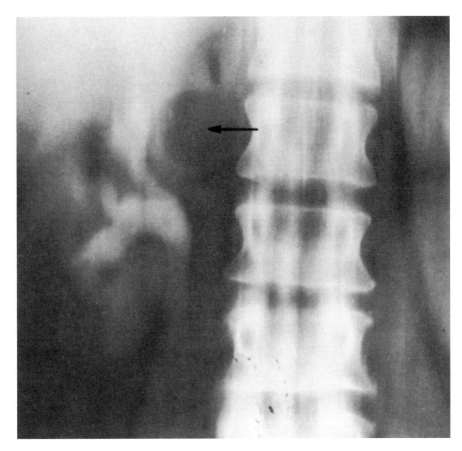

FIGURE 5.5 *Intravenous urogram shows a well-defined cyst on the medial border of the right kidney* (arrow). *(Reprinted with permission from NJ O'Higgins, GD Chisholm, RCN Williamson [eds]. Surgical Management [2d ed]. Oxford, UK: Butterworth–Heinemann, 1991;683.)*

Indications for this procedure are the same as for IVPs and IVUs. However, the retrograde pyelogram is used with patients who are allergic to iodine-bound contrast material; who have a nonfunctioning kidney incapable of concentrating and excreting contrast; if excretory urograms are unsatisfactory; or if other methods of imaging are unavailable or inappropriate. The contraindication to this procedure is allergy to cutaneous iodine-based cleansing agents.[1,3]

Procedure
The patient undergoing retrograde urography should fast from food and fluids after midnight before the procedure, and cathartics, suppositories, or enemas should be used for bowel preparation as with the IVU.

The examination is usually done in the surgical department or in a specially equipped cystoscopy suite at a urologist's office. Sedation and analgesia precede insertion of a local anesthetic into the urethra. General anesthesia may be required if the patient cannot fully cooperate with the

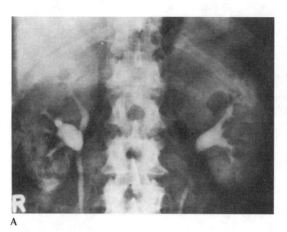
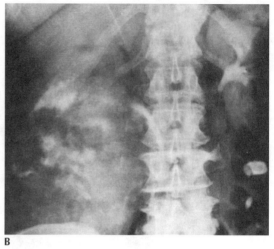

A   B

FIGURE 5.6 *(A)* *Intravenous urogram carried out because of hypertension with renal impairment. A large mass is in the left upper renal pole.* *(B)* *Intravenous urogram done because of hematuria. A large mass is destroying the right kidney, with extensive amorphous calcification—a renal carcinoma. (Reprinted with permission from NJ O'Higgins, GD Chisholm, RCN Williamson [eds]. Surgical Management [2d ed]. Oxford, UK: Butterworth–Heinemann, 1991;682.)*

procedure. The cystoscope is inserted and the ureteral catheter is then advanced through it, and placed in the lower ureteral segment. Contrast material is gently injected or infused by means of gravity into the upper urinary tract. A series of x-rays are performed as the contrast is infused.

Immediately after the procedure, the patient is observed for allergic reaction to iodine contrast. Urine output and appearance should be recorded for the first 24 hours after procedure. Hematuria or dysuria may be common after the examination. If hematuria does not clear and dysuria persists or worsens, the urologist should be notified. Analgesics may be required to treat dysuria for 24–48 hours post procedure.[2,3]

Postprocedural complications include urinary tract infection (UTI), pyelonephritis, and flank pain. Pyelonephritis is related to instrumentation and injection of material into a sterile body compartment. It is a potentially serious complication characterized by flank pain, dysuria, chills, and fever for 24–48 hours after the procedure. Urine for culture and analysis must be performed should these symptoms occur, and appropriate antibiotics administered as directed.

Overdistension of the renal collecting system by contrast material may produce flank pain and fever, mimicking pyelonephritis. This response typically is transient and disappears within 48 hours. However, a urinalysis and culture should be done as a precautionary measure to rule out infection.[3]

Clinical Implications

Abnormal results may reveal an intrinsic abnormality of ureters and kidney pelvis (such as congenital defects), an extrinsic abnormality of the ureters (such as an obstructive tumor causing ureteral constriction), or ureteral obstruction due to stone disease.[2]

Cystogram or Voiding Cystourethrogram

Background
A cystogram or voiding cystourethrogram (VCUG) requires catheterization and installation of contrast material into the bladder, thereby outlining the bladder cavity. A cystogram is a series of x-rays of the bladder during filling; VCUGs are radiograms of the bladder and urethra obtained during micturition.[1,3]

Procedure
These procedures are contraindicated in patients with allergy to cutaneous iodine-based cleansing solutions or current UTI.

The contrast medium is usually instilled via a transurethral catheterization. When necessary, the contrast medium can be administered via percutaneous suprapubic bladder puncture. During bladder filling, radiograms are taken using standard overhead x-ray tube equipment, or, less frequently, "spot" films are taken using real time, image-intensified fluoroscopy. During the VCUG, x-ray images of the bladder and urethra are taken during micturition.[1,3]

After the procedure, the patient is observed for complications. The principal complications of the cystogram/VCUG test are UTI and urethral or bladder discomfort.[3]

Clinical Implications
The VCUG is used to evaluate patients with recurrent UTI, febrile UTI, vesicoureteral reflux, and unexplained gross or microscopic hematuria.

The results may demonstrate a congenital anomaly of the urinary system, trauma or tumor of the lower urinary tract, and the degree or grade of vesicoureteral reflux.[3]

Retrograde Urethrogram

Background
The urethra can be imaged radiographically by retrograde injection of radiopaque fluid. The retrograde urethrogram (RUG) technique is useful for examining the urethra.[1]

Procedure
A RUG requires installation of a relatively small volume of iodine-bound contrast material into the male urethra. The fluid is instilled through a catheter-tipped syringe or Foley catheter snuggled into the fossa navicularis with the balloon inflated with approximately 1 ml of fluid. X-rays of the urethra are obtained after installation of approximately 15–30 ml of contrast material. Contraindications to this procedure include allergy to cutaneous iodine-based cleansing solutions and concurrent UTI that should be treated before a RUG whenever possible.[3]

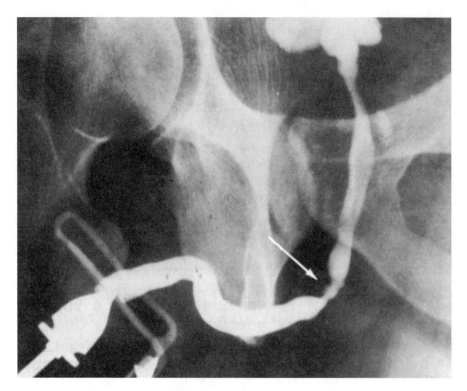

FIGURE 5.7 *This patient with prostatic calcification complains of difficulty voiding—the urethrogram shows a urethral stricture* (arrow). *(Reprinted with permission from NJ O'Higgins, GD Chisholm, RCN Williamson [eds]. Surgical Management [2d ed]. Oxford, UK: Butterworth–Heinemann, 1991;687.)*

After the test, mild dysuria and urethral burning may occur, but these are typically transient.[3] Mild analgesics may be required.

Clinical Implications
RUG is performed to evaluate for urethral stricture, fistula, trauma, diverticulum, or tumor (Figure 5.7).[3]

Angiography

Background
Angiography refers to radiographic visualization of blood vessels through the use of radiopaque contrast media. Angiographic study of the urinary tract is almost exclusively used to visualize vascular renal structures. The renal arteriogram is a moderately invasive procedure that usually requires a hospital stay. Increasing use of ultrasonography, CT and MRI scanning, and digital angiography has resulted in a decrease in the use of angiography for the diagnosis of urologic problems.[1]

Procedure
A renal arteriogram may be performed, assuming the patient does not have allergy to intravenous, iodine-bound contrast material.[3]

Angiographic study of the kidneys requires percutaneous needle puncture and catheterization of a common femoral artery. The catheter is advanced into the aorta to the level of the renal arteries. Rapid serial radiograms are obtained during and after bolus injection of radiopaque contrast medium into the aorta at the level of the renal arteries (aortorenal arteriogram), or directly into one of the renal arteries (selective renal arteriogram). Radiographic images obtained over the first 2–4 seconds after injection allow visualization of the renal arterial system. The next 15–20 seconds are marked by opacification of contrast in the renal parenchyma; this is the nephric phase.

After satisfactory x-rays have been obtained, the catheter is removed. Direct pressure is held on the puncture site until bleeding is controlled, after which a pressure dressing is applied. The patient is required to remain at completely flat bed rest for the next 6 hours, with restriction of flexion or bending of the joint adjacent to the puncture site. The pressure dressing should be assessed for signs of frank bleeding until the dressing is removed 24–48 hours after the procedure.[1–3]

Clinical Implications

In urologic practice, renal arteriography is most often performed to investigate renal tumors, to obtain vascular maps before surgery is performed, to evaluate the suitability of potential kidney donors, to assess renal trauma, and to assess renal vascular lesions that may be precipitating hypertension.[1,3]

Adenocarcinomas of the kidney are generally hypervascular, whereas transitional cell carcinomas are poorly vascularized and difficult to identify by angiography (Figure 5.8). Benign renal cysts are avascular, with displacement of normal vessels around the sharply outlined lesion. Renal abscesses can mimic renal cysts on angiography.[1]

Although CT scans readily demonstrate renal tumors, many surgeons obtain renal arteriograms as preoperative vascular maps to determine the vascular limits of the tumor, its degree of hypervascularity, and whether it has any other blood supplies in addition to its renal artery.[1]

Ultrasound Studies

Ultrasonography is a noninvasive procedure for visualizing soft-tissue structures of the body by recording the reflection of ultrasonic waves directed into the tissues (echo reflection maps).[4]

Ultrasound uses high-frequency sound waves to characterize the position, size, shape, and consistency of soft-tissue organs.[4]

Ultrasound waves for imaging are generated by transducers, devices that convert electrical energy to sound energy and, conversely, generate an electrical potential when struck by reflected sound waves. Thus, they act as both sound transmitters and sound receivers. In imaging, repeated bursts of ultrasound emanate from the transducer and are transmitted through tissues. Between transmissions, the transducer acts as a sound detector.[1]

Ultrasound imaging is based on the principle that tissues of varying density differentially reflect acoustic energy. Ultrasound images are

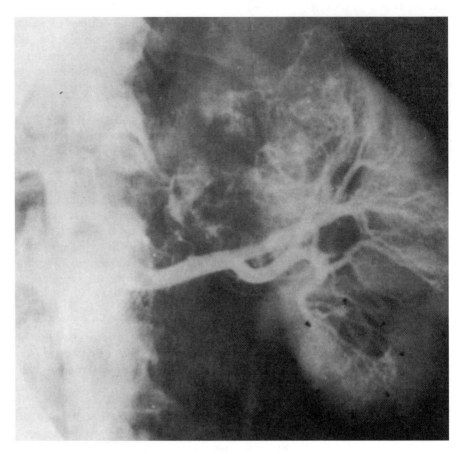

FIGURE 5.8 *Selective renal arteriogram—there is an extensive abnormal vascular pattern in a mass at the left upper renal pole. A second carcinoma is in the lower renal pole (arrowheads). (Reprinted with permission from NJ O'Higgins, GD Chisholm, RCN Williamson [eds]. Surgical Management [2d ed]. Oxford, UK: Butterworth–Heinemann, 1991;683.)*

reflected sounds picked up by the transducer. These sounds vary in intensity and time according to the nature and location of the tissues from which they are reflected. The reflected sound energies received by the transducer are converted into electrical signals that are amplified and then converted by the computer into analog echo images of the acoustic profile of the tissues being examined. The images can be viewed directly in real time or permanently recorded on hard copy, film, or videotape.[1]

Therefore, the basic physical principles of clinical ultrasonography are as follows:

1. An ultrasound beam is directed into the patient's body.
2. Body tissues with different acoustic impedance reflect the sound waves with varying degrees of intensity.
3. The various echo (reflection) waves are electronically processed and displayed in real time.

4. Recordings of these displays may be made for documentation purposes on a variety of media.
5. Pathologic processes are detectable because lesions often contain tissues with acoustic properties different from the acoustics of normal, surrounding tissues.[4]

Sonography produces good images of the urinary tract. It is useful as the initial screening procedure in suspected urinary tract disease, particularly when exposure to x-rays is undesirable or intravenous contrast medium is contraindicated due to allergy or poor renal function.[1]

The renal calyces produce strong sonographic echoes, those from the renal cortex are of intermediate strength, and echoes from the renal pyramids are the least intense. Fluid-filled structures, including uncomplicated cysts, distended bladder, dilatated ureter, or hydronephrotic kidney, are anechoic. In contrast, renal tumors, complicated cysts, and abscesses produce echoes of varying degrees ranging from minimal to intense.[1]

The advantages of diagnostic ultrasound include its safety and noninvasiveness. No contraindications to this procedure, no radiation risk for both patient and examiner, and no harmful cumulative effect with repeated examinations exist. Diagnostic ultrasound does not require the injection of contrast materials or isotopes or ingestion of opaque materials. Because ultrasound studies demonstrate structure, rather than function, they may be useful for patients with renal failure who cannot tolerate the intravenous contrast media required for IVU or arteriography.[1,3,4] It is a relatively inexpensive test, whose equipment is small and mobile in comparison with other imaging equipment. It requires little, if any, patient preparation and aftercare. Studies can be performed on an outpatient basis, obviating the need for extended hospitalization.[1,4]

The major disadvantages of sonography are that structures behind bones or bowel gas cannot be imaged, air-filled structures cannot be studied, and extremely obese patients are often difficult to study. A skilled operator is required to operate the transducer. The scans must be read immediately by a specially trained radiologist and interpreted for adequacy. If they are unsatisfactory, the examination must be repeated.[1,4]

Sonography is the method of choice in many types of urinary tract abnormalities. The urinary tract may be visualized using renal, abdominal, bladder, and prostate ultrasonographic examinations.

Kidney Sonogram

Background
Renal ultrasonography is used to visualize the kidney parenchyma and associated structures. Renal ultrasound is particularly valuable in visualizing the kidneys in patients with iodine hypersensitivity.[4]

Procedure
Scans are usually performed with the patient in the decubitus position. Fasting is not necessary. A gel or lubricant, which helps conduct sound waves, is applied to the skin over the area to be examined. The ultra-

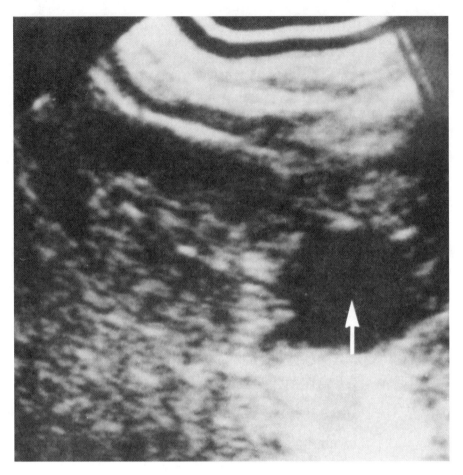

FIGURE 5.9   *Longitudinal ultrasound scan. A sharply demarcated echo-free lesion is in the lower renal pole—cyst (arrow). (Reprinted with permission from NJ O'Higgins, GD Chisholm, RCN Williamson [eds]. Surgical Management [2d ed]. Oxford, UK: Butterworth–Heinemann, 1991;680.)*

sonographer moves the transducer over the right or left flank, producing a display that is viewed on the monitor, and selected images are recorded for documentation purposes. The test usually takes 20–45 minutes.[4]

Clinical Implications
Abnormal findings may reveal cysts (Figure 5.9), masses (Figure 5.10), hydronephrosis (Figure 5.11), obstructed ureters, or calculi (Figure 5.12).[4]

Results provide information on the size and internal structure of a non-functioning kidney. The renal ultrasound images can easily differentiate between bilateral hydronephrosis; polycystic kidneys; the small, end-stage kidneys of glomerulonephritis or pyelonephritis. Solid lesions can be differentiated from cystic lesions.[4]

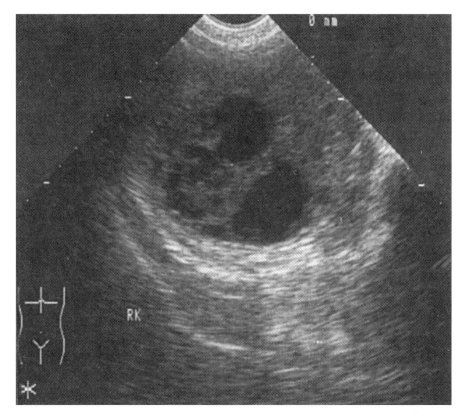

FIGURE 5.10   *Ultrasound shows a solid, cystic mass in a nonfunctioning right kidney identified by intravenous urogram. This was a hypernephroma. (Reprinted with permission from A Cuschieri, GR Giles, AR Moosa [eds]. Essential Surgical Practice [3d ed]. Oxford, UK: Butterworth–Heinemann, 1995;1469.)*

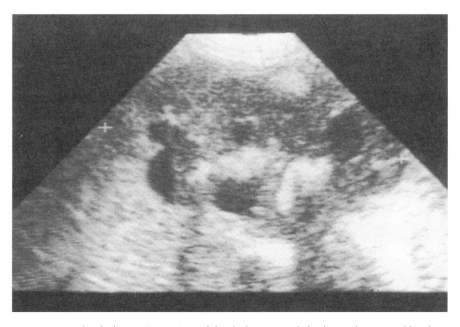

FIGURE 5.11   *Longitudinal ultrasonic section of this kidney reveals hydronephrosis and bright areas with acoustic shadows within the kidney. (Reprinted with permission from BO O'Donnell, SA Koff [eds]. Pediatric Urology [3d ed]. Oxford, UK: Butterworth–Heinemann, 1996;42.)*

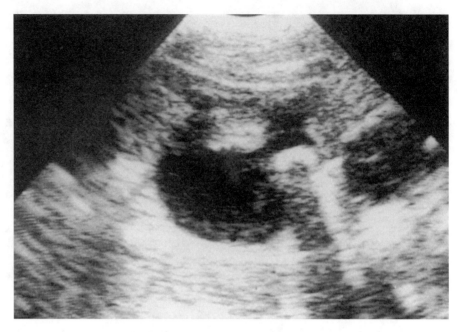

FIGURE 5.12 *Longitudinal ultrasonic section of a kidney reveals bright reflective areas with acoustic shadows, suggesting renal calculi. (Reprinted with permission from BO O'Donnell, SA Koff [eds]. Pediatric Urology [3d ed]. Oxford, UK: Butterworth–Heinemann, 1996;42.)*

Abdominal Ultrasound

Background
Abdominal ultrasonography can be used to visualize all solid organs of the upper abdomen, including the kidneys. It can be a valuable tool in detecting a variety of pathologic processes, including fluid collections, masses, infections, and obstructions.[4]

Procedure
Scans are generally performed in supine and decubitus positions. The patient should have nothing by mouth for 12 hours before the examination to improve anatomic visualization of abdominal structures. Intestinal gas overlying the area of interest interferes with sonographic visualization (air is a strong reflector of sound). If a patient has a large amount of gas in the bowel, the examination should be rescheduled.

Scans cannot be done over open wounds or through dressings, and obesity adversely affects tissue visualization.[4]

Clinical Implications
Kidney abnormalities that may be seen include hydronephrosis, cysts, tumors, masses, abscesses, calculi, and perirenal fluid collections.[4]

Urinary Bladder Sonogram

Background
The bladder sonogram examination is done as part of the investigation of a possible bladder tumor. It also provides a simple method of estimating postvoid residual urine volume, thus reducing the need for urinary catheterization with its inherent risk of subsequent UTI. The patient may experience some discomfort during the sonogram from maintaining a full urinary bladder, necessary for this test.

Procedure
The patient with a fully distended bladder is instructed to lie supine on an examination table, and the bladder is then scanned. When the bladder scan is completed, the patient voids, after which additional images are then taken to check for residual volume.

Clinical Implications
Abnormal results may reveal tumors of the bladder, cancerous extension of other tumors to urinary bladder, or masses posterior to the bladder. Urinary retention with high postvoid residual volumes may also be demonstrated.[4]

Transrectal Prostate Sonogram

Background
The transrectal prostate sonogram is a valuable tool used in the diagnosis of prostate cancer. It is particularly effective when used in association with rectal examination and laboratory testing of blood samples for levels of prostate-specific antigen and acid phosphatase.

Sonography can be used to evaluate the prostate and surrounding tissues. Small, subclinical tumors may be identified using this method. It is also useful in evaluating palpable nodules, as a guide to biopsy, to help stage a known carcinoma, and to assist in radiation "seed" placement. The volume of the prostate can be determined, making transrectal sonography useful in the evaluation of some micturition disorders (i.e., overflow incontinence due to benign prostatic hypertrophy).[4]

Procedure
Immediately before the study, a self-administered enema is used to eliminate fecal material from the rectum, which would otherwise interfere with results. The patient then lies on his or her left side with knees bent, and a draped and lubricated rectal probe is inserted. Advances in technology have allowed the development of small transducers capable of being placed within body orifices. Water may be introduced into the sheath surrounding the transducer. Scans are performed in various planes by slightly rotating the transducer.[4]

Clinical Implications
Abnormal results may be associated with prostatitis, benign prostatic hypertrophy, or carcinoma of the prostate.[4]

Computed Tomography or Computed Axial Tomography Scans

Background

CT scans, or computed axial tomography scans, produce x-rays similar to those used in conventional radiography, but are taken with a special scanner system.[2]

Conventional x-ray machines produce a flat picture with the body's organs superimposed over one another. The result is a two-dimensional image of a three-dimensional body. With CT scanning, an interconnected x-ray source and detector system is rapidly rotated around a supine patient within a gantry. Detectors record the number of transmitted x-rays during the scan period. Digital computers integrate the collected information, which is reconstructed into a cross-sectional image (tomogram) that is displayed directly on a television screen. The image can be photographed or stored for later retrieval.[1,2]

Therefore, CT produces cross-sectional images ("slices") of anatomic structures without superimposing tissues on one another. Additionally, CT can differentiate tissue characteristics within a particular solid organ.[2]

Radiograms and CT scans are reflections of the amount of x-rays passing through body tissues and reaching the respective detectors. Tissues that absorb much of the x-ray beam (e.g., bone) appear as white (radiopaque) shadows on the CT scan, just as they do on conventional x-rays; tissues that absorb little photon energy, (e.g., fat and gas) record as black (radiolucent) shadows; soft tissues record as various shades of gray. Body tissues of varying density have their own radio-attenuating values, which are denoted by CT numbers. Water has been assigned a CT number of 0; fat and gas have negative CT numbers; bone and metal have positive CT numbers; and soft tissues have varying positive CT numbers greater than 0 (the CT number of water), but less than the CT number of bone. Any tissue on the CT slice can easily be assigned a CT number by the machine.[1]

A CT abdominal scan provides axial images of the abdominal contents, including the kidneys, ureters, bladder, major renal vessels, and pelvic lymph nodes (Figure 5.13). The advantages of CT scanning of the urinary tract are that it demonstrates organ morphology exceptionally well, is relatively easy to interpret, and can be done on an outpatient basis. Its disadvantages are its basis in ionizing radiation, the size and immobility of the equipment, and cost of the studies.[1,3]

Procedure

The patient lies supine and immobile on a motorized couch that moves into a doughnut-shaped gantry. X-ray tubes within the gantry move around the patient, generating pictures that are simultaneously projected onto a monitor screen. The patient should remain still during the procedure so that adequate serial images can be obtained. Sedation and analgesics may help the uncooperative or anxious patient lie quietly during the test.

CT abdominal examination is often preceded by having the patient drink a contrast preparation, which helps outline the bowel so it can be readily differentiated from other structures during the study. Should a questionable area need further clarification during the examination, iodine contrast substance can be injected intravenously and more pic-

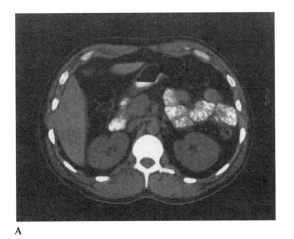
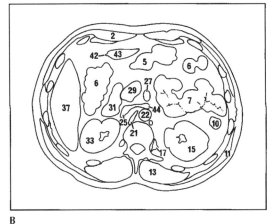

A   B

FIGURE 5.13   **(A)** *Computed tomography scan section, which passes through the body of the first lumbar vertebra. The kidneys are embedded in a mass of fatty connective tissue termed the* perirenal *(perinephric)* fat. **(B)** *Key to scan section: 2 = rectus abdominus, 7 = jejunum, 13 = erector spinae, 15 = left kidney, 22 = aorta, 25 = inferior vena cava, 33 = right kidney, 37 = right lobe of the liver. (Reprinted with permission from H Ellis, B Logan, A Dixon [eds]. Human Cross-Sectional Anatomy: Pocket Atlas of Body Sections and CT Images. Oxford, UK: Butterworth–Heinemann, 1994;105.)*

tures taken. An allergy to iodine is a contraindication to its use.

Pelvic CT examinations usually require both intravenous and rectal (barium enema) contrast administration. To help delineate the vaginal wall, female patients may be required to insert vaginal tampons before undergoing pelvic CT scans. Hypersensitivity reactions may occur when contrast materials are injected. The patient may experience warmth, flushing of the face, salty taste, and nausea with IV injection of contrast material. An emesis basin should be available as a precaution. After injection of contrast material, the patient must be monitored for untoward signs and symptoms such as respiratory difficulty, heavy sweating, palpitations, or progression to an anaphylactic reaction. Resuscitation equipment and drugs should be readily available.[2]

Clinical Implications

Abnormal abdominal and pelvic CT scan findings may reveal tumors (Figure 5.14), cysts, retroperitoneal lymphadenopathy, skeletal bone metastases, and abdominal masses. Renal cysts have CT numbers close to that of water and lower than those of tumors, complicated cysts, and abscesses.[1,2] CT demonstration of the extent and spread of genitourinary tumors is useful for staging.[2,3] Vertebral abnormalities, including lumbar herniated disks, spinal stenosis, and tumors that can contribute to neuropathic bladder dysfunction, can be defined through spinal CT imaging.

Magnetic Resonance Imaging

Background

It is generally agreed that MRI is probably the most powerful and versatile imaging technique in medicine. Clinical MRI has its basis in the nuclear prop-

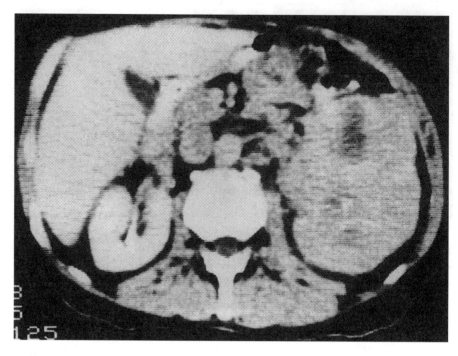

FIGURE 5.14 *Computed tomography scan of the abdomen shows a large left renal mass—a renal carcinoma. (Reprinted with permission from NJ O'Higgins, GD Chisholm, RCN Williamson [eds]. Surgical Management [2d ed]. Oxford, UK: Butterworth–Heinemann, 1991;729.)*

erties of hydrogen atoms within the body. The nucleus of a hydrogen atom consists of a single proton. Any atom containing an odd number of protons has the nuclear property of spin, with its nucleus behaving like a tiny magnet. Ordinarily, the axis of spin of each hydrogen nucleus within the body is randomly oriented. However, if the whole body or part of it is placed in a strong magnetic field (like that produced by the large magnets housed in magnetic resonance [MR] imagers), the hydrogen nuclei of the body part within that field wobbles like a top around the lines of magnetic force. If these nuclei are then additionally stimulated by short pulses of radio waves of appropriate frequency, the nuclei absorb the energy and invert their orientation within the magnetic field (they are elevated to a state of higher energy). Once the short radio-frequency pulse terminates, the hydrogen nuclei return at various speeds (depending on the density of the tissues they reside in) to their original low-energy orientation in the magnetic field. Energy is emitted in the form of radio waves as this process occurs, a phenomenon called *nuclear magnetic resonance*. The emitted radio wave energies from the resonating hydrogen nuclei are collected by the MR units, converted to digits, coded spatially, and the information is then reconstructed into tomographic body images that resemble CT scans.[1] In other words, when the radio waves generated by the MR scanner are discontinued, the protons within the body rapidly return to a lower energy state, producing a signal (tiny radio waves) that a computer can detect and convert into an image.[3]

MR tomographic images are reflections of the varying hydrogen densities in different body organs and diseased tissues.[1] Rigidly bound hydrogen nuclei, such as those in compact bone and calcified structures, register as black zones on the MR image. They are said to be MR silent (they do not generate radio wave energy). Hydrogen nuclei that move too rapidly are also MR silent and register as black zones on the image. Thus, moving blood, for example, is imaged in various shades of black, depending on the rate of blood flow.

Loosely bound hydrogen nuclei within fat generate stronger radio waves during MR testing and appear white on the MRI scan. Thus, fat is demonstrated by MR as a bright, intense, white image, the opposite of the black image it gives on radiograms and CT scans.

Tissues of the brain, spinal cord, viscera, and muscles produce MR signals of intensities between the brightest white images of fat and the black images of cortical bone.[1]

The MRI study is useful for visualizing the kidneys, prostate and other structures within the pelvis. Views can be generated in coronal, sagittal, and transaxial planes.[3]

MRI has many advantages. It uses no ionizing radiation; no harmful genetic effects have been attributed to the energy ranges used for MRI; no bowel preparation or fluid and food restrictions are necessary; contrast media are not required to distinguish the gastrointestinal tract or vascular structures; and the images produced by MRI provide better information about soft tissues than any other method of imaging.

MRI has the following disadvantages. The equipment is large and expensive, resulting in studies that cost more than other imaging procedures. Patients with metallic implants, including surgical clips, joint replacements, pacemakers, spinal cord stimulators, cardiac defibrillators, and morphine pumps, cannot be exposed to the powerful magnetic field used in MRI. Respiratory motion causes severe artifacts in abdomen and thoracic imaging. Severely obese persons may not fit into the gantry opening, and last, claustrophobic patients may be unable to tolerate MRI.[1]

Procedure

Although no special patient preparation is required before an MRI, there are numerous safety factors that must be considered. Absolute contraindications to MRI include the presence of implanted devices (pacemakers, cochlear implants, some prosthetic devices, drug-infusion pumps, neurostimulators, bone-growth stimulators, and certain intrauterine contraceptive devices), internal metallic objects (metallic fragments, bullets, shrapnel, surgical clips, pins, plates, screws, metal sutures, or wire mesh). Electronic implants are at risk for damage from both the magnetic fields and the radiofrequency pulses. Pregnancy and epilepsy are relative contraindications.

Before entering the MR suite, patients should be advised to remove dental bridges, hearing aids, credit cards, keys, hair clips, shoes, belts, jewelry, clothing with metal fasteners, hair pins, wigs, and hairpieces. Fasting or drinking clear liquids several hours before examination for abdominal or pelvic MRI may be necessary.[5]

When performing the MR examination, the patient is positioned on a movable examination couch, which is moved into the tunnel-shaped gantry. The patient is asked to remain still during the procedure. The gantry is narrow and may frighten some individuals. Sedation may be required if the patient is claustrophobic or otherwise unable to hold still during the procedure. In some instances, gadolinium diethylenetriamine pentaacetic acid (DPTA), a noniodinated contrast, is injected into a vein for better visualization of anatomy. Gadolinium has low toxicity and fewer side effects than x-ray contrast agents. Throughout the procedure, the patient hears a rhythmic knocking sound. No discomfort is associated with the MR examination.[5]

Clinical Implications

MRI of the abdomen and pelvis may demonstrate retroperitoneal structures, neoplasms (especially useful in staging tumors), evaluation of renal transplants, an abdominal or pelvic mass, or a genitourinary system tumor. Renal transplants can be serially evaluated by this modality.[3,5]

Spinal MRI may demonstrate pathology that could contribute to lumbosacral nerve damage and neuropathic bladder (spinal or metastatic tumor, lumbar herniated disk, spinal stenosis, or other arthritic changes) (Figure 5.15).

MRI of the prostate may demonstrate an enlarged hyperplastic prostate gland that indents the bladder or a focus of carcinoma, which would appear as a small area of more intense MR signal then normal surrounding tissue.[1]

Radionuclide Imaging (Nuclear Imaging)

Background

Nuclear imaging of urinary tract structures is obtained by means of intravenous or intravesical infusion of a radionuclide tracer substance. A radionuclide is an atom that has an unstable nucleus within its orbital electrons. In an attempt to reach stability, the radionuclide emits radiation, the most common types being alpha, beta, and gamma electromagnetic radiation particles. In nuclear medicine, gamma radiation is used in diagnostic procedures, as it is easy to detect and is the least ionizing type.[3,6]

Computerized scintillation detectors detect gamma radiation by giving off a light flash or scintillation. Collectively, the scintillations appear on the imaging device, outlining the organs under study, providing information on their size, shape, position, and functional activity.[6]

The radioactive materials used in nuclear medicine diagnostic imaging are called *radiopharmaceuticals*.[6] The most common radiopharmaceuticals are technetium 99m DPTA, and technetium 99m dimercaptosuccinic acid (DMSA).

DPTA is injected in an intravenous bolus, and sequential, computer-generated images are obtained at 30 seconds, and at 1, 5, 10, 15, and 20 minutes. During this time frame, DPTA images the kidneys, ureters, and bladder. DPTA is principally excreted through glomerular filtration, and the initial 30-second image can be used to determine cortical blood flow.[3]

DMSA radionuclide is also injected as an intravenous bolus, after which computer-generated, serial images of the renal parenchyma are obtained (Figure 5.16). DMSA binds to the basement membrane of the proximal renal tubule, and the serial images allow evaluation of the renal cortex.[3]

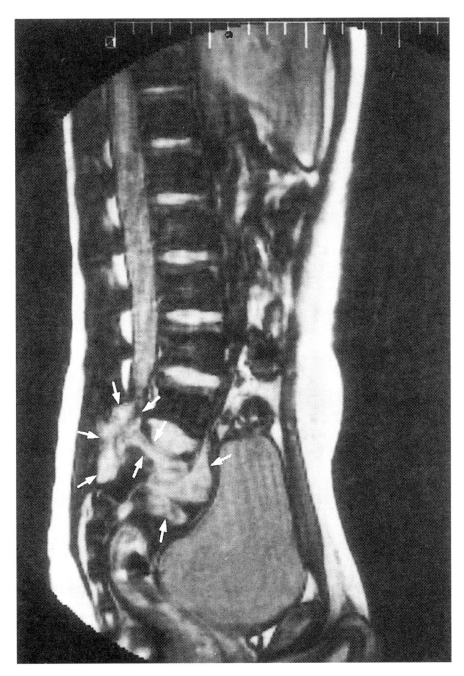

FIGURE 5.15 *Neurogenic bladder from sacral tumor. This 12-year-old boy presented with difficulty with micturition and low back pain. Sagittal midline magnetic resonance image shows a large pear-shaped flaccid neurogenic bladder. This is due to the presence of a Ewing sarcoma, which is arising in the upper sacrum. The tumor is outlined by small arrows. It has a dumbbell shape with the isthmus lying in the sacrum. Extension exists anteriorly, with a soft-tissue mass lying between the sacrum and the bladder. Extension also exists posteriorly, with tumor seen extending superiorly and inferiorly within the spinal canal. The advantage of magnetic resonance imaging in this patient is the ability to image in the sagittal plane, its ability to show the total extent of the three components of the tumor, and also the ability of magnetic resonance imaging to provide excellent contrast between the tumor and the adjacent tissues. (Reprinted with permission from BO O'Donnell, SA Koff [eds]. Pediatric Urology [3d ed]. Oxford, UK: Butterworth–Heinemann, 1996;35.)*

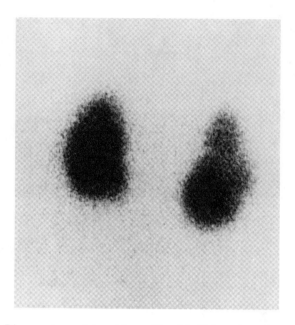

FIGURE 5.16 *Dimercaptosuccinic acid scan. The right kidney shows homogeneous distribution of isotope, but there is decreased uptake of isotope in the lower pole of the left kidney. (Reprinted with permission from BO O'Donnell, SA Koff [eds]. Pediatric Urology [3d ed]. Oxford, UK: Butterworth–Heinemann, 1996;88.)*

Several types of imaging devices are used in the field of nuclear medicine. The most basic is the gamma camera, an instrument placed over the target area, which it views in two dimensions. The major limitation of the gamma camera is that it is two-dimensional and lacks depth perception. Today, through single photon emission computed tomography, gamma cameras have achieved the third dimension, increasing the diagnostic ability of nuclear medicine imaging.[6]

There are several types of genitourinary radionuclide studies, including the renal blood flow scan, used to assess the arterial, capillary, and venous blood flow in both kidneys; the renal structural scan, used to assess size, shape, position, and function of the kidneys; the renogram, used to assess kidney function; and the nuclear cystogram, used to evaluate vesicoureteral reflux in patients who are allergic to intravesical iodine-bound contrast agents.[3, 6]

The major disadvantage of radionuclide studies is the radiation hazard to the patient, who retains the radioactivity for relatively short periods until it either dissipates on its own, or is eliminated in urine and feces, or both. These tests may be harmful to a fetus or infant and are contraindicated during pregnancy or lactation.[6]

In almost all instances, radionuclide imaging exposes the patient to less radiation than would be received if he or she were undergoing more traditional diagnostic x-ray studies (i.e., IVU). Additionally, the test is safe and painless, and side effects, such as nausea, are minimal.[6]

Procedure

The radiopharmaceutical dose is derived from calculations that include the age and weight of the patient and is administered intravenously. A sufficient time interval is allowed for the radioactive material to concentrate in the specific tissue to be studied. An imaging device records the position and concentration of the radiation that emerges from the radionuclide; the data are then processed by computer.[6]

The DPTA scan is used to evaluate glomerular filtration. When furosemide (Lasix) is injected during the DPTA scan, analysis of the washout of radionuclide from the kidneys provides an assessment of obstruction of the upper urinary tract.[7]

The DMSA scan uses a radionuclide that is filtered at the glomerulus and concentrated in the renal tubule. This scan allows both accurate evaluation of glomerular filtration and identification of focal renal scarring within the renal parenchyma (areas where functioning nephrons have been destroyed and replaced by fibrous tissue).[7,8]

Clinical Implications

Abnormal results could indicate a space-occupying "cold" or nonfunctioning area caused by a renal stone, tumor, cyst, or abscess (Figure 5.17). In contrast, increased blood flow to a vascular tumor may also be visualized. Decreased blood flow is observed with renal transplant rejection, nonfunctioning kidneys, infarction, and severe renal insufficiency.[6]

Abnormal pattern results may be indicative of hypertension, obstruction by stones or tumors, renal failure or decreased renal function, diminished renal blood flow, or renal transplant rejection.[6]

The nuclear cystogram can demonstrate vesicoureteral reflux. It is useful for patients who are allergic to intravesical iodine-bound contrast materials. However, it lacks the anatomic detail of the voiding cystogram.[3]

Radionuclide scans are also valuable in the investigation of incontinence when a dysfunctional voiding state compromises upper urinary tract function.[7] For example, the incontinent patient is often prone to frequent UTIs. If pyelonephritis occurs repeatedly, renal scarring occurs over time, and kidney function deteriorates. Additionally, the patient with overflow incontinence due to prostatic hypertrophy may develop chronic upper tract damage due to increased intravesical pressure and vesicoureteral reflux.

Endoscopic Studies

Endoscopy is the general term for examination of body organ cavities by means of endoscopes, rigid or flexible tubes that have a lighted lens system, used for direct visual examination of certain internal body structures. The fiberoptic flexible instruments redirect and transmit light around twists and bends in cavities and hollow organs. Both rigid and fiberoptic endoscopes have a light source that allows visualization at the distal tip of the scope and a separate port for installation of drugs, lavage, suction, and insertion of brushes, forceps, or other instruments used for excision, sampling, or other diagnostic and therapeutic work. The fiberoptic scope is used in areas of the body that are not easily accessible or directly visualized by rigid scopes.

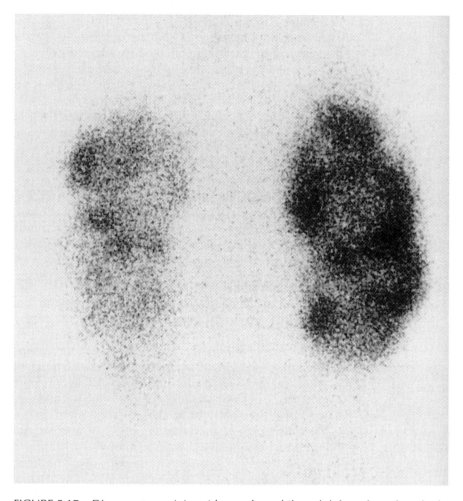

FIGURE 5.17   *Dimercaptosuccinic acid scan shows bilateral defects throughout both kidneys; the left is involved to a greater extent than the right. The cause of this abnormal scan was multiple renal stones. (Reprinted with permission from BO O'Donnell, SA Koff [eds]. Pediatric Urology [3d ed]. Oxford, UK: Butterworth–Heinemann, 1996;42.)*

Endoscopic procedures are done within the genitourinary system both for diagnosis of pathologic conditions and for therapy, such as removal of tissue or urinary calculi. Biopsy tissue is submitted to the pathology laboratory for histologic examination.[9] Genitourinary system endoscopic procedures include nephroscopy, ureteroscopy, and cystourethroscopy.

Nephroscopy

Nephroscopy is a procedure that allows visualization of the renal pelvis and calyces from an antegrade perspective. Nephroscopy is performed after a percutaneous tract has been established through the flank, accessing the renal pelvis. Spinal or general anesthesia is needed for this procedure.[3]

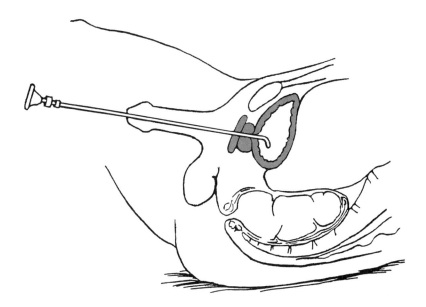

FIGURE 5.18   *Rigid cystourethroscopy requires introduction of the metal scope into the bladder via the urethra.*

Ureteroscopy

Ureteroscopy allows direct visualization of ureters and ureterovesical junctions. This procedure is performed from the retrograde perspective. The ureteroscope is a flexible instrument designed to dilate and visualize each ureter. Ureteral dilatation is extremely painful, and the procedure requires significant sedation or anesthesia. Ureteroscopy can be done to determine the cause of hematuria, to detect tumors and stones, and to remove ureteral calculi.[3,9]

Cystourethroscopy

Cystourethroscopy is the most commonly used urologic endoscopic procedure. The urethra, bladder urothelium, trigone, and ureterovesical junctions are visualized from a retrograde perspective. Rigid or flexible instruments may be used. Rigid cystourethroscopy requires introduction of the metal scope into the bladder via the urethra (Figure 5.18). Images are obtained during insertion or withdrawal of the endoscopie. Flexible cystoscopy uses a flexible sheath containing a fiberoptic system attached to a powerful light source. Fiberoptic images may not be as clear as those produced by rigid instruments.[3] Cystourethroscopy may be used for both diagnostic and therapeutic purposes. It is diagnostically useful to identify and biopsy suspicious lesions. Therapeutically, the cystoscope may be used to perform meatotomy (incision of urinary sphincter to enlarge the opening), to crush and retrieve small stones from the urethra, bladder, and ureter, and to fulgurate bladder tumors.[9]

Indications

Indications to perform genitourinary endoscopy include the evaluation of urinary calculi, recurrent UTI, febrile UTI, vesicoureteral reflux, bladder outlet obstruction, urethral stricture, urethral or bladder fistula, urinary incontinence, neuropathic bladder, and congenital abnormalities of the urinary system. Current UTI is a relative contraindication.[3]

Procedure

A surgical consent must be obtained before cystoscopic procedures. Nothing-by-mouth guidelines are followed if spinal or general anesthesia is necessary. Otherwise, an intravenous, conscious, sedative medication, such as diazepam (Valium) or midazolam (Versed), is administered to relax the patient.

The examination can be performed in an operating room or in the urologist's office. After preparing the external genitalia with an antiseptic solution, the patient is placed in the lithotomy position with legs in stirrups and is properly grounded, padded, and draped. Then a local anesthetic jelly is instilled into the urethra, where it is retained for 5–10 minutes before passage of the cystoscope. Glycine solution or sterile water is instilled through the scope, which is connected to an irrigation system. This distends the bladder for the purpose of better visualization.[9]

After the cystourethroscopy, voiding patterns should be monitored and fluids encouraged. Blood clots and localized edema may cause the patient difficulty in voiding, with urinary retention, hesitancy, weak urinary stream, or urinary dribbling anytime within the first several days post procedure. Warm sitz baths and mild analgesics may be helpful. However, an indwelling catheter may sometimes be necessary to facilitate urinary drainage.[9]

Urinary frequency, dysuria, pink to light red urine color, and urethral burning are common after cystoscopy. However, frank bleeding, clots, or difficulty with urination must be reported to the urologist promptly.[9]

Antibiotics are typically prescribed before and after cystoscopy to prevent infection. The potential for gram-negative shock is always present with urologic procedures. The urethra, a highly vascular organ, can allow bacteria to enter the bloodstream directly through any break in its endothelial lining. The onset of symptoms can be rapid. After the endoscopic procedure, the patient should be observed for chills, fever, tachycardia, hypotension, and back pain. These are indicators of septic shock, which should be promptly reported to the physician. Blood cultures can then be ordered, followed by an aggressive regimen of antibiotic therapy.[9]

References

1. Palubinskas AJ. Imaging of the Urinary Tract. In DR Smith (ed), General Urology (11th ed). Los Altos, CA: Lange Medical Publications, 1984;55–108.
2. Fischbach F. X-Ray Studies. In Fischbach F (ed), A Manual of Laboratory and Diagnostic Tests. Philadelphia: Lippincott–Raven, 1996;683–743.
3. Gray M. Diagnostic Procedures. In M Gray (ed), Genitourinary Disorders. St. Louis: Mosby, 1992;32–51.

4. Fischbach F. Ultrasound Studies. A Manual of Laboratory and Diagnostic Tests. Philadelphia: Lippincott–Raven, 1996;828–866.
5. Fischbach F. Special System and Organ Function Studies. A Manual of Laboratory and Diagnostic Tests. Philadelphia: Lippincott–Raven, 1996; 930–986.
6. Fischbach F. Nuclear Medicine Studies. A Manual of Laboratory and Diagnostic Tests. Philadelphia: Lippincott–Raven, 1996;617–682.
7. Gray M. Assessment of Patients with Urinary Incontinence. In DB Doughty (ed), Urinary and Fecal Incontinence: Nursing Management. St. Louis: Mosby, 1991;47–94.
8. Fine EJ, Blaufox MD. Urological Applications or Radionuclides. In HM Pollack (ed), Clinical Urography (Vol 1). Philadelphia: WB Saunders, 1990.
9. Fischbach F. Endoscopic Studies. A Manual of Laboratory and Diagnostic Tests. Philadelphia: Lippincott–Raven, 1996;787–827.

6   Urodynamic Studies

Jack L. Rook

Urodynamic study is an important part of the evaluation of patients with urinary incontinence. Before the development of urodynamics, the examiner simply observed the act of voiding, noting the strength of the urinary stream and drawing inferences about the possibility of obstruction of the bladder outlet versus pelvic floor weakness. Fluoroscopy, with the capability to observe the lower urinary tract during the act of voiding, became available in the 1950s. In the 1960s, the principles of hydrodynamics were applied to lower urinary tract physiology, and the field of urodynamics was introduced.[1]

The term *urodynamics* refers to a series of tests that measure the transport, storage, and elimination functions of the urinary tract.[2] Urodynamic study of the lower urinary tract can provide useful clinical information about the voiding pattern and function of the urinary bladder and sphincteric mechanism.[1]

Symptoms elicited by the history and signs from the physical, endoscopic, and/or radiographic examination must often be further investigated by urodynamic testing so that specific therapy can be devised that is based on the altered physiology of the lower urinary tract.[1]

Bladder function can be studied using cystometry. Sphincteric function is assessed using urethral pressure profile (UPP) studies, and voluntary sphincter activity can be recorded by electromyography (EMG).

The act of voiding is a function of the interaction between bladder and sphincter. The result is the flow rate, which can be simultaneously recorded along with bladder activity (by intraluminal pressure measurements) and sphincteric activity (by EMG). Integrating all three of these tests in a simultaneously recorded comparative manner provides a more complete physiologic picture. This comprehensive approach may involve synchronous recording bladder pressure, flow rate, volume voided, and electrical activity around the urinary sphincter (EMG), along with fluoroscopic imaging of the lower urinary tract.[1] Access to urodynamic testing is essential for the clinician who gives care to patients with incontinence.[2]

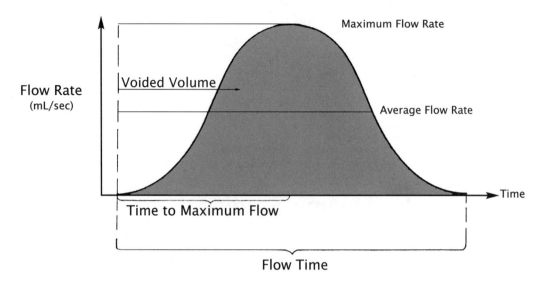

FIGURE 6.1   *Parameters for flow rate include flow time, time to maximum flow, maximum flow rate, average flow rate, and voided volume. The shaded area seen under the curve represents the total volume.*

Urine Flow Studies (Uroflowmetry)

Uroflowmetry is an objective measure of the rate and force of bladder evacuation. The test is noninvasive and easily performed. Accurate evaluation requires that the patient void with a full bladder, and the patient should arrive at the testing situation with a strong desire to urinate.[2]

The flow rate is recorded electronically: The patient voids into a container connected to a transducer that records urine weight and converts it to volume, which is recorded on a chart in milliliters per second.[1]

Indications for urine flow studies include all patients with voiding dysfunction. In these patients, abnormal urine flow rates may result from deficient detrusor contractility, internal or external sphincter dysfunction, or structural obstruction, as with prostate enlargement or stricture. Uroflowmetry cannot, however, differentiate between these causes. More complete urodynamic evaluation would be required. Uroflowmetry is, however, a useful screening tool for the identification of voiding pathology. Uroflowmetry is also useful in the pre- and post-treatment evaluation of patients who have had urethral dilation procedures for urethral stricture disease and in the assessment of the effect of pharmacologic agents on urethral sphincteric resistance and voiding efficiency. Uroflowmetry's main use is as an integral part of multifunction voiding studies, which also include intravesical pressure analysis and sphincter EMG. It typically precedes the invasive instrumentation required for detailed testing.[3]

Parameters for flow rate include (Figure 6.1)[3]

1. *Flow time:* the time over which measurable flow occurs
2. *Time to maximum flow:* the time elapsed from the onset of flow to maximum rate

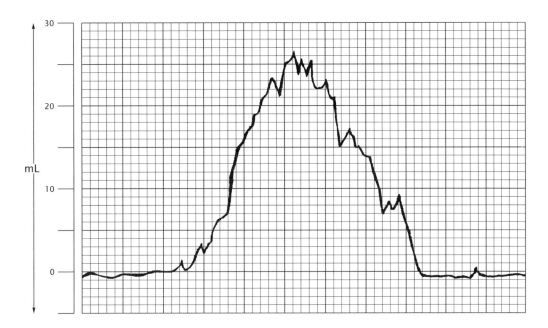

FIGURE 6.2   *The normal flow pattern is represented by a bell-shaped, irregular curve. Here, flow rate is approximately 25 ml per second.*

3. *Maximum flow rate or peak flow (Qmax)*: the maximum measured value of the flow rate
4. *Voided volume*: the total volume expelled by way of the urethra
5. *Average flow rate (Qavg)*: voided volume divided by flow time
6. *Voiding time*: total duration of micturition
7. *Flow pattern*: may be continuous, interrupted, or specifically described

Considerable sex and age variation in normal maximum flow rates exists. The rates tend to be significantly higher in females and decrease with age in both sexes. The normal maximum flow rate values are[3,4]

- Males younger than 50 years, greater than 22 ml per second
- Males 40–60 years, greater than 18 ml per second
- Males older than 60 years, greater than 13 ml per second
- Females younger than 50 years, greater than 25 ml per second
- Females older than 50 years, greater than 18 ml per second

A normal flow pattern is represented by a bell-shaped curve that is rarely completely smooth (Figure 6.2).[1]

Postvoid residual volume measurements may be undertaken via either catheterization or ultrasonic scanning. This can provide valuable adjunctive information.[2]

Normal voiding with a normal flow rate is the product of both detrusor activity and outlet resistance. Sphincteric relaxation usually precedes detrusor contraction by a few seconds, and when relaxation is maximal, detrusor activity starts and is sustained until the bladder is empty.

Outlet resistance is the primary determinant of flow rate. It varies according to functional or mechanical factors. Functionally, outlet resistance is primarily related to sphincteric activity. If the sphincter does not relax during detrusor contraction, partial obstruction occurs. Overactivity of the sphincter is usually a neuropathic phenomenon. However, it can also result from irritative phenomena such as infection, or, even more commonly, it could represent a psychological phenomena.

In women, mechanical factors resulting in obstruction to urine flow may take the form of cystoceles, urethral kinks, or, most commonly, iatrogenic scarring, fibrosis, and compression from previous vaginal or periurethral procedures. The classic mechanical factor in men is an enlarged prostate (benign prostatic hypertrophy, prostate tumor).[1]

Variations in Flow Rate

The graphic data are displayed as a flow "curve," which falls into one of four characteristic patterns, including normal, explosive, intermittent, and obstructive. Interpretation of the results requires evaluation of both numeric and graphic data.

Normal Flow Pattern

The normal flow pattern resembles a bell curve (see Figure 6.2). In men, maximum bladder contraction produces a Qmax greater than 12 ml per second, and the mean or average flow (Qavg) exceeds 8 ml per second. In women, the corresponding flow measurements tend to be greater. The normal adult voided volume should exceed 250 ml, and the postvoid residual volume is expected to be less than 25% of the total bladder volume. A normal flow pattern implies that the individual empties his or her bladder efficiently and completely.[2]

Explosive Flow Pattern

The explosive flow pattern has a steeper tracing of greater amplitude than the normal pattern, with a shorter voiding time (Figure 6.3). The Qmax and Qavg values are greater than those in the normal pattern. An explosive flow pattern is often seen in cases of stress urinary incontinence, although in women, an explosive flow pattern may represent a variant of normal, unobstructed voiding.[2]

Intermittent Flow Pattern

The intermittent flow pattern is characterized by a sawtooth configuration (Figure 6.4). The Qmax is often normal (more than 12 ml per second), although the Qavg or mean flow is usually less than 8 ml per second, and the voiding time is prolonged. The patient with an intermittent flow pattern, then, has significant residual volume present.[2]

Intermittent flow pattern may occur with voluntary sphincter overactivity, detrusor sphincter dyssynergia, or lower motor neuron neurogenic bladder. Figure 6.4A demonstrates voluntary sphincter overactivity. The flow time is greatly prolonged, flow rate fluctuates due to variations in voluntary sphincter activity (at one point reaching 32 ml per second), and the Qavg is low. Figure

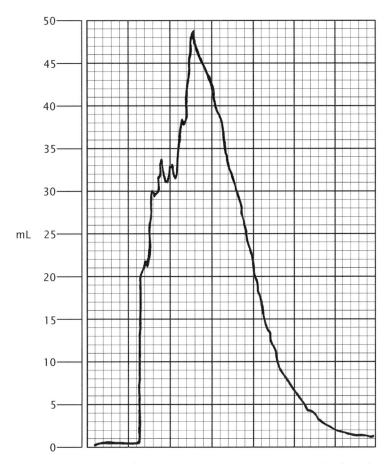

FIGURE 6.3   *The explosive flow pattern tracing has a greater amplitude and a shorter voiding time than the normal pattern.*

6.4B demonstrates the urine flow study for detrusor sphincter dyssynergia. With this pattern, the maximum flow rate never exceeds 15 ml per second and Qavg is low, indicative of obstruction. The urine flow is almost completely interrupted in the middle. This fluctuating pattern reflects sphincteric hyperactivity. Figure 6.4C demonstrates the classic flow rate pattern of the patient with lower motor neuron bladder and abdominal straining. Here the patient is voiding without the aid of detrusor contractions, primarily by abdominal straining. The flow rate pattern demonstrates spurts of urine with complete interruption between them, because the patient cannot sustain increased intra-abdominal pressure.[1]

Obstructive Flow Pattern
The obstructive flow pattern is a depressed curve with low peak (Qmax less than 12 ml per second) and mean (Qavg less than 8 ml per second) flow values (Figure 6.5A and B). The volume voided may be small and voiding time prolonged, which is associated with incomplete emptying. Postvoid residual volumes often exceed 25% of total bladder capacity. The obstructive flow pattern implies the presence of bladder outlet obstruction or deficient detrusor

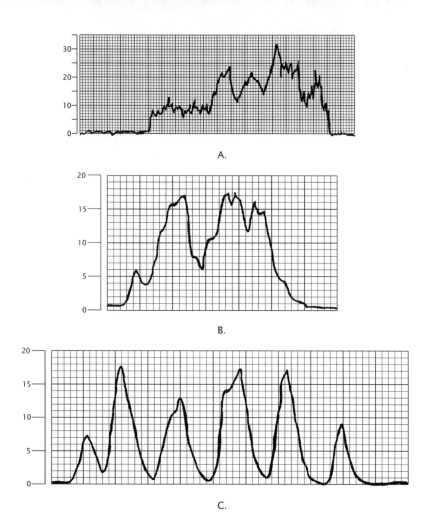

FIGURE 6.4   *The intermittent flow pattern is characterized by a sawtooth configuration. With voluntary sphincter overactivity **(A)**, flow time is greatly prolonged, flow rate fluctuates due to variations in voluntary sphincter activity, and the average flow rate is low. With detrusor sphincter dyssynergia **(B)**, the maximum and average flow rates are low and urine flow may be completely interrupted, reflecting sphincteric hyperactivity. The classic flow rate pattern of the patient with lower motor neuron bladder **(C)** demonstrates spurts of urine with complete interruption between them, and urination occurring due to abdominal straining only.*

contraction. Pressure flow analysis via cystometry is required to determine which of these conditions is causing the poor flow pattern.[2]

In early obstruction due to benign prostatic hypertrophy, the flow rate is low (5–6 ml per second), flow time is prolonged, and there is sustained low flow with minimal variation (see Figure 6.5A). In later mechanical obstruction, flow studies demonstrate markedly prolonged flow time associated with a fluctuating curve due to attempts at improving urine flow by increasing intra-abdominal pressure (see Figure 6.5B).[1]

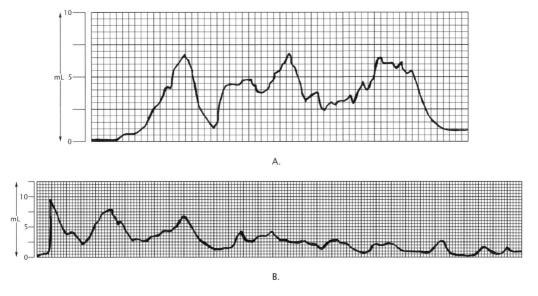

A.

B.

FIGURE 6.5   *The obstructive flow pattern is a depressed curve with low peak flow and average flow rate values. In early obstruction (A) due to benign prostatic hypertrophy, there is sustained low flow with minimal variation. In later mechanical obstruction (B), flow studies demonstrate markedly prolonged flow time with a fluctuating curve.*

Reduced flow rate in the absence of mechanical obstruction is due to some impairment of detrusor activity. Figure 6.6 demonstrates this poor flow pattern.[1]

Although many variations are possible in the shape of the flow curve, by itself, it can be one of the most valuable urodynamic studies undertaken to evaluate voiding dysfunction. Flowmetry is not only of diagnostic value, but is also helpful in follow-up studies to evaluate the effectiveness of a particular treatment. In some cases, however, flowmetry alone does not provide enough data about the abnormality causing incontinence. More information must then be obtained by evaluation of bladder function.[1]

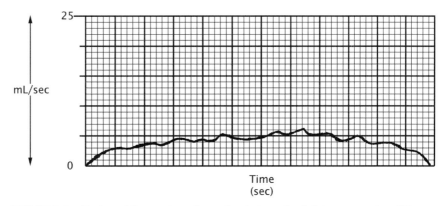

FIGURE 6.6   *Reduced flow rate pattern due to impaired detrusor contractility.*

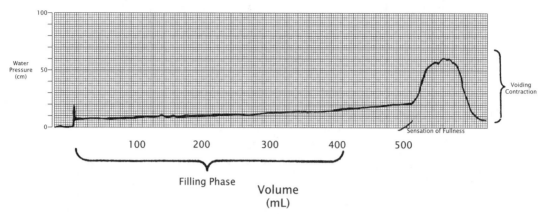

FIGURE 6.7   *The normal cystometrogram is a graph that plots intravesical pressure against the volume of liquid instilled via catheter into the bladder in a retrograde manner.*

Cystometrogram

A cystometrogram (CMG) is a dynamic test of bladder filling that compares volume and intravesical pressure by means of a computer-generated graph (Figure 6.7). To perform the CMG, one or more catheters are introduced through the urethra, into the bladder of the supine patient.[5] Liquid is then instilled in a retrograde manner to fill the bladder. Sterile water, a saline solution, or water-soluble radiographic contrast material is commonly used.[2]

Two catheters or a single multilumen catheter is placed in the bladder. Typically, one tube is for filling, while the other one measures intravesical- or total-bladder pressure (Pves). The two-catheter technique offers the advantage of allowing removal of the filling tube, thereby enhancing quality of the pressure-flow study.[2,5]

The pressure inside the bladder is actually a function of both intra-abdominal and intravesical pressure. Thus, true detrusor pressure (Pdet) is the value obtained after subtracting the intra-abdominal pressure (Pabd) from the Pves. Intra-abdominal pressure is usually recorded by a small balloon catheter inserted into the rectum and connected to a separate transducer.[1] In women, an intravaginal balloon device may be substituted for the rectal balloon (Figure 6.8).[5]

The rectal/vaginal and urethral catheters are connected to transducers, and the respective pressure values are recorded on a polygraph or computer. Three measurements are displayed, including Pves, Pdet, and Pabd. Pves is the sum of two sources: The detrusor muscle produces pressure (Pdet) via its smooth muscle bundles in the bladder wall, and the Pabd is produced by the abdominal musculature and the effect of gravity. It is the simultaneous determination of Pabd and Pves that allows subtraction of abdominal influences on intravesical pressure and calculation of the Pdet. The Pdet is that portion of intravesical

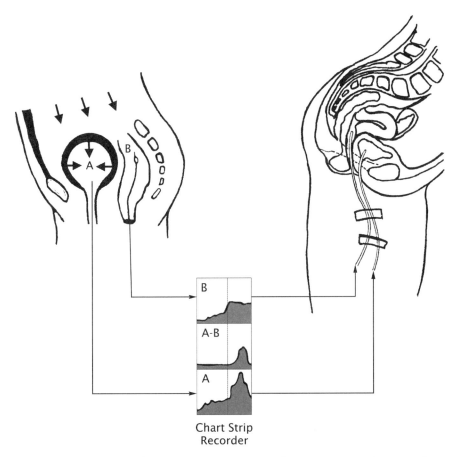

Chart Strip
Recorder

FIGURE 6.8   *When performing a cystometrogram, the true intravesical pressure is a function of both intra-abdominal and intravesical pressure. True detrusor pressure (A-B) is the value obtained after subtracting the intra-abdominal pressure (B) from the intra-vesical pressure value (A). Intra-abdominal pressure can be recorded using a rectal (left) or intravaginal (right) balloon catheter device.*

pressure produced by detrusor contractility during bladder filling and evacuation (Figure 6.9).[2]

Figures 6.10 and 6.11 demonstrate simultaneous recording of intra-abdominal and intravesical pressures. In Figure 6.10, if one considers only intravesical pressure (top recording), one might assume adequate detrusor contraction. However, comparison with the intra-abdominal pressure (lower recording) shows that, in fact, there is no detrusor contraction at all. In contrast, in Figure 6.11, the difference between the two can be clearly seen as being pure detrusor contraction.[1]

Indications for testing include the evaluation of urinary urgency or incontinence, neuropathic bladder dysfunction, bladder outlet obstruction, and urinary retention of unknown cause.

A urinary tract infection is a relative contraindication to urodynamic testing. Before CMG testing, the urinary system should be rendered ster-

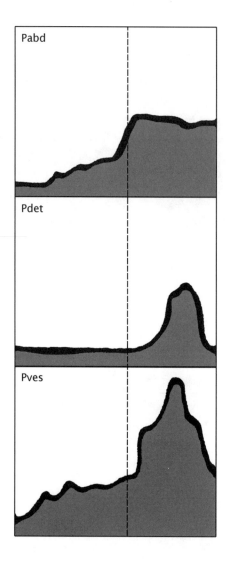

FIGURE 6.9   *The total intravesical pressure (Pves) is the sum of the detrusor muscle pressure (Pdet) and the abdominal pressure (Pabd). The Pdet is that portion of intravesical pressure produced by detrusor contractility during bladder filling and evacuation.*

ile by appropriate antibiotic coverage. An absolute contraindication is an acute debilitating illness.

After the test, the patient is monitored for discomfort related to urethral instrumentation, and for infection.[5]

Bladder Function and the Normal Cystometrogram

The basic bladder functions evaluated by CMG include sensation, accommodation, compliance, bladder capacity, contractility, and voluntary control.

The CMG (see Figure 6.7) is performed during bladder filling and micturition. It measures the volume of fluid in the bladder plotted against intravesical pressure. The normal CMG curve shows a fairly constant low intravesical pressure until the bladder nears capacity, a moderate rise as

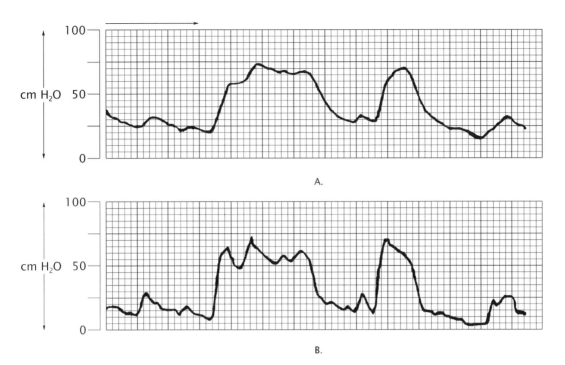

FIGURE 6.10   *Simultaneous recording of intravesical (**A**) and intra-abdominal pressure (**B**). Comparison of (**A**) and (**B**) shows that there is no detrusor contraction occurring and that all intravesical pressure generated is due to increased intra-abdominal pressure.*

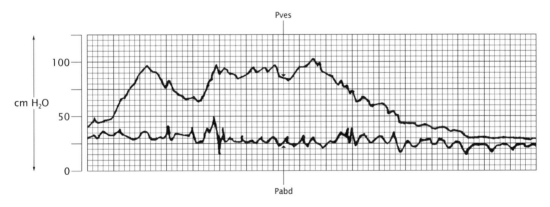

FIGURE 6.11   *Simultaneous recording of intra-abdominal pressure (Pabd) and bladder pressure (Pves). Here, the difference between the two can be clearly seen as being pure detrusor contraction.*

capacity is reached, and then a sharp rise when voiding is initiated. Normally, a sensation of fullness is first perceived when the bladder contains 100–200 ml of fluid, and is strongly felt as an urge to void as the bladder nears capacity (400–500 ml). The bladder normally shows no evidence of contractility or activity during the filling phase. This represents bladder stability. Bladder instability occurs when contractions of the detrusor muscle are not under volitional control.[1]

The bladder has the power of accommodation. It accommodates to increasing volume by maintaining an almost constant intraluminal pressure throughout its filling phase, regardless of the volume present. The property of accommodation is a reflection of the transitional epithelium lining the bladder lumen, which thins out while the underlying detrusor muscle bundles stretch. This allows the bladder to accommodate the higher volume of fluid without a significant change in intraluminal pressure. Accommodation directly influences compliance. As the bladder progressively accommodates larger volumes with little change in intraluminal pressure, the compliance values become higher as compliance equals change in volume (by change in pressure).[1]

Figure 6.12 schematically depicts six frequently seen CMG filling tracings that demonstrate variations of compliance. Tracing number one is from a normal CMG, demonstrating capacity to 350–500 ml, normal compliance, and no involuntary contractions. Tracing number two is the large capacity bladder, with capacity greater than 1,000 ml, and abnormally high compliance due to little increase in bladder pressure despite the high-volume filling. This tracing is typical of the overdistended bladder, as may result from neurogenic denervation (the so-called lower motor neuron bladder), or chronic outlet obstruction with myogenic injury.

Tracing number three demonstrates a poorly compliant bladder, with low capacity and a steep pressure rise with filling. Here, the bladder is converted into a poor storage organ, whose etiologic implications include: an artifactually induced tracing caused by too rapid filling during CMG; a myogenic variety due to muscle hypertrophy from detrusor overactivity (as with early obstruction); the fibrotic bladder caused by chronic bladder wall inflammation; and, last, one frequently obtains the poorly compliant CMG tracing in a patient who has had a chronic indwelling Foley catheter.

The hypersensitive bladder is seen in tracing number four. The capacity is small, but compliance remains normal, with little pressure rise during filling. This bladder, although having no involuntary contractions, has decreased capacity due to sensory phenomena. This bladder tracing is typically found with idiopathic female frequency syndrome or in the inflamed bladder. Tracing number five demonstrates involuntary contractions occurring spontaneously during filling. Compliance is also reduced due to detrusor hypertrophy, resulting from the frequent involuntary contractions. This low-capacity, hypersensitive bladder may be idiopathic, or such gross instability may be due to outlet obstruction. However, neurogenic causes most frequently result in this tracing (as with an upper motor neuron spinal cord lesion).

The sixth tracing describes a bladder with reduced capacity and involuntary contraction occurring at low-filling volumes. Steepness of the

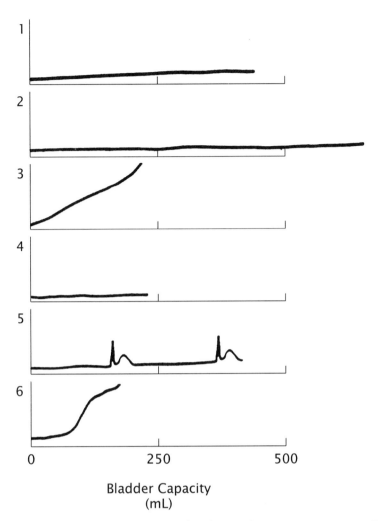

FIGURE 6.12   *Schematic representation of six frequently seen cystometrogram (CMG) filling tracings that demonstrate variations of compliance: (1) the normal CMG; (2) the large capacity bladder; (3) a poorly compliant bladder; (4) the hypersensitive bladder; (5) the low capacity, hypersensitive bladder with involuntary contractions; (6) the reduced-capacity bladder with an involuntary contraction at low filling volumes.*

curve is due to muscle contraction and indicates poor compliance. Frequently, this curve is seen with upper motor neuron injury, although it may result from outlet obstruction in the male.[3]

Once the bladder is filled to capacity, and the subject perceives the desire to urinate and consciously allows urination to proceed, strong bladder contractions occur and are sustained until the bladder is empty. This voluntary detrusor control is assessed as part of the cystometric study to rule out uninhibited bladder activity. Included in this assessment is a determination as to whether the patient can inhibit urination while voiding.[1]

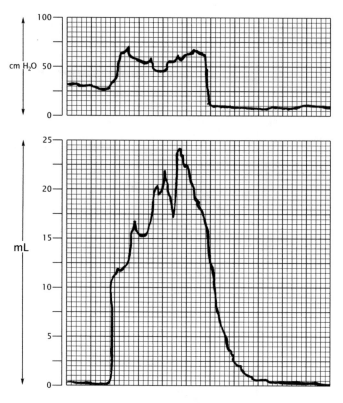

FIGURE 6.13   *This figure demonstrates simultaneous recording of a normal detrusor contraction (Pdet) and a normal flow rate study (bottom tracing).*

Normally, voiding contractions are in the range of 20–40 cm of water, a pressure magnitude that is generally adequate to deliver a normal flow rate of 20–30 ml per second and completely empty the bladder if it is well sustained. A higher voiding pressure is indicative of an increase in outlet resistance in the face of healthy detrusor musculature. Figure 6.13 shows a normal flow rate associated with normal detrusor contraction that is well sustained and of short duration, resulting in complete bladder emptying.[1]

The urodynamic study typically consists of filling and voiding cystometry. Four cystometric phases (I, II, III, and IV) exist, with I through III found in filling cystometry, and phase IV being the voiding CMG (Figure 6.14).

During filling cystometry, phase I demonstrates a mild rise in pressure due to influence of the initial fluid infusion; during phase II, there is minimal increase in pressure as the bladder accommodates to the continual increase in volume; in phase III, there is a further rise in pressure as the bladder wall is stretched to its functional limit or capacity, and control over voiding is maintained with urgency; and in phase IV, the voiding CMG demonstrates the voluntary detrusor contraction that results in efficient voiding.[6]

In summary, the filling cystometry determines capacity, sensation, compliance, and detrusor stability. *Capacity* refers to the total amount of fluid the bladder holds during cystometric evaluation, with the normal

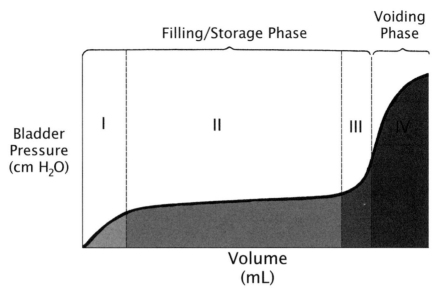

FIGURE 6.14 *The cystometrogram can be broken down into four cystometric phases (I, II, III, and IV), with I–III found in filling cystometry and phase IV being the voiding cystometrogram.*

adult capacity being 400–550 ml. Sensation includes the subjective assessment of "first sensation" or the first desire to void (90–150 ml), "second sensation," or the normal desire to void (200–300 ml), and "third sensation," which refers to a strong desire to void (400–550 ml or maximum capacity). Compliance measures the bladder's ability to adjust to increasing volumes, calculated as the change in volume over the change in detrusor pressure; and *detrusor stability* refers to the bladder's ability to remain relaxed and inactive during filling. The filling CMG is followed by the intravesical pressure assessment during voluntary voiding.

Cystometrogram and Pathologic Changes

Pathologic Changes in Bladder Capacity
Cystometric bladder capacity is determined either by the patient's subjective report of a sense of bladder fullness or when an unstable contraction causes early emptying.[2] The bladder capacity, normally 400–500 ml (see Figure 6.7), can be reduced or increased in a variety of disorders.

Abnormally small cystometric capacity is caused by sensory urgency or detrusor instability. Bladder hypersensitivity is caused by irritant disorders that inflame the bladder wall, which causes decreased tolerance to filling. Urinary tract infection, chemotherapy, radiotherapy-induced cystitis, interstitial cystitis, and bladder calculi or tumors all cause irritation and inflammation of the bladder wall with sensory urgency and compromised cystometric capacity.[2] Detrusor instability with small capacity provoked by bladder filling might also indicate a neuropathic bladder due to an upper motor neuron lesion. Incontinence and chronic renal failure are other

TABLE 6.1   Causes of reduced or increased bladder capacity*

Causes of reduced bladder capacity
    Enuresis or incontinence
    Bladder infections
    Bladder contracture due to fibrosis (from tuberculosis, interstitial cystitis, etc.)
    Upper motor neuron lesions
    Defunctionalized bladder
    Postsurgical bladder
Causes of increased bladder capacity
    Sensory neuropathic disorders
    Lower motor neuron lesions
    Megacystis (congenital)
    Chronic urinary tract obstruction

---

*Normal capacity in adults is 400–500 ml.

causes of reduced bladder capacity, as both conditions are associated with a contracted bladder (Table 6.1).[1]

Increased bladder capacity may occur in women who train themselves to retain large volumes of urine, causing chronic overdistension of the bladder due to the infrequent voiding. It is also increased in sensory neuropathic disorders (peripheral neuropathy, lower motor neuron lesions), and chronic obstruction with progressive detrusor muscle damage.[1] Complete absence of sensation of filling is commonly observed with sacral spinal cord lesions caused by trauma, multiple sclerosis, transverse myelitis, or congenital defects (spina bifida and myelomeningocele).[2]

What is usually of greatest significance is the bladder with reduced capacity and increased cystometric pressure, or large capacity associated with decreased pressure.[1] Such situations promote vesicoureteral reflux and upper tract damage.

Pathologic Changes in Sensation
The patient subjectively reports the sensation of bladder filling. Usually, the adult first sensation occurs at a bladder volume of 90–150 ml, and the sensation of fullness occurs at a volume of 300–600 ml.[2] A slight rise in intravesical pressure on cystometry (phase III) signifies that the bladder is filled to capacity and that the patient perceives it.[1]

Abnormally early sensation indicates an irritative bladder disorder or marked anxiety; repeat filling studies along with patient reassurance should help the clinician distinguish between these factors. Abnormally delayed sensation of filling indicates chronic bladder overdistension or partial sensory loss resulting from peripheral neuropathy, sacral nerve root injury, or idiopathic causes. Total absence of sensation of filling usually indicates sacral spinal cord or cauda equina abnormality.[2] In such cases, the cystometric sign of bladder fullness (phase III) is delayed (sensory neuropathy, overdistension) or absent (lower motor neuron lesion).

Pathologic Changes in Accommodation and Compliance
Accommodation is a reflection of intravesical pressure changes in response to filling. In a bladder with a normal power of accommoda-

tion, intravesical pressure does not vary with progressive bladder filling until capacity is reached. Whenever detrusor tonicity is increased, however, intravesical pressure progressively increases at small volumes, suggesting a loss of accommodation with reduced bladder capacity.[1]

Bladder wall compliance is determined by measuring the change in intravesical pressure during a change in volume. Normally, the bladder fills to capacity at a relatively low pressure, and, as a result, the slope of the line showing detrusor pressure generated during the CMG remains nearly flat (see Figure 6.7), and the compliance value is high.[2] Compromised compliance is seen as a steady increase in the slope of the detrusor pressure line proportional to volume (see Figure 6.12, curves 3, 5, 6), lowering compliance calculations. Poor bladder wall compliance places the patient at greater risk for infection and vesicoureteral reflux with upper tract dilatation and compromised renal function.[2,7]

Pathologic Changes in Stability and Contractility

Bladder instability occurs when detrusor muscle contractions are not under volitional control.[8] Such unstable contractions are seen on CMG as a spontaneous rise in intravesical pressure (indicating detrusor muscle contraction), followed by a decline (muscle relaxation) (Figure 6.15). These contractions are associated with urinary leakage, compromised capacity, and sensations of urgency.[2]

Unstable contractions may be associated with neurologic diseases of the brain and suprasacral spinal cord segments, bladder outlet obstruction, irritative disorders, and idiopathic causes.[2]

Cystometric study may disclose complete absence of detrusor contractility due to motor or sensory deficits or conscious inhibition of detrusor activity. Low pressure with a large capacity may signify sensory loss, a lower motor neuron lesion, a chronically distended bladder, or a large bladder due to myogenic damage.[1]

Detrusor hyperactivity due to suprasacral (upper motor neuron) lesions occurs because of interruption of neural connections between the sacral spinal cord and higher (mid-brain and cortical) centers of micturition (Table 6.2). Typically, an upper motor neuron lesion results in uninhibited contraction activity on CMG during bladder filling in association with detrusor sphincter dyssynergia and variations in voiding pressure and flow rate (Figure 6.16).[1]

Sphincter Electromyography

The filling CMG is most valuable when done in conjunction with EMG of pelvic floor muscles (sphincter EMG). A sphincter EMG measures electrical activity of the striated voluntary pelvic floor musculature during bladder filling and micturition.[5]

Several techniques for electromyographic study of the urinary sphincter exist, including use of either surface or needle electrodes. Surface electrode recordings can be obtained either from the anal sphincter by using an anal plug electrode, or with electrocardiogram patches placed over the perineal

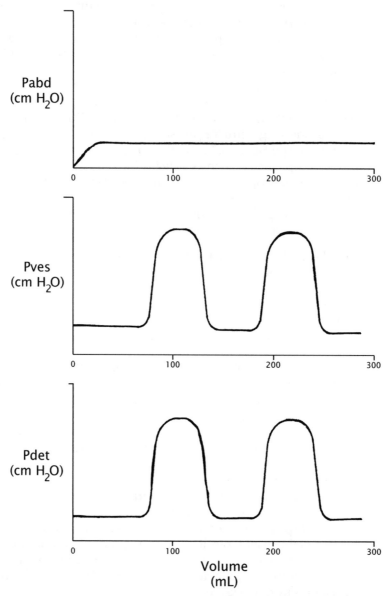

FIGURE 6.15   *Schematic representation of bladder instability demonstrates detrusor muscle contractions that are not under volitional control. The intravesical pressure changes (Pves) are seen to be due to pure detrusor contractions (Pdet) without contribution from any rise in intra-abdominal pressure (Pabd).*

TABLE 6.2   Variations in detrusor contractility

Normal contractions (normal volume, well-sustained contractions)
Uninhibited contractions
    Upper motor neuron lesions
    Cerebrovascular lesions
Absent or weak contractions
    Sensory neuropathic disorders
    Conscious inhibition of contractions
    Lower motor neuron lesions

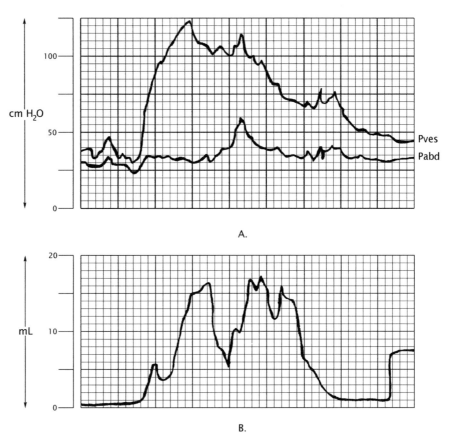

FIGURE 6.16 *The cystometrogram (CMG) and pressure flow study of a patient with an upper motor neuron lesion and detrusor sphincter dyssynergia. The CMG study (**A**) reveals variations in voiding pressure with the maximum pressure reaching high levels. This is associated with variations in flow rate (**B**). (Pves = intravesical pressure changes; Pabd = intra-abdominal pressure.)*

area. The surface electrode technique offers the advantages of patient mobility during testing and decreased discomfort with the use of noninvasive electrodes. It provides assessment of only gross muscle action during bladder filling and micturition, however, and it is limited by significant artifact. Recording via percutaneous needle electrodes inserted into the anal or urethral sphincter provides a more artifact-free analysis of gross muscle action during bladder filling and micturition (Figure 6.17).[1,5]

During the electromyographic study, the electrical activity present within the pelvic floor and external urinary sphincter increases progressively with bladder filling. During bladder contraction for voiding, the electrical activity ceases completely, permitting free flow of urine. Electrical activity then resumes at the termination of detrusor contraction to secure closure of the bladder outlet (Figure 6.18).[1]

Persistence of electromyographic activity during detrusor contraction interferes with the voiding mechanism. This lack of coordination between

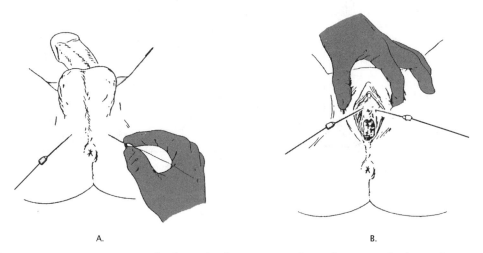

FIGURE 6.17 *Percutaneous needle electrode placement into the anal (A) or urethral (B) sphincters as part of the needle electromyographic examination.*

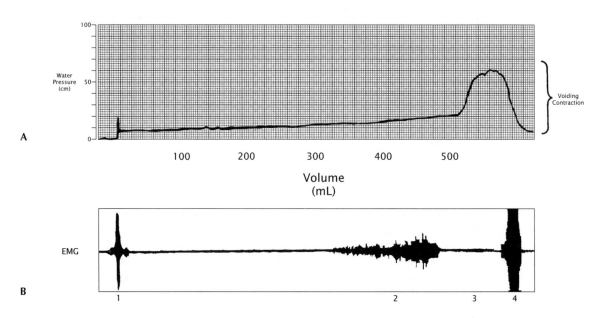

FIGURE 6.18 *Simultaneous recording of the cystometrogram (A) and electromyogram (EMG) (B). During bladder contraction for voiding, the electrical activity ceases completely and then resumes on the termination of detrusor contraction to help secure closure of the bladder outlet. (1 = bulbocavernosus reflex; 2 = progressively increasing electrical activity [contraction] of pelvic floor muscles during later phase of filling; 3 = abrupt electrical silence during voiding; 4 = electrical activity after completion of voiding to secure closure of the bladder outlet.)*

detrusor and sphincter, known as *detrusor sphincter dyssynergia*, interferes with the free flow of urine. This is best demonstrated through simultaneous recording of flow rate, CMG, and EMG. Therefore, the sphincter EMG typically is performed during the filling CMG and voiding flow study.[1,5]

The sphincter response to bladder filling is characterized by a phenomenon called *recruitment*. Muscle recruitment implies that as the bladder fills, motor units of sphincter muscle fibers are progressively added in response to the greater workload. The polygraph recorder of the EMG machine detects electric signals from these motor units, and a pen sweeps back and forth as they occur. The wider the sweep of the pen, the greater the muscle's tone. As a result of recruitment, the EMG recording pen sweeps more vigorously as the bladder approaches capacity (see Figure 6.18).[2]

The electromyographic recording demonstrates only the activity of the external sphincter mechanism or the pelvic floor musculature, or both, under voluntary control. It gives no information about the smooth involuntary muscle component of the sphincter.[1]

Urethral Pressure Studies

The UPP is a graphic recording of pressure within the urethra at each point along its length. The procedure requires specially designed catheters with multiple side holes and an occluded tip. Infusion catheters vary in size between 8 and 10 French, and most have four diametrically opposed perfusion orifices some distance from the catheter tip.[3,9]

Fluid infused into the catheter escapes through its side holes. The UPP measures the resistance of the urethral walls to distension caused by this escaping fluid. This resistance is expressed in terms of the pressure necessary to maintain a steady flow of fluid through the catheter system.[3]

The UPP recording commences in the bladder, after which the catheter is withdrawn through the entire length of the urethra, with 0.5 mm per second being the ideal withdrawal rate. The initial pressure recorded on the recording strip is the intravesical pressure. As the catheter is withdrawn, the UPP demonstrates a positive deflection at the bladder neck and a progressive increase in urethral pressure until the midportion of the urethra in the female (Figure 6.19) and the membranous urethra in the male (Figure 6.20) is reached. Beyond this point, the pressure progressively decreases again until the external meatus is reached.[3]

Nomenclature for UPP study parameters include: maximum urethral pressure, the maximum pressure of the profile curve; maximum urethral closure pressure, which is the difference between the maximum urethral pressure and bladder pressure; and functional profile length, the length of the urethra along which the pressure exceeds bladder pressure (Figure 6.21).[3,10]

Anatomic variations lead to a significant difference between the appearance of the male and female UPP curve. Contributing to normal urethral compliance are smooth and striated muscle activity, a fibroelastic component of the urethral wall, and vascular tension due to the rich, spongy network about the urethra. Extrinsic compressions, as with

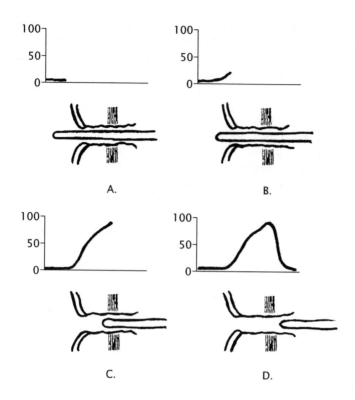

FIGURE 6.19 *The urethral pressure profile recording in women commences in the bladder, after which the catheter is withdrawn through the entire length of the urethra. The initial pressure recorded represents the intravesical pressure (**A**). As the catheter is withdrawn, the urethral pressure profile demonstrates a positive deflection at the bladder neck and a progressive increase in urethral pressure until approximately the mid-portion of the urethra (**B** and **C**) is reached. Beyond this point (**D**), the pressure progressively decreases again until the external meatus is reached.*

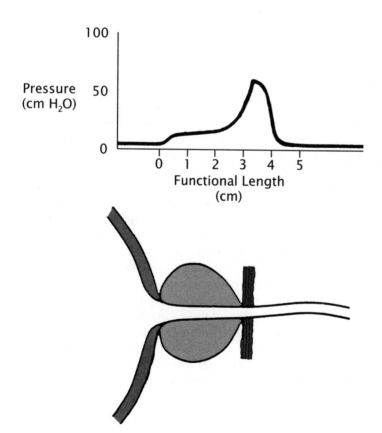

FIGURE 6.20 *The urethral pressure profile tracing in the male varies from that seen in the female. There is a slight elevation in pressure corresponding to the normal prostate with a greater elevation occurring at the level of the external sphincter.*

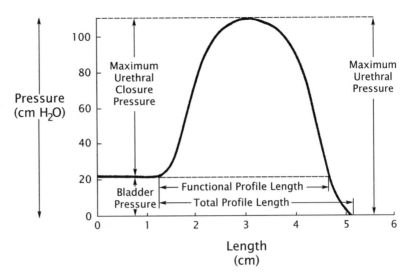

FIGURE 6.21   *Nomenclature for the urethral pressure profile study is seen in this schematic representation.*

enlarged prostatic tissue, add to urethral compliance by varying degrees. Alteration in any of these variables may significantly alter the appearance of the UPP curve.[3]

Profilometry studies require the simultaneous recording of external sphincter activity to ensure that unintentional external sphincter contraction has not caused artifactual increases in maximum closing pressure (Figure 6.22). Many patients with hypersensitive urethras and neurogenic bladder dysfunction find it impossible to inhibit the external sphincter during the perfusion-withdrawal process.[3]

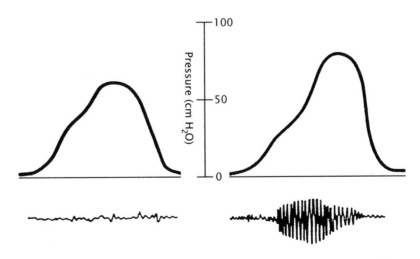

FIGURE 6.22   *Simultaneous recording of external sphincter electromyographic activity and the urethral pressure profile study. The recording on the left is performed without sphincter contraction. The recording on the right had an artifactual increase in maximum closing pressure due to simultaneous contraction of the external sphincter seen as increased electromyogram activity (lower tracing).*

TABLE 6.3 Clinical applications of urethral pressure studies

Urinary incontinence
Bladder outlet obstruction
Neuropathic urethra
Monitoring drug therapy
Monitoring sphincter surgery and its results
Effects of nerve stimulation/block

The UPP study may also include simultaneous measurement of rectal and bladder pressures. Simultaneous measurement of rectal pressure is advocated as a means to identify unintentional abdominal straining, which might alter the normal profile curve. Simultaneous measurement of bladder pressure requires the use of special catheter techniques. Whereas simple perfusion profilometry has poor diagnostic yield, its value may be improved by the performance of more elaborate studies (profilometry with varying degrees of bladder fullness, in varying postures, and under stress), in conjunction with the simultaneous measurement of rectal pressure and external sphincter EMG.[3,11,12]

Indications

Urethral pressure studies in conjunction with other urodynamic studies, such as EMG, cystometry, and pressure flow studies, can provide useful information in a variety of lower urinary tract dysfunctions (Table 6.3).

UPP studies are useful in the evaluation of female urinary incontinence. In patients with stress urinary leakage, a decrease in maximum closing pressure and alteration in functional profile length is seen.[13–16] With benign prostatic hypertrophy, an increase in functional profile length, and the presence of a prostatic peak has been shown to correlate with obstruction.[17,18] Urethral sphincter hypoactivity as a result of neurogenic disease may result in a poor profile, with a markedly decreased maximal urethral pressure. Neurogenic hyperactivity of the sphincter (sphincter dyssynergia) is generally a phenomenon of voiding, hence not amenable to profile measurement.[3]

The UPP is also a useful method to assess the results of external sphincterotomy performed in patients with dyssynergic sphincters and to assess the effectiveness of the various uropharmacologic agents that are given to alter urethral compliance. Internal sphincter augmentative therapy using alpha-adrenergic agents, and alpha-adrenergic–blocking sphincter muscle relaxant medications may be assessed.[19–24] Last, urethral pressure profilometry may be of value during surgical placement of prosthetic sphincters, in which by intraoperative monitoring, the prosthesis may be adjusted to provide optimal urethral compression pressure.[3,25]

Complete Urodynamic Assessment

Measurement of each physiologic variable described (uroflowmetry, UPP, EMG, CMG) gives useful clinical information. At a minimum, a proper urodynamic study should include recordings of intravesical pressure, intra-abdominal pressure, EMG, flow rate, and voided volume. For greatest clinical usefulness, all data should be recorded simultaneously. Machines of varying complexity are available for recording urodynamic studies. Some are simple, limited to one or two channels, whereas more complex machines may have as many as eight channels.[1]

The data derived from urodynamic studies are descriptive of urinary tract function. Simultaneous visualization of the lower urinary tract by means of video fluoroscopy provides more precise information about pathologic changes underlying the symptoms. With video fluoroscopy, the examiner can observe the configuration of the bladder, bladder base, and bladder outlet during filling, and changes in pelvic floor support during voiding. Combined cinefluoroscopy and pressure measurements thus represent the ultimate in urodynamic studies.[1]

The pressure flow study combines data from the CMG, sphincter EMG, and uroflowmetry to provide a detailed analysis of micturition events. The simultaneous recording of these three tests is necessary to completely evaluate the voiding cycle.

Using the double catheter cystometry technique, a small 4-French pressure catheter may be left in the urethra at the completion of cystometry to allow for the monitoring of intravesical pressure during voiding. This catheter is of such small caliber that it does not significantly interfere with voiding dynamics and produces little artifact.[3]

Filling cystometry, during which time bladder pressure and sphincter EMG are monitored, precedes the voiding study. When the bladder is full, the urethral-filling catheter is removed, and the small pressure-measuring catheter remains in place. The patient is then asked to void in a normal manner, without abdominal straining. During voiding, urine flow rate, sphincter EMG, and detrusor pressure are monitored.[3]

Under normal circumstances, the onset of voiding is preceded by sphincter relaxation, evident on the EMG tracing. Detrusor contractions follow, and, with progressive increases in intravesical pressure, opening pressure for the system is then reached and urine flow commences. Urine flow rate rises to a rapid peak, and the intravesical pressure is maintained until emptying is complete. At this point, the detrusor slowly relaxes, and there is a return of external sphincter activity seen on the EMG tracing.[3,26]

The following sections describe pressure-flow analysis for some of the more common urologic problems associated with incontinence.

Explosive Flow Pattern and Stress Incontinence

Explosive flow pattern is often associated with low micturition pressure and weak sphincter muscle contraction. It occurs in women with stress urinary incontinence (Figure 6.23). With this pattern, low urethral resistance allows the bladder to empty itself rapidly even at low intravesical pressures.[2]

Poor Flow Pattern

Bladder outlet obstruction produces a poor flow pattern. Pressure flow analysis of the poor flow pattern either reveals abnormally high or low

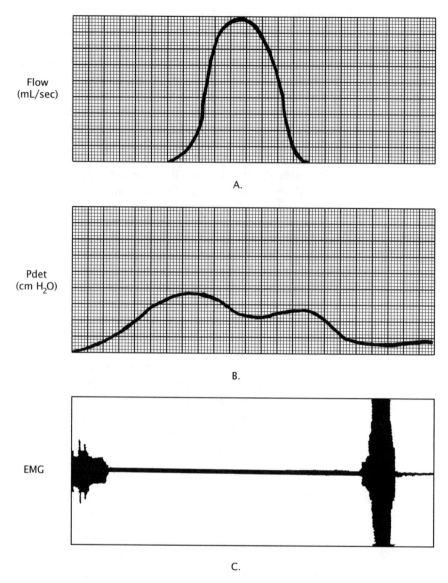

Flow
(mL/sec)

A.

Pdet
(cm H$_2$O)

B.

EMG

C.

FIGURE 6.23   *The explosive flow pattern (**A**) occurs in women with stress urinary incontinence. The cystometrogram demonstrates a low micturition pressure (**B**), and the electromyogram (EMG) response (**C**) is normal. (Pdet = detrusor pressure.)*

contraction pressures, depending on the longevity of the obstruction, with appropriate sphincter relaxation.

In early bladder outlet obstruction, contraction pressure is high and the flow pattern poor. The bladder is producing greater than normal energy despite the compromised flow. Quieting of the sphincter EMG indicates appropriate relaxation of pelvic floor muscles. This pattern should alert the examiner to search for the source of obstruction.[2]

In contrast, with long-standing bladder outlet obstruction, chronic stretching of the bladder wall causes an increased capacity bladder with decreased sensitivity and weakened detrusor musculature. Here, a low contraction pressure and poorly sustained contraction accompany a poor flow pattern. In this case, the poor flow occurs because of deficient detrusor contractility in combination with the obstructed outflow. Therefore, with long-standing bladder outlet obstruction, CMG demonstrates an increased capacity bladder with a weak detrusor contraction pressure, flow pattern is poor, and the EMG response is normal.[2]

Peripheral neuropathy, autonomic neuropathy, or polyradiculopathy secondary to lumbar spinal stenosis can also cause a poor flow pattern. In such cases, urine flow is poor, CMG demonstrates an increased capacity bladder with weak detrusor contraction, and the electromyographic response before micturition is slightly decreased. The decreased electromyographic response is indicative of the underlying neuropathic process affecting the somatic motor fibers and represents a decreased summation of electrical signals or action potentials. With this pattern, there may be a contribution of abdominal straining; therefore, one must follow the Pabd tracing of the CMG.

Intermittent Flow Pattern

An intermittent flow pattern can be associated with bladder outlet obstruction; an upper motor neuron bladder with detrusor sphincter dyssynergia; weak detrusor contractility; a lower motor neuron bladder, which requires abdominal straining to void; and an uninhibited neurogenic bladder.

Bladder outlet obstruction is characterized by intermittent flow with decreased Qmax and Qavg on flow studies, increased pressure on CMG, and a normal electromyographic study.

With upper motor neuron lesions, a dyssynergic sphincter may cause dynamic obstruction of the outlet, as it fails to relax in response to micturition, causing resistance to urinary flow.[2] The upper motor neuron bladder and detrusor sphincter dyssynergia study demonstrates intermittent flow with a decreased Qmax and Qavg. CMG testing reveals an increase in intravesical pressure occurring intermittently when the detrusor contracts against a closed sphincter (see Figure 6.16). Electromyographic testing demonstrates activity occurring during the detrusor contraction.

An intermittent flow pattern associated with low-voiding pressure and weak or absent detrusor contractility occurs with sacral spinal cord injury, cauda equina syndrome, or polyneuropathy. Supplementing a weak detrusor muscle by abdominal straining produces the intermittency seen with this flow pattern. The CMG's abdominal pressure channel (Pabd) documents the presence of abdominal enhancement in the face of poor quality bladder contraction (Pdet).[2] The lower motor neuron bladder cystometrically demonstrates increased capacity and absent detrusor pressure once abdominal pressure is subtracted (see Figure 6.10). Intermittent flow seen on flow studies matches the abdominal pressure readings. The EMG response is markedly diminished or absent due to the neuropathic process.

An uninhibited bladder occurs secondary to cerebrovascular accident, organic brain syndrome, closed head injury, or other neurodegenerative diseases, such as Alzheimer's or Parkinson's, all of which cause a lack of cerebral inhibition of the pontine micturition center. This results in incontinence secondary to the uninhibited bladder contractions with a normal CMG/EMG response. As the CMG begins, the pressure study appears normal. At a low capacity, however, there may be a detrusor contraction with a normal EMG response. As the bladder continues to fill, the patient continues to have detrusor contractions at seemingly low vesical volumes with a normal EMG response.

References

1. Tanagho EA. Urodynamic Studies. In DR Smith (ed), General Urology (11th ed). Los Altos, CA: Lange Medical Publications, 1984;424–443.
2. Gray M. Assessment of Patients with Urinary Incontinence. In DB Doughty (ed), Urinary and Fecal Incontinence: Nursing Management. St. Louis: Mosby, 1991;47–94.
3. Webster GD. Urodynamic Studies. In MI Resnick, RA Older (eds), Diagnosis of Genitourinary Disease. New York: Thieme-Stratton, 1982;173–206.
4. Abrams P, Torrens M. Urine Flow Studies. In R Turner-Warwick, CG Whiteside (eds), Urologic Clinics of North America. Philadelphia: WB Saunders, 1979;6:71.
5. Gray M. Diagnostic Procedures. In M Gray (ed), Genitourinary Disorders. St. Louis: Mosby, 1992;32–51.
6. The Fundamentals of Female Urodynamic Study Interpretation: Case Studies Using the LuMax Fiberoptic Cystometry System. Minneapolis: Med Amicus, 1997.
7. Hackler RH, Zampieri TA. Low compliant bladders in the spinal cord injured population (abstract). J Urol 1988;139:195A.
8. Abrams PH. Bladder instability: concept clinical associations and treatment. Scand J Urol Nephrol 1984;87(Suppl):7.
9. Brown M, Wickham JEA. The urethral pressure profile. Br J Urol 1969;41:211.
10. International Continence Society. First report on the standardization of terminology of lower urinary tract function. Br J Urol 1976;48:39.
11. Enhorning G. Simultaneous recording of intravesical and intraurethral pressure. Acta Chir Scand 1961;(Suppl)276:1.
12. Amussen M, Ulmstein U. Simultaneous urethrocystometry with a new technique. Scan J Urol Nephrol 1976;10:7.
13. Raz S, Kaufmann JJ. Carbon dioxide urethral pressure profile in female incontinence. J Urol 1977;117:765.
14. Sussett J, Plante P. Studies of the female urethral pressure profile. Part II. Urethral pressure profile in female incontinence. J Urol 1980;123:70.
15. Gershon CR, Diokno AC. Urodynamic evaluation of female stress incontinence. J Urol 1978;119:787.
16. Tangho EA. Urodynamics of female urinary incontinence with emphasis on stress incontinence. J Urol 1979;122:200.

17. Webster GD, Lockhart JL, Older RA. The evaluation of bladder neck dysfunction. J Urol 1980;123:196.
18. Abrams PH. Sphincterometry in the diagnosis of male bladder outflow obstruction. J Urol 1975;116:489.
19. Abel BJ, Cosbie-Ross J, Gibbon NO, et al. Urethral pressure measurement after division of the external sphincter. Paraplegia 1975;13:37.
20. Bourne RB, El Ghatit AZ, Anderson JT. Carbon dioxide urethral pressure profilometry before and after external sphincterotomy in spinal cord injury patients. J Urol 1977;117:655.
21. Awad SA, Downie JW, Lywood DW, et al. Sympathetic activity in the proximal urethra in patients with urinary obstruction. J Urol 1976;115:545.
22. Donker PJ, Iranovici F, Noach EL. Analysis of the urethral pressure profile by means of electromyography and administration of drugs. Br J Urol 1972;44:180.
23. Olsson CA, Siroky MB, Krane RJ. The phentolamine test in neurogenic bladder dysfunction. J Urol 1977;117:481.
24. Whitfield HN, Doyle PT, Mayo ME, et al. The effect of adrenergic blocking drugs on outflow resistance. Br J Urol 1975;47:823.
25. Scott FB, Attia SL. Urethral Pressure Profile Studies, Before, During, and After Surgical Treatment of Incontinence. Glasgow: International Continence Society, Annual Conference, 1976.
26. Blaivas JG, Labib KL, Bauer SB, et al. A new approach to electromyography of the external urethral sphincter. J Urol 1977;117:773.

7 Electromyography and Pudendal Nerve Conduction Studies in the Neuro-Urologic Workup

Jack L. Rook

Pudendal Nerve Conduction Studies

Traditionally, incontinence was a medical problem evaluated with techniques, such as uroflowmetry and cystometry, based solely on function. Such studies do not address etiology of the incontinence. Electrophysiologic techniques introduced since the 1980s provide etiologic information for patients with incontinence. Needle electromyography (EMG) examination of the sphincters and pelvic musculature has been done for quite some time, but conduction studies of the nerves governing pelvic function have not been done until recently. In the early 1980s, pudendal nerve distal latency measurements to the urinary sphincter became an important addition to needle EMG examination of the sphincter muscles in evaluation of patients with urinary incontinence.[1]

Pudendal latency nerve conduction studies were first described in 1984 when eight articles were published in a single year using this new technique to investigate the causes of urinary and fecal incontinence.[2–9] The procedure involved recording urinary sphincter contraction induced by pudendal nerve stimulation. Sphincter contraction was recorded by electrodes mounted on a Foley catheter.[5–7,10,11] The catheter-mounted ring electrodes consist of two lengths of platinum wire wound onto a thin, plastic-coated cylinder that fits onto the Foley catheter (Figure 7.1). This special catheter electrode is used to record the voluntary (striated) sphincter compound motor action potentials with pudendal nerve conduction studies.[12]

In 1988, a disposable "St. Mark's stimulating electrode" was devised and sold by Dantec Medical (Figure 7.2). The electrode has an adhesive backing that allows it to be applied to a routine nonsterile glove. A special connector allows it to plug into all regular EMG machines. The ground is affixed to the patient's thigh.[1,13]

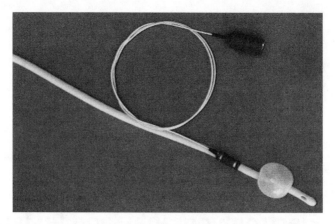

FIGURE 7.1   *Foley catheter-mounted ring electrode. (Reprinted with permission from MB Chancellor, JG Blaivas. Practical Neuro-Urology: Genito-Urinary Complications in Neurologic Disease. Boston: Butterworth–Heinemann, 1995;76. Courtesy of Medtronic Functional Diagnostics, Shoreview, MN.)*

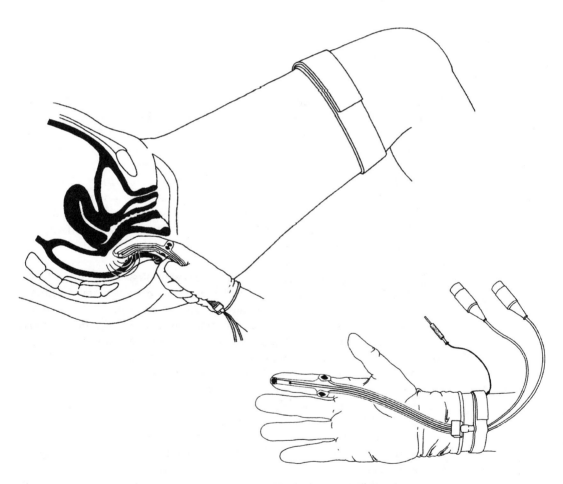

FIGURE 7.2   *St. Mark's electrode. (Reprinted with permission from MB Chancellor, JG Blaivas. Practical Neuro-Urology: Genito-Urinary Complications in Neurologic Disease. Boston: Butterworth–Heinemann, 1995;89. Courtesy of Medtronic Functional Diagnostics, Shoreview, MN.)*

Technique for Pudendal Nerve Stimulation

The EMG machine settings are the same as with standard motor nerve conductions. The sweep speed should be set at 1–2 milliseconds per division, and sensitivity (gain) at 200 μV per division.

With palm down, the examiner's index finger is inserted into the patient's rectum to the base of the finger. The lithotomy position is usually more comfortable for the patient. The physician's finger should sweep along the anterior sacrum to the patient's right to feel the bony ridge that makes up the lower curve of the lesser sciatic notch. Just over this ridge (in the notch itself), is the best place to stimulate. Once familiar with the pelvic anatomy, it is not difficult to find the lesser sciatic notch in a patient.[1]

When the electrode is in the right position, 15–30 mA of stimulating current of 100-millisecond duration is usually required. After stimulation, the physician should feel the rectal sphincter and pelvic musculature contract around the inserted finger. The right side waveform should be up-going, with a normal latency being approximately 2 milliseconds. Next, the physician sweeps his or her finger to the patient's left, finds the left sciatic notch, and repeats the stimulation. It may be necessary to use the left hand for this stimulation. The waveform on the left is usually inverted or down-going, but may be of similar orientation to the right-sided waveform.[1]

Normal values of pudendal distal latency for men and nulliparous women are 2.0 milliseconds (0.5 SD) on the right side, and 1.9 milliseconds (0.3 SD) on the left. Normal values for women who have had at least one vaginal delivery on both sides are 2.3 milliseconds (0.4 SD).[1,3,14]

Clinical Use of Pudendal Nerve Conduction Velocity Studies in Relation to Incontinence

Pudendal nerve distal latencies are delayed to the urinary sphincter immediately after vaginal delivery. These measurements improve over time, but never return to the same range as those in nulliparous women or women who have delivered by cesarean section.[1,9,14–19] This pudendal nerve injury that occurs during vaginal delivery may be the cause of delayed urinary or fecal incontinence that develops in women after menopause. The reason for the delayed appearance of the symptoms is not known, but may have to do with the additional pelvic muscle weakness that develops as a consequence of the reduced hormonal trophic effect of estrogen on pelvic muscles after menopause.[1,8,20] Last, women who experience stress urinary incontinence after vaginal delivery are usually found to have prolonged pudendal distal latency measurements to the urinary sphincter.[1,5–7,10,11]

Pelvic Floor Needle Electromyography

Urethral sphincter needle EMG is a valuable diagnostic tool in the evaluation of women with urinary incontinence and voiding dysfunction.[21–33] As discussed in Chapter 6, sphincter EMG plays an important role as part of the urodynamic testing. However, although conventional urodynamic studies may demonstrate the pathophysiologic behavior of the bladder, such investigations do not probe the neurologic basis of the disorder.[34,35]

In pelvic floor disorders, EMG can provide useful objective clinical information about the integrity and innervation of the pelvic floor musculature, particularly the external urinary sphincter. Taken together with the clinical urodynamic data, EMG data are indispensable in determining a precise diagnosis and in management planning.[34]

The motor supply to the striated urethral sphincter arises from anterior horn nerve cell bodies located in spinal segments S2 through S4. The pudendal nerve carries these fibers to the urethral sphincter and superficial perineal muscles.[21]

Nerve damage causing incontinence and voiding dysfunction can occur at any level in the central or peripheral nervous system and includes disorders causing dysfunction in central regulation (i.e., cerebrovascular accident, organic brain syndrome, brain tumor, normal-pressure hydrocephalus, upper motor neuron spinal cord injury), radiculopathy from disk disease or lumbar spondylosis involving the cauda equina, lesions of the lumbosacral plexus, pudendal neuropathy from injury due to vaginal delivery, and denervation of the pelvic plexus as a consequence of radical pelvic surgery.[21]

Technique

EMG of the pelvic floor and sphincters can be performed as part of two distinct assessments. EMG is used in the urodynamic laboratory to examine sphincter activity during bladder filling and voiding. In the neurophysiology laboratory, EMG has been performed to assess the integrity of innervation of pelvic floor musculature.[34] The latter is discussed in this chapter.

The changes in electrical potential produced by contraction of the striated muscles may be measured by needle electrodes.[34,36,37] Needle electrodes may sample anal sphincter, periurethral, or urethral sphincter muscle. The most common needle electrodes used in electromyographic assessments are concentric and monopolar.

The concentric needle electrode consists of steel wire contained within a thin, pointed canula. The wire electrode is separated from the canula needle by an insulating substance. The recording surface is the bare tip of the wire electrode, and the reference electrode is the outside of the canula itself. The uptake area of this electrode is relatively small, and includes parts of several motor units in normal muscles. Because of the close association of active and reference electrodes, the concentric needle offers the possibility of selective recordings from individual muscles with minimal artifact associated with the recording.[34,38]

The monopolar needle electrode consists of a solid steel electrode, which is insulated to just below its tip. The reference electrode is placed on the skin at some distance from the muscle being tested, and a simple ground electrode is required. This technique usually leads to greater artifact than would be seen with concentric needles.[34]

Given the sensitive nature of the area being tested, it is important to optimize patient comfort and reduce anxiety by ensuring optimal privacy, explaining each step of the examination, and using an anesthetic cream on the area tested. An anesthetic cream containing 2.5% lidocaine and 2.5% prilocaine is applied over the perineal mucosa for 20 minutes before the procedure. A small amount of 1% lidocaine without epinephrine can be injected intradermally for additional anesthesia if necessary.[21]

Before inserting the needle electrode, the bladder is emptied using a 14-French Foley catheter. This enables optimal determination of both electrical activities of the urethral sphincter at rest and appropriateness of motor unit recruitment with filling of the bladder.[21]

For the periurethral approach, the patient rests in the dorsal lithotomy position with the hips flexed and the legs abducted. The physician inserts a 1-in., 30-gauge concentric needle electrode. In women, the needle is inserted approximately 5-mm anterior to the urethral meatus (at 12 o'clock). In the male, with the examining finger to the rectum, the needle is inserted percutaneously 2 cm lateral to the midline halfway between the anus and the lower border to the scrotum. The needle is advanced toward the apex of the prostate until the individual motor unit action potentials (MUAPs) characteristic of skeletal muscle are detected audibly or are visualized on the oscilloscope screen. The audio output of the EMG machine is used to guide electrode placement into the bulk of the sphincter muscle. An amplifier gain of 50 μV per division is used for the duration of the needle examination because urethral sphincter MUAPs are smaller than those of other skeletal muscle.[21,34]

Needle EMG techniques have a number of disadvantages, including artifact due to muscle tightening and incomplete relaxation from the pain of the needle insertion; some patients are embarrassed and afraid of perineal and introitus needle insertion and may simply refuse the needle EMG studies, and the localized sample may not be representative of the whole muscle bulk constituting the external urethral sphincter and pelvic floor.[34]

The needle EMG examination of the urethra is similar to that of other skeletal muscles and includes determination of insertional activity, spontaneous activity at rest, recruitment, and MUAP wave form characteristics.

Normal Findings

On insertion of the needle electrode into the urethral sphincter, there is a burst of activity (insertional activity) that then fades to a resting interference pattern made up of three or four tonically firing units.[34] Insertional activity is caused by muscle fiber depolarization with needle electrode insertion and repositioning. In normal sphincters, this usually lasts for less than 500 milliseconds.[21]

Spontaneous activity is determined with the EMG needle maintained in one position with the patient at rest and the bladder empty. Recording of spontaneous activity in the pelvic floor muscles (unlike other skeletal muscle) is difficult to evaluate as the periurethral sphincter muscle shows a continuous tonic contraction.[34,39] This activity has been shown to present even during sleep. This phenomenon is necessary as it is crucial that the urinary sphincter be closed except during volitional urination. During volitional micturition, the activity of the sphincter ceases.[34,40]

Therefore, the urethral sphincter is tonically active at all times except just before, and for the duration of, voiding.[21] The external urethral sphincter at rest usually demonstrates one or two motor unit action potentials firing per second. During bladder filling, there is a gradual increase in EMG activity that reaches maximum just before voiding.[34] This continuous electrical activity can make the detection of fibrillation potentials and positive sharp waves difficult. The best way to overcome this problem is to evaluate spontaneous resting activity just after the patient empties his or her bladder. This should minimize the tonic electrical activity.[21]

Assessment of motor unit recruitment can be accomplished in several ways: by filling the bladder with water or carbon dioxide gas, by asking the patient to cough, and by asking him or her to squeeze as if he or she was trying to stop from passing gas or stop urine flow in mid stream. A normal response to these provocative maneuvers is an increase in the firing rate of active motor unit potentials and recruitment of additional motor unit potentials.[21,41]

In neuro-urology, EMG generally is performed simultaneously with cystometry. During bladder filling, there usually is a gradual increase in EMG activity that reaches maximum just before micturition. Then, sphincter relaxation persists throughout the detrusor contraction, and EMG activity resumes at the end of voiding. Often, a strong contraction of the external urethral sphincter is seen just at the end of the detrusor contraction. If the patient is asked to voluntarily stop voiding, there should be an abrupt increase in EMG activity representing a voluntary sphincter contraction.[34]

MUAP waveform analysis is also useful in the determination of nerve injury. The normal parameters for MUAP waveform duration and amplitude include

1. A number of studies have determined the MUAP urethral sphincter waveform duration in control subjects is between 3.0 to 5.7 milliseconds (plus or minus 1.0 SD).
2. The mean amplitude of the normal MUAP potential is between 50 to 1,500 μV.[21,42,43]

Clinical Correlation

The electrophysiologic abnormalities seen in four different types of urinary incontinence (overflow, uninhibited, stress, and instability) are summarized in Table 7.1.

Stress Urinary Incontinence

Stress urinary incontinence (SUI) is one type of urinary incontinence. Typically, women with SUI have involuntary loss of urine with increased intra-abdominal pressure in the absence of a detrusor contraction. In general, women with SUI have MUAPs of large amplitude, increased duration, and polyphasic potentials.[21] Neurophysiologic studies have

TABLE 7.1 Urodynamic and electrophysiologic features in different types of urinary incontinence

Type of incontinence	Lesion location	Etiology	Urodynamic features	Pudendal NCV findings	EMG findings
Overflow incontinence due to impaired detrusor contractility	Lower motor neuron, spinal nerve root, sacral plexus, peripheral nerve	Sacral SCI Cauda equina injury Lumbar-sacral nerve root injury Pelvic plexopathy Polyneuropathy	Large-capacity bladder Weak or absent detrusor contraction with normal-to-absent EMG response during micturition Diminished urine flow on uroflowmetry	Increased latency	Variably abnormal EMG Denervation potentials Decreased insertional activity Polyphasia
Uninhibited bladder incontinence	Suprapontine cortical lesions	CVA Brain tumor Normal-pressure hydrocephalus Organic brain syndrome Alzheimer's disease	Uninhibited coordinated detrusor contraction, usually at low capacities	Normal pudendal NCV	Normal EMG
Stress urinary incontinence	Pudendal nerve Impaired integrity of pelvic floor and external sphincter	Childbirth Gynecologic surgery TURP in men	Elevated maximum and average flow on uroflowmetry Low-amplitude CMG contraction Normal EMG relaxation during micturition	Increased latency	Abnormal sphincter EMG
Instability incontinence	Upper motor neuron lesion between pons and sacral spinal cord	SCI between pons and conus medullaris	CMG shows detrusor hyperreflexia High-pressure contractions (against a closed bladder outlet) DSD on CMG/EMG Irregular flow on uroflowmetry	Normal pudendal NCV	DSD on EMG/urodynamic testing No denervation potentials

CMG = cystometrogram; CVA = cerebrovascular accident; DSD = detrusor sphincter dyssynergia; EMG = electromyography; NCV = nerve conduction velocity; SCI = spinal cord injury; TURP = transurethral prostatectomy.

demonstrated partial denervation of the anal sphincter and pubococcygeus in women with SUI.[34]

SUI occurs with either a lower motor neuron lesion in the sacral canal (i.e., spinal stenosis, herniated intravertebral disk) or pelvic nerve injury after radical pelvic surgery. Such patients have evidence of partial denervation and abnormal motor units recorded from the urethral sphincter and pubococcygeus muscles.[34] Snooks et al.[44] also reported prolongation of the perineal terminal motor latency in women with SUI.

Women with SUI associated with pelvic prolapse have also been shown to have partially denervated pelvic muscles. The extent of urinary incontinence is determined by the degree of damage affecting the urethral sphincter reflected in prolongation of the terminal motor latency.[34,45]

Lower Motor Neuron Lesion

Classically, the behavior of a decentralized lower motor neuron bladder has been described as areflexic, hypotonic, or flaccid. On EMG, sharp waves and fibrillation potentials are seen at rest, and an incomplete interference pattern with polyphasic activity are seen on volitional testing. Lower motor neuron bladder occurs with myelodysplasia, cauda equina injury, polyneuropathy, and after radical pelvic surgery.[34,46]

Upper Motor Neuron Lesion

In upper motor neuron disease with the lesion above the pontine micturition center, all of the urethral reflexes are intact, and the EMG results are normal, except for a lack of voluntary control. When the neurologic lesion is above the brain stem, there usually is a detrusor hyperreflexia associated with complete relaxation of the external urethral sphincter. Thus, in a physiologic sense, these patients void normally but simply lack control.[34,47]

When the neurologic lesion is between the brain stem and the sacral spinal cord, there is discoordination between the detrusor and external sphincter. Persistent EMG activity during voiding may occur. When this occurs during an involuntary detrusor contraction, it is known as a *detrusor sphincter dyssynergia*, a pathologic condition in which micturition is uncoordinated. Detrusor sphincter dyssynergia is always due to a neurologic lesion of the spinal cord.[34,48,49]

References

1. Gominak SC. Pudendal Nerve Distal Latency. In 1997 AAEM Course C: The Electrophysiologic Evaluation of Bladder and Bowel Dysfunction. Rochester, MN: Johnson Printing Company, 1997;13–17.
2. Kiff ES, Barnes PRH, Swash M. Evidence of pudendal neuropathy in patients with perineal descent and chronic straining at stool. Gut 1984;25:1279.
3. Kiff ES, Swash M. Slowed conduction in the pudendal nerves in idiopathic (neurogenic) faecal incontinence. Br J Surg 1984;71:614.
4. Kiff ES, Swash M. Normal proximal and delayed distal conduction in the pudendal nerves of patients with idiopathic (neurogenic) faecal incontinence. J Neurol Neurosurg Psychiatry 1984;47:820.

5. Snooks SJ, Barnes PRH, Swash M. Damages to the innervation of the voluntary anal and periurethral sphincter musculature in incontinence: an electrophysiologic study. J Neurol Neurosurg Psychiatry 1984;47:1269.
6. Snooks SJ, Swash M. Abnormalities of the innervation of the urethral striated sphincter musculature in incontinence. Br J Urol 1984;56:401.
7. Snooks SJ, Swash M. Perineal nerve and transcutaneous spinal stimulation: new methods for investigation of the urethral striated sphincter musculature. Br J Urol 1984;56:406.
8. Snooks SJ, Swash M, Henry MM. Electrophysiologic and manometric assessment of failed postanal repair for anorectal incontinence. Dis Colon Rectum 1984;27:733.
9. Snooks SJ, Swash M, Setchell M, Henry MM. Injury to innervation of pelvic floor sphincter musculature in childbirth. Lancet 1984;ii:546.
10. Smith ARB, Hosker GL, Warrell DW. The role of the pudendal nerve damage in the aetiology of genuine stress incontinence in women. Br J Obstet Gynaecol 1989;96:29.
11. Snooks SJ, Badenoch DF, Tiptaft RC, Swash M. Perineal nerve damage in genuine stress urinary incontinence. An electrophysiologic study. Br J Urol 1985;57:422.
12. Benson JT. Pelvic floor neurophysiology—An AAEM Workshop. American Association of Electrodiagnostic Medicine. Rochester, MN: Johnson Printing Company, 1998.
13. Lubowski DZ, Nicholls RJ, Burleigh DE, Swash M. Internal anal sphincter in neurogenic fecal incontinence. Gastroenterology 1988;95:997.
14. Benson JT, McClellan E. Clinical Neurophysiological Technique and Urinary and Fecal Incontinence. In DR Ostergard, AE Bent (eds), Urogynecology and Urodynamics Theory and Practice (4th ed). Baltimore: Williams & Wilkins, 1996;225–250.
15. Allen RE, Hosker GL, Smith ARB, Warrell DW. Pelvic floor damage and childbirth: a neurophysiological study. Br J Obstet Gynaecol 1990;97:770.
16. Snooks SJ, Henry MM, Swash M. Faecal incontinence due to external anal sphincter division in childbirth is associated with damage to the innervation of the pelvic floor musculature: A double pathology. Br J Obstet Gynaecol 1985;92:824.
17. Snooks SJ, Swash M, Henry MM, Setchell M. Risk factors in childbirth causing damage to the pelvic floor innervation. Int J Colorectal Rectal Dis 1986;1:20.
18. Snooks SJ, Swash M, Mathers SE, Henry MM. Effect of vaginal delivery on the pelvic floor: A 5-year follow-up. Br J Surg 1990;77:1358.
19. Sultan AH, Kamm MA, Hudson CN. Pudendal nerve damage during labour: Prospective study before and after childbirth. Br J Obstet Gynaecol 1994;101:22.
20. Laurberg S, Swash M, Henry MM. Delayed external sphincter repair for obstetric tear. Br J Surg 1988;75:786.
21. Olsen AL. Methodology of Urethral Needle EMG in Women. In 1997 AAEM Course C: The Electrophysiologic Evaluation of Bladder and Bowel Dysfunction. Rochester, MN: Johnson Printing Company, 1997;21–24.

22. Buchthal F, Pinelli P. Analysis of muscle action potentials as a diagnostic aid in neuro-muscular disorders. Acta Med Scan 1953;142(Suppl 266):315.
23. Chantraine A. EMG Examination of the Anal and Urethral Sphincters. In JE Desmedt (ed), New Developments in Electromyography and Clinical Neurophysiology. Basel: Karger, 1973;421–432.
24. DiBenedetto M, Yalla SV. Electrodiagnosis of striated urethral sphincter dysfunction. J Urol 1979;122:361.
25. Diokno AC, Koff SA, Anderson W. Combined cystometry and perineal electromyography in the diagnosis and treatment of neurogenic urinary incontinence. J Urol 1976;151.
26. Fowler CJ, Kirby RS. Abnormal electromyographic activity (decelerating burst and complex repetitive discharges) in the striated muscle of the urethral sphincter in 5 women with persisting urinary retention. J Urol 1985;57:67.
27. Fowler CJ, Kirby RS. Electromyography of urethral sphincter in women with urinary retention. Lancet 1986;28:1456.
28. Fowler CJ, Kirby RS, Harrison MJG, et al. Individual motor unit analysis in the diagnosis of disorders of urethral sphincter innervation. J Neurol Neurosurg Psychiatry 1984;47:637.
29. Franksson C, Peterson I. Electromyographic investigation of disturbances in the striated muscle of the urethral sphincter. Br J Urol 1955;27:154.
30. Gunasekera WSL, Richardson AK, Eversden ID. Urethral function in neurological disorders of the lower urinary tract. Surg Neurol 1983;20:239.
31. Jesel M, Isch-Treussard C, Isch F. Electromyography of Striated Muscle of Anal and Urethral Sphincters. In JE Desmedt (ed), New Developments in Electromyography and Clinical Neurophysiology. Basel: Karger, 1973;406–420.
32. Mayo ME: The value of sphincter electromyography in urodynamics. J Urol 1979;122:357.
33. Vereecken RL, Verduyn H. The electrical activity of the paraurethral and perineal muscles in normal and pathological conditions. Br J Urol 1970;52:457.
34. Chancellor C, Mandel S, Manon-Espaillat R. Electromyography in Neuro-Urology. In MB Chancellor, JG Blaivas (eds), Practical Neuro-Urology. Boston: Butterworth–Heinemann, 1995;75–83.
35. Fowler CJ. Pelvic floor neurophysiology. Methods Clin Neurophysiol 1991;2:1.
36. Blaivas JG. The neurophysiology of micturition: a clinical study of 550 patients. J Urol 1982;127:958.
37. Bradley WE, Scott FB, Timm GW. Sphincter electromyography. Urol Clin North Am 1974;1:69.
38. Rosenfaick P. Electromyography: Sensory and Motor Conductions. Findings in Normal Subjects. Copenhagen, Denmark: Rikshospitalet Laboratory of Clinical Neurophysiology, 1975.
39. Floyd WF, Walls EW. Electromyography of the sphincter ani externus in man. J Physiol 1953;122:500.

40. Eardley I, Fowler CJ. Urethral sphincter electromyography. Int Urogynecol J Pelvic Floor Dysfunct 1993;4:282.
41. Benson JT. Clinical Neurophysiological Techniques in Urinary and Fecal Incontinence. In DR Ostergard, AE Bent (eds), Urogynecology and Urodynamics: Theory and Practice. Baltimore: Williams & Wilkins, 1996;239.
42. Fowler CJ. Pelvic floor neurophysiology. Methods Clin Neurophysiol 1991;2:1.
43. Fowler CJ. Pelvic Floor Neurophysiology. In Osselton JW (ed), Clinical Neurophysiology. Oxford, UK: Butterworth–Heinemann, 1995;241.
44. Snooks SJ, Barnes PRH, Swash M. Abnormalities of the innervation of the voluntary anal and urethral sphincters in incontinence: An electrophysiological study. J Neurol Neurosurg Psychiatry 1984;47:1269.
45. Smith ARB, Hosker GL, Warrell DW. The role of partial denervation of the pelvic floor in the aetiology of genitourinary prolapse and stress incontinence of urine: A neurophysiological study. Br J Obstet Gynaecol 1989;96:24.
46. Rockswold G, Bradley WE. The use of evoked electromyographic responses in diagnosing lesions of the cauda equina. J Urol 1977;118:629.
47. Blaivas JG, Sinha HP, Zayed AAH, Labib KB. Detrusor external sphincter dyssynergia: a detailed electromyographic study. J Urol 1981;125:545.
48. McGuire EM, Brady S. Detrusor-sphincter dyssynergia. J Urol 1979;121:774.
49. Kaplan WE, Firlit CF, Schoenberg HW. Female urethral syndrome. External sphincter spasm as etiology. J Urol 1980;124:48.

8 Laboratory Assessment of Urinary Function

Jack L. Rook

The laboratory assessment of urinary function may yield important clues as to the cause of urinary incontinence, as well as provide information on genitourinary (GU) system pathology and overall systemic health.

A number of factors that contribute to incontinence can be identified through clinical and laboratory evaluation. For example, increased urine production (due to diabetes mellitus, diabetes insipidus, and other disorders of water metabolism, and hypercalcemia), and irritated bladder mucosa due to urinary infections may contribute to incontinence. Each disorder has characteristic laboratory abnormalities.

Chronic urinary tract disorders can adversely affect overall renal function. For example, those patients who have chronic urinary tract infections that develop into pyelonephritis can develop scarring of renal tissue that over time, can result in chronic renal failure. Patients who have vesicoureteral reflux, chronic obstruction due to stone disease, or prostatic hypertrophy can develop chronic hydronephrosis (enlargement of kidneys) that over time damages renal tissue, contributing to chronic renal failure.

Laboratory data can provide information about neoplastic disorders affecting the GU system: serum markers for prostate cancer are available; the presence of hematuria, an abnormal finding, could represent neoplasia anywhere along the GU pathway; elevated serum calcium may signify metastatic disease.

Last, pressure ulcers, osteomyelitis, and soft-tissue infection often occur concomitantly with urinary incontinence in debilitated and spinal cord–injured patients. These disorders have characteristic laboratory abnormalities. The laboratory assessment of urinary infections, stones, prostatic disease (benign or malignant), and chronic GU dysfunction of any kind can help lead to prompt and appropriate treatment of the respective disorder.

This chapter reviews common urine and serum laboratory studies used in evaluation of the urinary system (Table 8.1). The urine studies include

TABLE 8.1   Common urine and serum laboratory studies used in evaluation of the urinary system

Laboratory test	Normal adult values
Chemstrip	
pH	4.5–8.0
Protein	Absent
Glucose	Absent
Hb	Absent
Urine nitrite	Negative
Specific gravity	1.003–1.030
Urinalysis	
Specific gravity	Extreme range: 1.003–1.035
	Normal range: 1.010–1.025
Color	Pale to darker yellow
Clarity	Clear
pH	Normal pH: 4.6–8
	Average pH: 6
Blood/Hb	Absent
Protein	Absent
Glucose	Absent
Bilirubin	Negative
Microscopic examination of urine sediment	
RBC count	0–2/HPF
RBC casts	0/LPF
WBC count	0–4/HPF
WBC casts	0/LPF
Urine epithelial cells	
Renal	0–2/HPF
Bladder	Common
Squamous	Common
Hyaline casts	0–2/LPF
Crystals	Interpreted by physician
Bacteria	None/HPF
Urine culture and sensitivity*	
24-Hour urine collection	
Volume	600–2,500 ml/24 hrs
Osmolality	300–900 mOsm/kg/24 hrs
Protein	10–140 mg/liter/24 hrs
Glucose	Less than 0.3 g/24 hrs
Chloride	140–250 mEq/liter/24 hrs
Sodium	40–220 mEq/liter/24 hrs
Potassium	25–125 mEq/24 hrs (markedly intake-dependent)
Urine creatinine	Men: 0.8–1.8 g/24 hrs
	Women: 0.6–1.6 g/24 hrs
Creatinine clearance	Men: 85–125 ml/min/1.73 m^2
	Women: 75–115 ml/min/1.73 m^2
	Geriatric: 96.9 ± 2.9 ml/min/1.73 m^2
24-Hour urine studies of stone constituents	
Uric acid	250–750 mg/24 hrs
Calcium	100–300 mg/24 hrs
Oxalate	7–44 mg/24 hrs (male)
	4–31 mg/24 hrs (female)
Cystine	Less than 38 mg/24 hrs
Complete blood cell count	
WBC count	5,000–10,000/μl
RBC count	Men: 4.2–5.4 × 10^6/μl
	Women: 3.6–5.0 × 10^6/μl
Hematocrit	Men: 46% ± 3.1%
	Women: 40.9% ± 3%

TABLE 8.1   continued

Laboratory test	Normal adult values
Hb	Men: 14.0–17.4 g/dl
	Women: 12.0–16.0 g/dl
Mean corpuscular volume	82–100 μm^3
Sedimentation rate	
Erythrocyte sedimentation rate (Westergren)	Men: 0–15 mm/hr
	Women: 0–20 mm/hr
Renalytes	
Chloride	98–106 mEq/liter
Potassium	3.5–5.3 mEq/liter
Sodium	135–145 mEq/liter
Glucose	65–110 mg/dl
Blood urea nitrogen	7–20 mg/dl
Creatinine	0.6–1.3 mg/dl
Other serum tests	
Calcium	Total: 8.6–10.0 mg/dl
	Ionized: 4.65–5.28 mg/dl
Oral glucose tolerance test	Fasting adult: 70–110 mg/dl
	30 mins: 110–170 mg/dl
	60 mins: 120–170 mg/dl
	2 hrs: 70–120 mg/dl
	3 hrs: 70–120 mg/dl
Uric acid	Men: 3.5–7.2 mg/dl
	Women: 2.6–6.0 mg/dl
Acid phosphatase	0–3.1 ng/ml
Prostate-specific antigen	Men: 0–4 ng/ml

Hb = hemoglobin; HPF = high-powered field; LPF = low-powered field; RBC = red blood cell; WBC = white blood cell.
*Done to identify the exact organism present and to predict which drugs will be effective in treating the infection.

the chemstrip, urinalysis (UA), urine culture and sensitivity, various 24-hour urine tests, and microscopic evaluation of urine. Serum tests reviewed include the complete blood cell (CBC) count, renalytes, cancer markers, diabetic, and renal stone disease studies.

This chapter applies the various laboratory tests available to aid in the evaluation of various clinical GU disorders, including urinary tract infection, stone disease, diabetes mellitus, and disorders of water metabolism, including diabetes insipidus, renal damage with proteinuria, hematuria, and chronic renal failure.

Urologic Laboratory Examination

Examination of urine specimens aids the urologic workup and frequently helps establish the diagnosis and treatment needs of patients with urologic disease.

UA is unquestionably one of the most cost-effective and useful screening tests available. It is best to examine urine that has been properly obtained. The importance of the method of urine collection cannot be overstated. Urine must be collected by a strictly uniform method in the physician's office, laboratory, or hospital. The specimen should be obtained before a genital or rectal examination to prevent contamination from the introitus or expressed prostatic secretions. Urine obtained from a drainage bag is not a proper specimen for UA. First-voided morning specimens are helpful for qualitative protein testing and for specific gravity assessment. Urine specimens that have been left standing for a few hours become alkaline in pH and may contain lysed red cells, disintegrated casts, or rapidly multiplying bacteria. A freshly voided specimen obtained a few hours after the patient has eaten is most reliable.

It is usually simple to collect a clean-voided, midstream urine sample from most men. The procedure should include foreskin retraction, cleansing of the meatus with povidone-iodine (Betadine), and passing the first 15–30 ml of the stream without collection. The next portion 50–100 ml of urine is collected in a sterile specimen container, which is capped immediately afterwards. In adult males, it is rarely necessary to collect urine by catheterization unless urinary retention is present or assessment of residual urine is required.

It is virtually impossible for a woman to obtain a satisfactory, clean-voided, midstream specimen without help. A voided specimen from an unprepped patient is not useful unless it is completely normal. If results of an initial UA specimen in a nonsterile container are normal, no further study is indicated. If abnormal, a urine specimen must be obtained by a more exacting technique whereby the patient is placed in a lithotomy position, the vulva and urethral meatus are cleansed with povidone-iodine, the labia are separated, and she is then instructed to void into a container held close to the vulva. After passing 10–20 ml of urine, the next 50–100 ml is collected in a sterile container that is immediately capped. If a satisfactory specimen cannot be obtained by this method, the clinician should not hesitate to obtain a specimen by catheterization.[1]

Urine Dipstick (Chemstrip)

Dipstick tests are available for UA outside the laboratory setting. They can be used and read directly by patients and health care providers. The dipstick is impregnated with chemicals that react with specific substances in the urine to produce color-coded visual results. Color controls are provided against which the actual color produced by the urine sample, at the correct elapsed time, can be compared with the control chart.[2]

The chemstrip procedure is as follows:

1. The chemstrip is dipped into a well-mixed fresh urine sample (within 1 hour of collection).
2. After removal, each reagent area on the dipstick is compared with the corresponding color-controlled chart within established time frames. If not timed correctly, color changes may produce invalid results.
3. If reagent chemicals on the impregnated pad become mixed, readings will be inaccurate. To avoid this, excess urine must be shaken off after withdrawing the dipstick from the sample.

Dipsticks actually function as miniature laboratories. These chemically impregnated reagent strips provide quick determination of pH, protein, glucose, ketones, bilirubin, hemoglobin (Hb) (blood), nitrite, leukocyte esterase, urobilinogen, and specific gravity.[2]

pH
The pH of urine is important in only a few clinical situations. Patients with uric acid stones rarely have a urinary pH over 6.5, as uric acid is soluble in alkaline urine. Patients with calcium stones or nephrocalcinosis are unable to acidify urine below pH 6.0. Urinary tract infections caused by urease-splitting organisms (most commonly proteus species) tend to have urinary pH over 7.0. Last, urine obtained within 2 hours of a large meal, or left standing at room temperature for several hours, tends to be alkaline.[1]

Protein
Dipsticks can be used to determine the presence of protein in urine. Persistent abnormalities require quantitative (24-hour urine protein) testing to rule out significant disease (glomerulopathy or cancer).[1]

Glucose
The glucose tests used in chemstrips are quite accurate and specific for urinary glucose. False-positive results may be obtained when patients have ingested large doses of aspirin, ascorbic acid, or cephalosporins. However, most patients with a positive reading have diabetes mellitus.[1]

Hemoglobin
The chemstrip test for Hb is not specific for red cells in the urine (free myoglobin from muscle breakdown may give a false-positive reading), and should only be used to screen for hematuria. Microscopic analysis of the urinary sediment is then required for confirmation.[1]

Urine Nitrate
The urine nitrate test is an indirect method for detecting bacteria in the urine. With dipstick testing, the nitrate area in a multiple reagent strip is calibrated so that any shade of pink that develops within 30 seconds indicates significant bacteriuria. A first-morning specimen is preferred for this test and is more likely to yield a positive result than a random urine sample that may have been in the bladder for only a short time. Even a faint pink hue is a reliable indicator of significant bacteriuria and is a cue for performing urine culture. However, a negative result in the presence of clinical symptoms should never be interpreted as indicating complete absence of bacteriuria: If an overnight sample is not used, there may not have been enough time for the nitrate to convert to nitrite (the chemical that causes the "pink" dipstick reaction) in the bladder. Additionally, some urinary tract infections are caused by organisms that do not convert nitrate to nitrite.[2]

Specific Gravity
The specific gravity of urine (normal, 1.003–1.030) is often important for diagnostic purposes. Patients with primary diabetes insipidus usually have specific gravity less than 1.010. Urine-specific gravity via dipstick is a simple test for evaluating hydration status in postoperative patients. Occasionally, urine osmolality determination is required to confirm the specific gravity findings.[1]

TABLE 8.2   Urinalysis

Normal values
  General characteristics and measurements
    Color: pale yellow to amber
    Appearance: clear to slightly hazy
    Specific gravity: 1.015–1.025 with a normal fluid intake
    pH: 4.5–8.0—average person has a pH of approximately 5–6
    Volume: 1,500 ml/24 hrs
  Chemical determinations
    Glucose: negative
    Ketones: negative
    Blood: negative
    Protein: negative
    Bilirubin: negative
    Urobilinogen: 0.1–1.0
    Nitrate for bacteria: negative
    Leukocyte esterase: negative

Urinalysis

The process of UA determines the following properties of urine: color, odor, turbidity, specific gravity, pH, glucose, ketones, blood, protein, bilirubin, urobilinogen, nitrate, and leukocyte esterase (Table 8.2). A 10-ml urine specimen is usually sufficient for conducting these tests. The results of UA vary according to the time of day the specimen is collected. Significant cellular abnormalities that show up in a morning specimen may be missed in dilute urine collected later in the day.[2]

For a UA procedure, the patient voids directly into a clean, dry container. All specimens are covered tightly, labeled, and immediately sent to the laboratory. If the specimen is not evaluated (or refrigerated) within 1 hour of collection, changes in urinary composition may occur: bacteria in the urine "split" urea (converting it to ammonia) producing an alkaline urine, urine casts decompose, and red blood cells (RBCs) may be lysed. A clean-voided specimen must be obtained. Feces, prostatic discharges, vaginal secretions, and menstrual blood contaminate the urine specimen.[2]

Urine Appearance

After urine collection, a quick-screen macroscopic examination can be done. Various medications, blood (hematuria), or pus (pyuria) often color urine. When red urine is seen, hematuria must be ruled out by microscopic analysis.

Fresh urine is normally clear to slightly hazy. Urine turbidity may result from urinary tract infections. Urine may be cloudy because of RBCs, white blood cells (WBCs), or bacteria. Pathologic urine is often turbid or cloudy. However, normal urine can also appear cloudy: Alkaline urine may appear cloudy because of large amounts of amorphous phosphates that can be made to disappear with the addition of acid. Acid urine may appear cloudy because of urates.[2]

Urine Color

Urine color is primarily a result of urochrome (pigments present in the diet or formed via metabolism). Urine specimens may normally vary in color from pale yellow to dark amber. The color of freshly voided urine is recorded as part of the UA. Normal urine color darkens on standing, a decomposition process starting approximately 30 minutes after voiding. Some foods and many medications alter the color of urine.

Near-colorless urine may be due to normal and to large fluid intake, reduction in perspiration, alcohol ingestion, diuretic therapy, or nervousness. It may also indicate pathology, including chronic interstitial nephritis, untreated diabetes mellitus, or diabetes insipidus.

Orange-colored urine may be due to concentrated urine caused by dehydration, fluid intake restriction, excessive sweating, or fever.

A brownish-yellow or greenish-yellow color may indicate bilirubin in the urine. Reddish to dark brown color may indicate Hb, porphyrins, or myoglobin in the urine. Milky urine is usually associated with the presence of pus (numerous WBCs).[2]

Urine-Specific Gravity

Specific gravity is a measurement of the kidneys' ability to concentrate urine. The test compares the weight of urine against the weight of distilled water, which has a specific gravity of 1.000. Because urine is a solution of minerals, salts, and compounds dissolved in water, the specific gravity is obviously greater than 1.000. The relative difference between the specific gravity of distilled water and the specific gravity of urine reflects the degree of concentration of the urine specimen.

The extreme range of urine-specific gravity (1.003–1.035) depends on the state of hydration. With normal hydration and volume, the specific gravity of urine is usually between 1.010 and 1.025.

Normally, specific gravity values vary inversely with amounts of urine excreted (decrease in urine volume equals increase in specific gravity). Consistently abnormal specific gravity is an indication of renal dysfunction.

Low specific gravity (1.001–1.010) occurs with diabetes insipidus, glomerulonephritis (kidney inflammation without infection), or pyelonephritis (kidney inflammation with bacterial infection).

Increased specific gravity (1.025–1.035) occurs with diabetes mellitus in which there is an abnormally large amount of urinary glucose, nephrosis in which there is an abnormally large amount of protein, or as a normal consequence of excessive nonrenal water loss via dehydration, fever, vomiting, or diarrhea.

Urine with a fixed low specific gravity (1.010) that does not vary from specimen to specimen is indicative of severe renal damage, with disturbance of both the concentrating and diluting abilities of the kidney.[2]

Urine pH

The symbol *pH* expresses the urine as an acid or a base solution and measures the free hydrogen ion concentration in the urine. The number 7 is the point of neutrality on the pH scale; the lower the pH, the greater the acidity; the higher the pH, the greater the alkalinity.

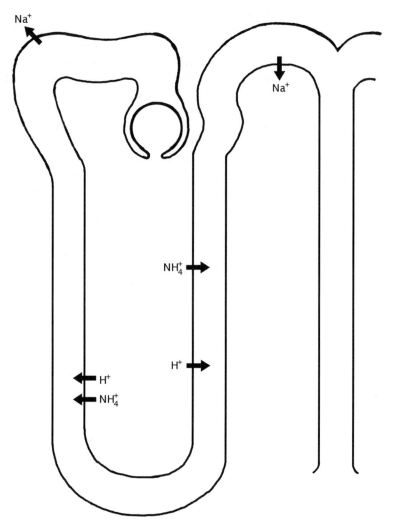

FIGURE 8.1 *The kidneys maintain normal acid-base balance primarily through the reabsorption of sodium (Na$^+$) and the tubular secretion of hydrogen (H$^+$) and ammonium (NH$_4^+$) ions.*

The urinary pH is an indicator of the renal tubule's ability to maintain normal hydrogen ion concentration in the plasma and extracellular fluid. The kidneys maintain normal acid-base balance primarily through the reabsorption of sodium and the tubular secretion of hydrogen and ammonium ions (Figure 8.1). Secretion of acid or alkaline urine by the kidneys is one of the most important mechanisms for maintaining a constant body pH.[2]

An accurate measurement of urinary pH can be done only on a freshly voided specimen. If the urine is kept for a prolonged length of time before analysis, the pH of the specimen becomes alkaline because bacteria split urea to produce ammonia (a base). Normal pH ranges from 4.6 to 8.0, with average pH being approximately 6 (acid). Acidic urine (pH less than 6) occurs with uncontrolled diabetes, diarrhea, starvation, dehydration, and with respiratory diseases in which CO_2 retention causes a systemic acidosis (emphysema). A diet high in meat or cranberry juice also keeps the urine acidic.

Alkaline urine (pH greater than 7) occurs with urinary tract infection, salicylate intoxication, renal tubular acidosis, chronic renal failure, and respiratory hyperventilation (blowing off CO_2 produces a systemic alkalosis). A diet that emphasizes citrus fruits and vegetables (particularly legumes) helps keep urine alkaline.[2]

Control of urinary pH is important in the management of renal calculi and urinary infection. Renal stone formation partially depends on the pH of urine. Patients being treated for renal calculi are frequently given diets or medication to change the pH of urine so that kidney stones will not form: Calcium phosphate and calcium carbonate stones develop in alkaline urine. In such instances, the urine must be kept acidic. Uric acid, cystine, and oxalate stones precipitate in acidic urine. In such cases, the urine should be kept alkaline. Last, urine should be kept acidic during treatment of urinary tract infections and persistent bacteriuria.[2]

Urine Blood or Hemoglobin

Normally, no blood or Hb is found in a urine sample. Blood may appear as intact red cells or as free Hb. The use of both a urine dipstick and microscopic examination of urine provides a complete clinical evaluation of hemoglobinuria and hematuria. Dipsticks dipped into the urine identify both hemoglobinuria and hematuria. To verify the presence of RBCs, a fresh urine specimen is centrifuged, and its sediment is examined microscopically.

The presence of free Hb in the urine is referred to as *hemoglobinuria*. Pure hemoglobinuria is usually related to conditions outside the urinary tract that causes such extensive or rapid destruction (hemolysis) of circulating erythrocytes that the reticuloendothelial system cannot metabolize or store the excess free Hb.

When intact RBCs and Hb are present in the urine, the term *hematuria* is used to indicate bleeding somewhere in the urinary tract. Hematuria occurs with lower urinary tract infections; urinary tract or renal cancers; urinary calculi; hemophilia or treatment with anticoagulants; glomerulonephritis; GU system trauma; or strenuous exercise. Any positive test for hematuria should be rechecked on a new urine specimen. If hematuria still appears, the patient should be further evaluated.

When urine dipstick gives a positive result for occult blood, but no RBCs are seen microscopically, myoglobinuria can be suspected. Myoglobinuria results from excretion of myoglobin, a muscle protein, into the urine as a result of traumatic muscle injury or a muscle disorder (muscular dystrophy). Aside from problems caused by the presence of myoglobin, false-positive results may occur with highly alkaline urine, which tends to cause hemolysis of red cells (producing hemoglobinuria without hematuria), and if menstrual blood contaminates a urine specimen.[2]

Urine Protein

Normally, UA should be negative for protein, as the glomerulus prevents passage of protein from blood to the glomerular filtrate. The persistent presence of protein in the urine is the single most important indication of renal disease. Detection of protein in urine (proteinuria), combined with a microscopic examination of urinary sediment, provides the basis for differential diagnosis of renal disease. To perform a qualitative protein UA, the urine is tested with a protein reagent dipstick. The test result color is compared to the color comparison chart provided on the reagent strip bottle. If more than a trace of protein is found in the urine, a quantitative 24-hour evaluation of protein excretion is necessary. However, a new second specimen should be tested qualitatively before the 24-hour specimen is collected.[2]

The clinical implications of proteinuria are reviewed in the urine protein for 24-hour collection section to follow.

Urine Glucose

Glucose is present in the glomerular filtrate but is normally reabsorbed by the nephron. The normal glucose UA value is "negative." In diabetes mellitus, the main cause of glycosuria, the blood glucose level exceeds the reabsorption capacity of the tubules, and glucose spills into the urine.

An enzyme-impregnated chemstrip, when dipped into urine, changes color according to the amount of glucose in the urine. The manufacturer's color chart provides a basis for comparison of colors between the sample and control values.

Urine glucose tests are used to screen for diabetes, to confirm a diagnosis of diabetes, or to monitor the degree of diabetic control. A single random sample positive test for urine sugar is not adequate for a diagnosis of diabetes. A urine glucose test combined with a blood glucose test provides even better information.[2]

Urine Bilirubin

Bilirubin, a breakdown product of Hb, is formed in cells of the spleen and bone marrow, and is then transported to the liver. Urine bilirubin aids in the diagnosis and monitoring of treatment for hepatitis and liver dysfunction. Urine bilirubin should be a part of every UA, because bilirubin may often appear in the urine before other signs of liver dysfunction become apparent (i.e., jaundice, weakness).

To perform this test, the urine sample should be examined using a chemically reactive dipstick within 1 hour of collection, because urine bilirubin is unstable, especially when exposed to light. Color changes are compared with controls on the bilirubin color chart. The results are interpreted as "negative" to "3+" or as "small, moderate, or large" amounts of bilirubin. Normally, there is no detectable bilirubin in the urine. Even trace amounts of bilirubin are abnormal and warrant further investigation.

Increased levels occur with hepatitis and liver diseases (caused by infections or exposure to toxic agents or drugs), and with obstructive biliary tract disorders (intrahepatic due to tumor, or extrahepatic obstruction due to stone disease or tumor).[2]

Microscopic Examination of Urine Sediment

Microscopic examination of urinary sediment is an essential part of all UAs, as the urine sediment provides information useful for both diagnoses and prognoses.[1,2]

TABLE 8.3   Microscopic examination of urine sediment

Urine sediment component	Clinical significance
Bacteria	Urinary tract infection
Casts	Tubular or glomerular disorders
Epithelial (renal) casts	Tubular degeneration
Red cell casts	Acute glomerulonephritis
White cell casts	Pyelonephritis
Epithelial cells	Damage to various parts of urinary tract
Renal cells	Tubular damage
Squamous cells	Normal or contamination
Erythrocytes (red blood cells)	Most renal disorders, menstruation, strenuous exercise
Leukocytes (white blood cells)	Most renal disorders, urinary tract infection, pyelonephritis

The urine sediment can be broken down into cellular elements (RBCs and WBCs and epithelial cells), casts, crystals, and bacteria, which may originate anywhere along the urinary tract. When casts occur, they may indicate tubular or glomerular disorders (Table 8.3), and they provide a direct sampling of urinary tract morphology.[2]

To perform a microscopic analysis of urine, the specimen should be examined immediately after collection. To prepare the sediment, a 10-ml specimen is centrifuged at 2,000 rpm for 5 minutes, following which 9 ml of the supernatant is removed. The sediment in the remaining 1 ml of urine is suspended by tapping the tube gently against a counter top. One drop of the remaining mixture is then placed on a microscope slide, covered with a cover slip, and examined under a low (10×) and then a high-power (40×) lens. Some significant sediment elements, particularly bacteria, are more easily seen if the slide is stained with methylene blue or Gram stain.[1]

Urine Red Blood Cells and Red Blood Cell Casts

The presence of even a few RBCs in the urine (hematuria) is abnormal. Although gross hematuria is more alarming to the patient, microscopic hematuria is no less significant. Persistent hematuria in an otherwise asymptomatic patient of either sex and any age signifies disease and requires further investigation.[1]

Normal values for RBCs are 0–2 per high-powered field. The finding of more than two RBCs is abnormal and can indicate infection, malignancy, or trauma anywhere along the GU system. Other causes of hematuria include renal stones, prostatitis, malignant hypertension, hemophilia, anticoagulant therapy overdose, and inflammation of organs near or directly adjoining the urinary tract (diverticulitis, appendicitis).[2]

Hematuria associated with infection (pyelonephritis, cystitis, or urethritis) generally clears after treatment of the underlying problem.[1] Vaginal bleeding might contaminate a urine specimen falsely, indicating hematuria.

Red cell casts normally should be absent when observing under low-field microscopy. They indicate hemorrhage and are always pathologic.

RBC casts also indicate acute inflammatory or vascular disorders of the glomerulus. Their presence in urine may be the only manifestation of acute glomerulonephritis, renal infarction, collagen disease, or renal involvement in subacute bacterial endocarditis. RBC casts and epithelial cell casts are frequently associated with systemic lupus erythematosus.[2]

Urine White Blood Cells and White Blood Cell Casts

Leukocytes (WBCs) may originate from anywhere in the GU tract. However, WBC casts always come from the kidney tubules. To evaluate for WBCs or WBC casts, urinary sediment is microscopically examined under high power for cells and low power for casts.

Normally, 0–4 WBCs may be seen per high power field. WBC casts should not be seen per low power microscopy. Large numbers of WBCs (50 cells or more per high-powered field) usually indicate acute bacterial infection somewhere within the urinary tract, whereas increased leukocyte levels are seen with all chronic renal or urinary tract diseases (chronic pyelonephritis, cystitis, prostatitis), fever, strenuous exercise, bladder tumors, or tuberculosis.[2]

WBC casts indicate renal parenchymal infection. Pyelonephritis is the most common cause.[2]

Urine Epithelial Cells and Epithelial Casts

Three kinds of urine epithelial cells can be found in urinary sediment, including renal tubule, bladder, and squamous epithelial cells.

Renal tubule epithelial cells are formed from cast-off nephron tubule cells that slowly degenerate. The presence of an occasional (0–2 per high-powered field) renal epithelial cell is not unusual because the renal tubules are continually regenerating. However, renal epithelial casts are always indicative of disease. Renal tubule epithelial cells are round, slightly larger than leukocytes, and contain a single large nucleus.[2]

Large numbers of epithelial casts are found when renal disease has damaged tubular epithelium. Mild-to-moderate numbers of renal tubule epithelium cells are found with acute tubular damage, acute glomerulonephritis, salicylate overdose, and in renal transplant patients with impending allograft rejection.[2]

It is not uncommon to find bladder transitional epithelial cells in normal urinary sediment. They range in shape from flat, to cuboidal, to columnar.[1,2] If bladder epithelial cells are present in large numbers or clumps and exhibit abnormal histology, they may be indicative of a malignant process affecting the urothelium.[1]

Squamous epithelial cells are common in normal urine sediment samples, indicating contamination of the specimen from the distal urethra in males and introitus in females. No significance should be placed on them. They are large, flat cells with irregular borders and a single small nucleus.[1,2]

Urine Hyalin Casts

Hyalin casts are clear, colorless casts formed when a specific protein within the renal tubules precipitates and gels. Their presence in urine depends on the degree of proteinuria. Urinary sediment is microscopi-

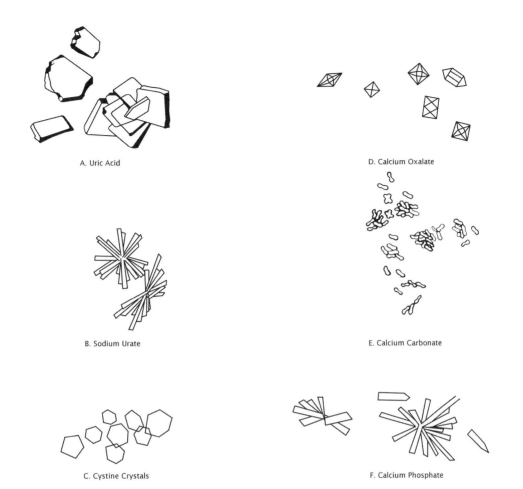

A. Uric Acid

D. Calcium Oxalate

B. Sodium Urate

E. Calcium Carbonate

C. Cystine Crystals

F. Calcium Phosphate

FIGURE 8.2   *Schematic representation of crystals that may appear in the urine. Each is identified by their specific appearance and solubility characteristics. Crystals that tend to form in acid urine include uric acid, sodium urate, cystine, and calcium oxalate. Crystals that tend to form in alkaline urine include calcium carbonate and calcium phosphate.*

cally examined for casts under low power. Normally, 0–2 hyalin casts are seen per low-powered field.

Hyalin casts indicate possible damage to the glomerular capillary membrane, which permits leakage of proteins through the glomerular filter system. Hyalin casts may be a temporary phenomenon in the presence of fever or strenuous exercise. However, the nephrotic syndrome may be suspected when large numbers of hyalin casts appear in the urine.[2]

Urine Crystals

A variety of crystals may appear in the urine; each identified by their specific appearance and solubility characteristics. Crystals that tend to form in acidic urine include uric acid, sodium urate, cystine crystals, and calcium oxalate. Crystals that tend to form in alkaline urine are calcium carbonate and calcium phosphate (Figure 8.2).[2]

Crystals in the urine may be present without clinical symptoms, or they may be associated with the formation of urinary tract calculi and give rise to clinical manifestations (colic) associated with partial or complete obstruction of urine flow.[2]

Bacteriuria

A presumptive diagnosis of bacterial infection may be made based on the results of microscopic examination of the urinary sediment. If several bacteria per high-powered field are found in a urine specimen obtained by suprapubic aspiration, catheterization in a woman, or in a properly obtained, clean-voided, midstream specimen from a man, a provisional diagnosis of bacterial infection can be made. However, these findings should be confirmed by bacterial culture.

Likewise, properly obtained urinary sediment that demonstrates more than five to eight WBCs per high-powered field is also considered abnormal (pyuria). If the patient has symptoms of a urinary tract infection, pyuria, and bacteriuria, one is justified in making a diagnosis of infection and initiating empiric therapy.[1]

Urine Culture and Sensitivity

The presumptive diagnosis of bacterial infection based on microscopic examination of the urinary sediment should be confirmed by culture. Urine itself is an excellent culture and growth medium for most organisms that infect the urinary tract. Formal culture techniques can be used to estimate the number of bacteria in the urine, to identify the exact organism present, and to predict which drugs will be effective in treating the infection. Cultures are particularly important in patients with recurrent or persistent infections, renal insufficiency, or drug allergies.[1,3]

The number of bacteria present in the urine (colony count) is influenced by the method of collection, the patient's hydration status, and whether the patient had been taking antimicrobial drugs.[1]

Special care must be taken when collecting specimens for urine culture. Whenever possible, early morning specimens should be obtained, as bacterial counts are highest at that time. A clean-voided urine specimen of at least 3–5 ml should be collected into a sterile container.

Specimen collection should be as aseptic as possible. The cleansing procedure must be done correctly to remove contaminating organisms from the vulva, urethral meatus, and perineal area so that any bacteria found in the urine can be assumed to have come only from the bladder and urethra.[3] The patient who is unable to comply with instructions should be assisted by health care personnel.

For females, general principles for specimen collection include

1. The area around the urinary meatus is cleaned from front to back using an antiseptic sponge.
2. While one hand spreads the labia apart, the other holds the sterile container using care not to contaminate the inside surface.

3. After voiding the first 25 ml into the toilet, a sufficient quantity of the remaining urine is directed into the sterile container.
4. The specimen container is then capped using care so as not to contaminate its inside surface.

For males, specimen collection is as follows[3]:

1. Any foreskin is completely retracted to expose the glans penis.
2. The area around the meatus is cleansed with antiseptic sponges.
3. After voiding approximately the first 25 ml of urine directly into the toilet, a sufficient amount of urine is directed into the sterile specimen container.
4. The specimen is then capped carefully.

Alternative methods for procuring urine specimens are catheterization or suprapubic aspiration. Catheterization heightens the risk of introducing a urinary tract infection and should be avoided if at all possible. Urine specimens for culture must never be retrieved from a urine collection bag that is part of an indwelling catheter drainage system.[3]

After collection, urine should be taken to the laboratory and examined as soon as possible. Ideally, specimens should be obtained before antibiotic or antimicrobial therapy begins.[3]

A count of 100,000 or more bacteria per ml indicates infection. A bacterial count of fewer than 10,000 bacteria per ml may indicate possible contamination.[3] Bacterial contamination comes from many sources, including perineal hair; hands; skin; clothing; bacteria beneath the prepuce in males; and bacteria from vaginal secretions, the vulva, or distal urethra in females. Cultures with growth of multiple organisms usually signify contamination, either due to improper collection method or improper laboratory technique.[1,3]

It is not always necessary to identify the specific organism causing infection in routine lower urinary tract infections; however, identification of the causative organism may be important in patients with recurrent or persistent symptoms and signs of urinary tract infection. Additionally, identifying the drugs to which the bacteria are sensitive may or may not be necessary, as *Escherichia coli*, which causes 85% of routine urinary tract infections, is known to be sensitive to numerous oral antimicrobial drugs. However, in patients with septicemia, renal insufficiency, diabetes mellitus, or suspected enterococcal, proteus, or *Pseudomonas* infections, it is important to determine the antibiotic sensitivity of the organism. Last, some bacteria (neisseriae, *Brucellaceae*, mycobacteria, anaerobes), fungi, and yeasts will not grow with common culture methods, and thus special culture techniques are required.[1]

24-Hour Urine Collection

Some diseases or conditions require a 24-hour urine specimen to evaluate kidney function accurately. Renal excretions of various substances may vary over time. Therefore, a random urine specimen might not give an accurate picture of the process taking place over a 24-hour period. More accurate information can be obtained from urine collected over a 24-hour period.

The 24-hour collection involves collecting the urine specimen in a suitable receptacle and either adding a preservative to it, keeping it refrigerated, or both. Most 24-hour urine specimen collections start early in the morning, usually approximately 7 AM. The first specimen is discarded and the time noted. All urine voided over the next 24 hours is collected into a large container labeled with the patient's name, time frame for collection, tests ordered, and other pertinent information. The last specimen should be obtained as closely as possible to the stated end time of the test. If refrigeration is necessary, the urine specimen must either be refrigerated immediately after the patient has voided, or the collection bottle must be placed into an iced container. Unless all urine is saved, results will not be accurate.

If other discharges, secretions, or heavy menstrual flow are present, the test may have to be postponed, or an indwelling catheter used to keep the specimen free of contamination. However, in some of these cases, thorough cleansing of the perineal or urethral area before voiding may be sufficient.[2]

Urine Volume

Urine volume measurements are indicated in the assessment of fluid balance and kidney function. A 24-hour urine volume is ascertained by measuring the entire urine amount in an appropriately calibrated receptacle. The total volume is recorded as urine volume in milliliters, or cubic cm (cc), per 24 hours. The normal volume of urine voided by the average adult in a 24-hour time period ranges from 600 to 2,500 ml. The amount voided over any period is directly related to the individual's fluid intake, body temperature, climate, and amount of perspiration that occurs.

Polyuria is an increase in the volume of excreted urine. It is a physiologic response to increased fluid intake, diuretic medications, chilling of the body, nervousness, large volume intravenous (IV) fluid infusion, or disease processes such as diabetes mellitus or diabetes insipidus.

Oliguria refers to decreased urinary output (less than 200 ml per 24 hours). It occurs due to various renal causes (ischemia, kidney disease caused by toxic agents, glomerulonephritis, nephritis), dehydration caused by prolonged vomiting, diarrhea, or excessive diaphoresis, mechanical obstruction of some area of the urinary tract, and cardiac insufficiency.

The extreme form of oliguria is anuria, a total lack of urine production. Anuria (less than 100 ml per 24 hours) may result from severe dehydration, complete urinary tract obstruction, acute cortical necrosis of the kidney, acute glomerulonephritis, acute tubular necrosis, or hemolytic transfusion reaction.[2]

Urine Osmolality

Osmolality, a more exact measurement of urine concentration than specific gravity, depends on the number of particles of solute in a unit of solution. Whenever a more precise measurement than specific gravity is indicated to evaluate the concentrating and diluting ability of the kidney, this test is done. A high urinary osmolality is seen with concentrated urine. With poor concentrating ability, urine osmolality is low. Normal osmolality values are 300–900 mOsm/kg per 24 hours.

Urine osmolality is increased in dehydration, IV fluid administration, congestive heart failure, Addison's disease, syndrome of inappropriate secretion of antidiuretic hormone (SIADH), and amyloidosis.

Osmolality is decreased in compulsive water drinking, aldosteronism, diabetes insipidus, hypokalemia, and hypercalcemia.[2]

24-Hour Urine Protein

Detection of protein in urine (proteinuria), combined with a microscopic examination of urinary sediment, provides the basis for differential diagnosis of renal disease. In a healthy renal and urinary tract system, the urine contains no protein or only trace amounts of protein. Normally, the glomerulus prevents passage of protein from the blood to the glomerular filtrate. The persistent presence of protein in the urine is the single most important indication of renal (glomerular) disease.

For qualitative protein assessment, a protein reagent dipstick is used, and the resultant color is compared with the color comparison chart on the reagent strip bottle. If more than a trace amount of protein is found in the UA, a new second specimen should be tested for positive results before the 24-hour specimen is collected. Normal adult 24-hour urine protein values are 10–140 mg/liter.

Proteinuria usually results from increased glomerular filtration of protein because of glomerular damage. Persistent proteinuria of any amount, in an apparently healthy person, usually indicates some renal disease. Renal diseases that are associated with proteinuria are glomerulonephritis, nephrosis, renal vein thrombosis, malignant hypertension, polycystic kidney disease, and chronic urinary tract obstruction.

Proteinuria may occur with nonrenal diseases and conditions, including fever or acute infection, trauma, leukemia, multiple myeloma, toxemia of pregnancy, diabetes mellitus, and hypertension. Postural proteinuria (orthostatic proteinuria) results from excretion of protein by patients who are standing or moving about all day. This type of proteinuria is intermittent and disappears when the person lies down. Postural proteinuria occurs in 3–15% of healthy young adults.

Proteinuria is associated with the finding of casts on the microscopic (low-powered field) sediment examination because protein is necessary for cast formation.[2]

Urine Glucose

Glucose is present in glomerular filtrate but is normally reabsorbed in the proximal convoluted tubule of the nephron. However, should the blood glucose level exceed the reabsorption capacity of the tubules, glucose spills into the urine (glucosuria, glycosuria). Normal urine glucose 24-hour specimen values should be less than 0.3 g per 24 hours.

Diabetes mellitus is the main cause of glycosuria. However, sugar in the urine is not necessarily abnormal. It may appear in urine after a heavy meal or during times of emotional stress.

Urine glucose tests are used to screen for diabetes, to help confirm a diagnosis of diabetes, or to monitor the degree of diabetic control. A random sample positive UA test or positive 24-hour urine sugar alone is not adequate for a diagnosis of diabetes. A urine glucose test combined with a blood glucose test provides more complete information.[2]

Quantitative 24-Hour Urine Chloride

The amount of chloride excreted in the urine in 24 hours is an indication of the state of electrolyte balance. Its measurement may be useful as a guide in adjusting fluid and electrolyte balance in dehydrated or postoperative patients and as a means of monitoring the effects of reduced-salt diets (which are of great therapeutic importance in patients with cardiovascular disease, hypertension, liver disease, and kidney ailments).

Urine chloride is often ordered, along with sodium and potassium, as a 24-hour urine test. Normal values for 24-hour urine chloride in the adult are 140–250 mEq/liter.

Decreased urinary chlorides occur with SIADH, vomiting, diarrhea, gastric suction, and diuretic therapy. Urinary chloride is also decreased by endogenous (Cushing's syndrome) or exogenous (mineralocorticoid therapy) corticosteroids.

Increased urinary chloride occurs with dehydration, renal tubular acidosis, and potassium depletion.[2]

Quantitative 24-Hour Urine Sodium

Sodium is a primary regulator for retaining or excreting water and maintaining acid-base balance. Sodium and potassium also influence nerve conduction and muscle irritability.

The 24-hour quantitative urine sodium test measures the amount of sodium excreted in a 24-hour period. It is done for diagnosis of renal, adrenal, water, and acid-base imbalances. The normal 24-hour urine sodium values are 40–220 mEq/liter per 24 hours.

Increased urinary sodium levels occur with adrenal failure (Addison's disease), salt-losing nephritis, renal tubular acidosis, SIADH, diuretic therapy, diabetes mellitus, hypothyroidism, and persistent vomiting.

Decreased urinary sodium levels occur with dehydration, congestive heart failure, liver disease, nephrotic syndrome, prerenal azotemia, and stress-induced diuresis.[2]

Quantitative 24-Hour Urine Potassium

Potassium acts as part of the body's buffer system and serves a vital function in the body's overall electrolyte balance. This balance is regulated by the urinary excretion of potassium by the kidneys. The 24-hour quantitative urine potassium test provides insight into electrolyte balance. Normal 24-hour urine potassium values are 25–125 mEq per 24 hours. This measurement is useful in the study of renal and adrenal disorders, and electrolyte and acid-base imbalances.

Elevated levels of urine potassium occur with diabetic and renal tubule disease, primary and secondary aldosteronism, Cushing's disease, and during treatment with adrenocorticotropic hormone or other exogenous steroids.

TABLE 8.4   Normal values for creatinine clearance

Age (yrs)	Males (ml/min)	Females (ml/min)
<20	88–146	81–134
20–30	88–146	81–134
30–40	82–140	75–128
40–50	75–133	69–122
50–60	68–126	64–116
60–70	61–120	58–110
70–80	55–113	52–105

Decreased levels of urine potassium occur in Addison's disease, and with severe renal disease (pyelonephritis, glomerulonephritis).[2]

Urine Creatinine and Creatinine Clearance

Creatinine is a substance that is normally easily excreted by the kidney. It is a by-product of muscle metabolism, produced at a constant rate according to the muscle mass of the individual. The normal serum creatinine is 0.4–1.5 mg/dl. The urine creatinine production for men is usually between 0.8 g to 1.8 g per 24 hours; for women, 0.6–1.6 g per 24 hours. Because all creatinine filtered by the kidneys in a given time interval is excreted into the urine, urinary creatinine levels can be used to determine the glomerular filtration rate. Disorders of kidney function prevent maximum excretion of creatinine.

The creatinine clearance test is a specific measurement of kidney function, primarily glomerular filtration. This test measures the rate at which the kidneys "clear" creatinine from the blood. *Clearance* of a substance refers to the imaginary volume (ml per minute) of plasma from which the substance (in this case creatinine) would have to be completely extracted for the kidney to excrete that amount in 1 minute. Creatinine clearance is measured in ml per minute per 1.73 m^2. Normal values for creatinine clearance by age can be seen in Table 8.4.[2]

The creatinine clearance test is used to evaluate renal function in debilitated individuals, to follow progression of renal disease, and to help adjust medication dosages for various treatments.

Decreased creatinine clearance is found with impaired kidney function (due to intrinsic renal disease, glomerulonephritis, pyelonephritis, nephrotic syndrome, acute tubular dysfunction, and amyloidosis), decreased renal perfusion (due to shock, hemorrhage, and congestive heart failure), and hepatic failure.

Increased creatinine clearance is found in states of high cardiac output, associated with burns, and with carbon monoxide poisoning. Additionally, exercise, pregnancy, and a diet high in meat may elevate urine creatinine clearance levels.[2]

24-Hour Urine Studies of Stone Constituents

Patients with recurrent urolithiasis may have an underlying abnormality in the renal excretion of calcium, uric acid, oxalate, magnesium, cystine, or citrate. Whenever a urinary tract stone is identified, 24-hour urine collections can be tested to determine abnormally high levels of each of the preceding constituents. Whenever a stone is recovered, a formal stone analysis is also recommended.[1]

Quantitative 24-Hour Urine Uric Acid

Uric acid is formed from the metabolic breakdown of nucleic acids, with its principal source being purines. This test evaluates uric acid excretion and is an important aid in diagnosis and evaluation of nephrolithiasis. It also reflects the effects of treatment with uricosuric agents by measuring the total amount of uric acid excreted within a 24-hour period after initiation of appropriate medications. Normal 24-hour urine uric acid values are 250–750 mg per 24 hours (with a normal diet).

Increased urine uric acid levels (uricosuria) occurs with gout, certain cancers (chronic myelogenous leukemia, polycythemia vera), after chemotherapy (particularly when treating lymphoma and leukemia), after strenuous exercise, and with a diet high in purines. A high urine uric acid concentration in the face of low urinary pH may produce the precipitation of uric acid stones in the urinary tract (even in patients who do not have gout).

Decreased urine uric acid levels are found with chronic kidney disease and folic acid deficiency.[2]

Urine Quantitative 24-Hour Calcium Levels

The 24-hour test for urinary calcium is most often ordered to determine parathyroid gland function. The parathyroid gland normally maintains the serologic balance between calcium and phosphorus by means of its hormone, parathyroid hormone. Hyperparathyroidism is a disorder of calcium, phosphate, and bone metabolism resulting from increased secretion of parathyroid hormone.

Hyperparathyroidism results in elevated serum calcium levels (hypercalcemia), and increased excretion of urinary calcium (hypercalciuria). Increased urinary calcium excretion almost always accompanies hypercalcemia. Whenever calcium is excreted in increasing amounts, the situation creates the potential for nephrolithiasis or nephrocalcinosis.

Normal 24-hour urine calcium values are 100–300 mg per day. Increased urine calcium levels are found in hyperparathyroidism, osteolytic bone cancers (primary cancers of breast and bladder, osteolytic bone metastases, and multiple myeloma), Paget's disease, renal tubular acidosis, glucocorticoid excess, vitamin D intoxication (due to excessive milk intake or sunlight exposure), idiopathic hypercalciuria, and after prolonged immobilization (particularly of children or adolescents). Hypercalcemia is also associated with diabetes mellitus, inflammatory bowel disease (Crohn's disease and some cases of ulcerative colitis), and thyrotoxicosis.

Decreased urine calcium levels are found in hypoparathyroidism, familial hypocalciuria, vitamin D deficiency (rickets), acute nephritis, and with metastatic carcinoma of the prostate (a blastic and not lytic tumor).[2]

TABLE 8.5   Complete blood cell count

Test (abbreviation)

White blood cell count (WBC)
Differential white cell count (Diff)
Red blood cell count (RBC)
Hematocrit (HCT)
Hemoglobin (Hb)
Red blood cell indices
    Mean corpuscular volume (MCV)
    Mean corpuscular hemoglobin (MCH)
    Mean corpuscular hemoglobin concentration (MCHC)
Stained red cell examination of peripheral blood smear
Platelet count (Plt)

Quantitative 24-Hour Urine Oxalate

Normal oxalate is derived from dietary oxalic acid (10%) and the metabolism of ascorbic acid (vitamin C) (35–50%) and glycine (40%). Patients who form calcium oxalate kidney stones appear to excrete a higher proportion of dietary oxalate in the urine. Normal values for 24-hour urine oxalate are 7–44 mg per 24 hours in males and 4–31 mg per 24 hours in females.

The 24-hour urine collections for oxalate are indicated in patients with surgical or physiologic loss of the distal small intestine, especially those with Crohn's disease whose incidence of nephrolithiasis approaches 10%. Hyperoxaluria and nephrolithiasis are also regularly present after jejunoileal bypass for morbid obesity. Vitamin C excess increases oxalate excretion and may be a risk factor for calcium oxalate nephrolithiasis. Increased urine oxalate values are also associated with ethylene glycol poisoning, primary hyperoxaluria (a rare genetic disorder), diabetes mellitus, cirrhosis, and vitamin B_6 deficiency.

Decreased urine oxalate values occur in renal failure and with hypercalciuria.[2]

24-Hour Urine Cystine

24-Hour urine cystine is useful for differential diagnosis of cystinuria, an inherited disease characterized by bladder calculi. Patients with cystine stones face recurrent urolithiasis and repeated urinary infections. Normal 24-hour urine cystine values are less than 38 mg per 24 hours in adults.

Cystine values in cystinuria are up to 20 times normal.[2]

Complete Blood Cell Count

The CBC count is a basic screening test and one of the most frequently ordered laboratory procedures. As it applies to the GU system, the CBC count is most useful in determining the presence or absence of infection and the degree of blood loss in a patient with hematuria. The CBC count consists of a series of tests that determine number, variety, percentage, and concentration of blood cells. They include the WBC count, WBC differential, the RBC count, Hb, hematocrit (HCT), and the mean corpuscular volume (MCV) (Table 8.5).[4]

TABLE 8.6 Differential white blood cell count

Cell	Normal adult values (%)
Band cells	3–6
Segmented neutrophils	50–62
Eosinophils	0–3
Basophils	0–1
Lymphocytes	25–40
Monocytes	3–7

White Blood Cell Count

WBCs or leukocytes fight infection and defend the body by a process called *phagocytosis* in which the leukocytes encapsulate and destroy foreign organisms. WBCs also produce, transport, and distribute antibodies as part of the immune response. Leukocyte and differential counts, by themselves, are of little value as diagnostic aids unless the results are related to the clinical condition of the patient.[4]

Normal WBC values are 5,000–10,000 per liter. Leukocytosis (WBC counts above 10,000 per liter) is usually due to an increase of only one type of white cell and is given the name of the type of cell that shows the main increase. Neutrophilic leukocytosis, or neutrophilia, occurs in acute infections. The degree of increase of white cells usually depends on the severity of the infection, the patient's general systemic health, the patient's age, and the marrow efficiency and reserve of WBCs. Neutrophilic leukocytosis may occur in an otherwise healthy person (physiologic leukocytosis) in response to excitement, stress, exercise, pain, or steroid therapy.[4]

Differential White Blood Cell Count

The total leukocyte count of the circulating WBCs is differentiated according to five types of leukocyte cells, each of which performs a specific function. The differential WBC count is expressed as a percentage of the total number of white cells. The percentage is the relative number of each type of leukocyte in the blood. Normal values are seen in Table 8.6. The differential count must always be interpreted in relation to the total leukocyte count.[4]

Neutrophils, also known as *segmented neutrophils, polymorphonuclear neutrophils,* "segs," or "polys," are the most numerous and important type of WBC in the body. They react to and constitute the primary defense against infection.[4] The neutrophil cell is 12–15 μm in diameter, has a characteristic dense nucleus (consisting of between two and five lobes), and has a pale cytoplasm (Figure 8.3).[5] Normal neutrophil differential values are 50–60% of the total WBC count.[4]

The neutrophil precursor cell (myeloblast) is formed and matures in the bone marrow (Figure 8.4). Before release into the bloodstream, its nucleus has a characteristic band-shape, and this cell is known as a *band cell.* Large numbers of band cells are held in the marrow as a "reserve pool," ready to be called on to fight infection.[5]

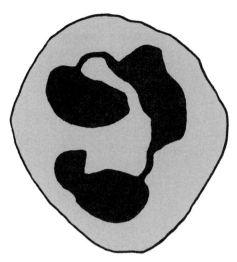

FIGURE 8.3 *The neutrophil cell is 12–15 μm in diameter, has a characteristic dense nucleus consisting of between two to five lobes, and has a pale cytoplasm.*

The normal function of neutrophils may be divided into three phases, chemotaxis, phagocytosis, and bacterial killing and digestion. *Chemotaxis* refers to neutrophil mobilization and migration in which the phagocyte is attracted to the bacteria by chemotactic substances released from damaged or inflamed tissues. Phagocytosis is the process by which the foreign material (bacteria) or dead or damaged cells of the host's body are engulfed, after which they are killed and digested.[5]

The test to determine segmented neutrophils evaluates the degree of neutrophilia or neutropenia. Neutrophilia is an increase of the absolute number of neutrophils, whereas neutropenia occurs when too few neutrophils are produced.[4]

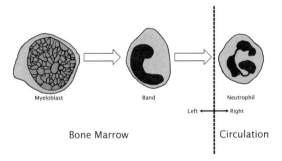

FIGURE 8.4 *The neutrophil precursor cell (myeloblast) is formed and matures in the bone marrow. As it matures, its nucleus develops a characteristic band shape; this cell, which is still in the bone marrow, is known as a* band cell. *The nucleus further matures into distinct lobes that are connected by thin fibers. This cell, known as the* mature neutrophil, *is then released into the circulation. The band forms are a reserved pool of white blood cells that can be released in cases of infection. A "shift to the left" occurs when an increase in white blood cells is required and there is a release of band forms from the bone marrow into the systemic circulation.*

An increase in circulating neutrophils is one of the most frequently observed blood count changes. Neutrophilia is often accompanied by fever due to the release of leukocyte pyrogen. Another characteristic feature of reactive neutrophilia is a "shift to the left" in the peripheral blood differential WBC count. This refers to the release of immature band forms of this leukocyte from the blood vessels where they are stored, a process known as *demargination*. The band forms are a reserve pool of WBCs that can be released in cases of infection. Therefore, a "shift to the left" occurs when an increase in WBCs is required and there is a release of band forms from the bone marrow (see Figure 8.4).[5]

Neutrophilia (increased absolute number and percentage of neutrophils) occurs in acute bacterial infections. It is also associated with inflammation, acute hemorrhage, myeloproliferative disorders (leukemia) and neoplasms of all types, tissue necrosis (due to myocardial infarction, tumors, burns, gangrene, carcinoma, or sarcoma), and metabolic disorders such as uremia.[4,5] Steroid administration is also associated with neutrophilia that tends to peak 4–6 hours after dosing.[4]

Neutropenia (decreased absolute number of neutrophils) occurs in viral infections, after myelosuppressive chemotherapy, and in some elderly patients or people of any age who are weak and debilitated. When a bacterial infection becomes overwhelming, the patient's resistance is exhausted and, as death approaches, the number of neutrophils decreases greatly.[4]

Red Blood Cell Count

Many tests look at the RBCs, including their number, size, amount of Hb, rate of production, and percentage composition of the blood. The RBC count, HCT, and Hb are closely related, but are different ways to look at the adequacy of RBC production. The same conditions cause respective rise and fall in each of these indicators.

The main function of the RBC (erythrocyte) is to carry oxygen from the lungs to the body tissues and to transfer carbon dioxide from the tissues to the lungs, a process achieved by means of the Hb molecule in red cells, which combines easily with oxygen and carbon dioxide. Oxygen binding to Hb gives arterial blood a bright red appearance, whereas venous blood appears dark red due to its low oxygen content. The red cell is shaped like a biconcave disk, affording more surface area for the Hb to combine with oxygen. The cell is also able to change its shape to permit passage through the smaller capillaries.[4]

With respect to evaluation of the GU system, the various RBC tests are most useful in evaluating for anemia. In this context, anemia may be a consequence of chronic renal failure, or it may occur secondary to blood loss or hemorrhage due to renal trauma, stone disease, or neoplasm somewhere within the GU tract.

The RBC test is performed by evaluating 7 ml of ethylenediaminetetraacetic acid venous blood with automated electronic devices that determine the number of RBCs. Normal RBC values in men are $4.2–5.4 \times 10^6$ per liter, and in women $3.6–5.0 \times 10^6$ per liter.[4]

Decreased RBC values occur in anemia, a condition in which there is a reduction in number of circulating RBCs, in the amount of Hb, or in the volume of packed cells (HCT), or a combination thereof. The anemia associated with end-stage renal disease occurs due to inadequate production of RBCs. This occurs because with renal organ failure there is a loss of the kidney-induced hormone erythropoietin. This hormone normally stimulates the production of RBCs. The anemia of chronic renal failure tends to be hypochromic (pale cytoplasm) and microcytic (small-sized RBCs).

Increased RBC values or erythrocytosis may occur in patients who are dehydrated. Hemoconcentration in dehydrated adults (caused by persistent vomiting or diarrhea) may actually obscure significant anemia.[4]

Hematocrit

The HCT test is part of the CBC count. This test determines RBC mass. The results are expressed as the percentage of packed red cells in a volume of whole blood (RBCs plus plasma). The HCT test is an important measurement in the determination of anemia. The word *hematocrit* means "to separate blood," which underscores the mechanism of the test, because the plasma and blood cells are separated by centrifugation.

To perform an HCT test, a capillary finger puncture is done after which the microcapillary tube is three-fourths filled with blood from the puncture site. The tube is then centrifuged, and the height of packed cells is measured and recorded as a percentage of the total amount of blood (RBCs plus plasma) in the capillary tube. The HCT test can also be done on automated hematology instruments using an anticoagulated venous blood sample.

Normal HCT values for adults are 36–48% (females) and 42–52% (males). The normal values for HCT vary with age and sex of the individual: HCTs in females are usually slightly lower than in males. A tendency toward lower values in men and women after age 60 years also occurs.

Decreased HCT values are an indicator of anemia, a condition in which there is a reduction in the HCT, amount of Hb, and the number of circulating RBCs. An HCT of 30 or less means the patient is moderately to severely anemic. HCT of less than 20% can lead to cardiac failure and death.

Usually, the HCT parallels the RBC count when the cells are of normal size (as the number of normal-sized erythrocytes increases, so does the HCT). The patient with chronic renal failure usually has microcytic anemia, however, and this relationship does not hold true. Microcytic anemia, with small red cells, produces a decreased HCT because the microcytic cells pack to a smaller volume. The RBC count, however, may be normal.[4]

Hemoglobin

Hb, the main component of erythrocytes, serves as a vehicle for the transportation of oxygen and carbon dioxide. The oxygen-combining capacity of blood is directly proportional to the Hb concentration, rather than to the number of RBCs (because some red cells contain more Hb than others).

The Hb determination is part of a CBC count. It helps to evaluate anemia, including its severity and response to treatment. Normal Hb values for adult females are 12.0–16.0 g/dl and 14.0–17.4 g/dl for adult males. Decreased levels of Hb are found in anemia (possibly due to chronic renal failure or GU hemorrhage) and with excessive fluid intake (fluid overload).

Increased levels of Hb are found with hemoconcentration due to dehydration, chronic obstructive pulmonary disease, congestive heart failure, polycythemia vera, smoking, and in people living at high altitudes. The panic Hb value in the anemic patient is less than 5.0 g/dl, which leads to heart failure and death.[4]

Mean Corpuscular Volume

Individual cell size is the best index for classifying anemias. The MCV expresses the mean volume occupied by a single red cell and is measured in cubic microns (μm^3). Normal MCV values are 82–100 μm^3. It is calculated from the RBC counts and from the HCT, and is expressed as a percentage via the following formula:

$$MCV = \frac{HCT\% \times 10}{RBC \times 10^{12}/liter}$$

The MCV indicates whether the RBC size appears normal (normocytic), smaller (microcytic), or larger (macrocytic). If the MCV is less than 82 μm^3, the red cells are microcytic. If the MCV is greater than 100 μm^3, the red cells are macrocytic. If the MCV is within the normal range, the RBCs are normocytic.

The MCV results are the basis of classification used in the evaluation of an anemia. Anemias are classified by size as being microcytic, normocytic, and macrocytic, and by color or appearance as hypochromic (pale pink) or normochromic.

Deficient Hb synthesis or chronic blood loss producing small, pale RBCs characterizes microcytic, hypochromic anemia (MCV 50–82 μm^3). This type of anemia occurs with iron deficiency (dietary inadequacy, malabsorption), increased iron loss due to chronic hemorrhage from the GU tract, and the anemia of chronic disease associated with renal end organ failure.

Normochromic normocytic anemia (MCV 82–100 μm^3) is anemia with an appropriate bone marrow response. It will occur immediately after GU trauma with acute hemorrhage (acute posthemorrhagic anemia). This type of anemia may also occur with decreased erythropoietin production in chronic renal disease.

Macrocytic anemias (MCV greater than 100 μm^3) typically do not occur as a consequence of renal disease unless there are concomitant nutritional deficiencies of vitamin B_{12} or folate. This can occur due to decreased ingestion (lack of animal products, strict vegetarian) or impaired absorption (intrinsic factor deficiency, pernicious anemia, gastrectomy, destruction of gastric mucosa by caustics, ileal resection, celiac disease) of vitamin B_{12}, and with folate deficiency (lack of vegetables, alcoholism).[4]

Erythrocyte Sedimentation Rate

The erythrocyte sedimentation rate (ESR) is the rate at which erythrocytes settle out of anticoagulated blood in 1 hour. This test is based on the fact that inflammatory and neoplastic processes cause an increase in blood proteins that attach themselves to RBCs, causing the red cells to aggregate. This makes them heavier and more likely to fall rapidly when placed in a special vertical test tube; the faster the settling of cells, the higher the ESR. The sedimentation rate is a nonspecific diagnostic laboratory finding that is indicative of some disease process that must be investigated further.

To perform the test, anticoagulated blood is suctioned into a graduated sedimentation tube and is allowed to settle for exactly 1 hour. The amount of settling is the patient's ESR. Normal Westergren ESR values for men are 0–15 mm per hour and in women 0–20 mm per hour.

Increased sedimentation rates are found with all infections, including osteomyelitis, inflammatory diseases, neoplasms, and with nephritis and nephrosis. In metastatic cancer and osteomyelitis, the ESR can be high, with values greater than 100 mm per hour.[4]

Renalytes

Renalytes are a series of serologic tests that provide information about hydration status, acid-base balance, and overall renal function. Renalyte tests include serum chloride, potassium, sodium, glucose, blood urea nitrogen (BUN), and creatinine.

Chloride

Chloride, a blood electrolyte, is an anion that exists predominantly in the extracellular spaces in combination with the cations sodium (sodium chloride) or hydrogen (hydrochloric acid). Chloride helps maintain cellular integrity through its influence on osmotic pressure, acid-base balance, and water balance.

Chlorides are excreted with cations (positive ions) during diuresis. Measurement of serum chloride is helpful in diagnosing disorders of acid base and water metabolism. Normal values in adults are 98–106 mEq/liter.

Decreased blood chloride levels occur in severe vomiting, chronic respiratory acidosis, burns, metabolic alkalosis, diabetes, Addison's disease, salt-losing diseases, overhydration, and with diuretic therapy. Increased blood chloride levels occur in dehydration, Cushing's syndrome, hyperventilation (which causes respiratory alkalosis), renal tubular acidosis, diabetes insipidus, and with excessive saline IV infusions.

Panic values for serum chloride are less than 70 mEq/liter or greater than 120 mEq/liter.[6]

Potassium

Potassium (K^+) is the principal electrolyte (cation) of intracellular fluid and the primary buffer within the cell itself. K^+ plays an important role in nerve conduction, muscle function, acid-base balance, and osmotic pressure, and K^+ helps control the rate and force of contraction of the heart and thereby the cardiac output.

The body is adapted for efficient K^+ excretion. Normally, 80–90% of the cells' K^+ is excreted in the urine by the glomeruli. The kidneys do not conserve K^+, and when an adequate amount of K^+ is not ingested, a severe deficiency can occur. K⁺ balance is maintained in adults on an average dietary intake of 80–200 mEq per day.

K^+ and sodium ions are important in the renal regulation of acid-base balance, because hydrogen ions are substituted for sodium and K^+ ions in the renal tubule. Normal K^+ values in adults are 3.5–5.3 mEq/liter.

The most frequent cause of K^+ deficiency is gastrointestinal loss (diarrhea, vomiting). Other causes of decreased blood K^+ (hypokalemia) levels are shifting of K^+ into cells (due to osmotic hyperglycemia or respiratory alkalosis), renal K^+ excretion (renal tubular acidosis, diuretic, antibiotic, and steroid administration), reduced K^+ intake (starvation, malabsorption), loss of K^+ through skin or damaged tissues (excessive sweating, draining wounds, severe burns), and IV fluid administration without adequate K^+ supplementation.

Panic values for hypokalemia are less than 2.5 mEq/liter, which could result in ventricular fibrillation. Hypokalemia enhances the effects of digitalis preparations, creating the possibility of digitalis intoxication and cardiac arrhythmia from even an average maintenance dose. Digitalis, diuretics, and hypokalemia are a potentially lethal combination. Such patients should be closely monitored.

Increased K^+ levels (hyperkalemia) occur when K^+ shifts from cells to extracellular fluid. This occurs with cell damage due to burns, accidents, surgery, chemotherapy, and disseminated intravascular coagulation. The damaged cells release K^+ into the blood. Hyperkalemia also occurs with inadequate renal excretion due to chronic renal failure, with excessive K^+ intake with metabolic diabetic ketoacidosis (acidosis drives K^+ out of cells), and with Addison's disease.

Panic values for hyperkalemia are greater than 7 mEq/liter. This could result in myocardial irritability, associated with electrocardiogram changes, including elevated T waves and flattened P waves. With severe hyperkalemia, ventricular fibrillation and cardiac arrest may ensue. Treatment for hyperkalemia includes sodium bicarbonate, glucose and insulin, diuretics, dialysis, and Kayexalate (a sodium-K^+ exchange resin), which can be administered orally, nasogastrically, or rectally.[6]

Serum Sodium

Serum sodium (Na^+) is the most abundant cation of the blood. Its primary functions include maintenance of osmotic pressure, acid-base balance, and to facilitate transmission of nerve impulses.

Normal adult serum Na^+ values are between 135 to 145 mEq/liter. Panic values for Na^+ are less than 120 mEq/liter and greater than 155 mEq/liter. Na^+ balance is maintained in adults with an average dietary intake of 90–250 mEq per day.

Reduced Na^+ levels (hyponatremia) are associated with severe burns, congestive heart failure, excessive fluid loss (severe diarrhea, laxative use, vomiting, sweating), excessive IV fluids without electrolytes, Addison's disease (lack of adrenal steroids impairs Na^+ reabsorption), severe nephritis or nephrotic syndrome, diabetic acidosis, edema, excess oral water intake, and as a consequence of diuretic use.

Hypernatremia (an increased Na^+ level) is uncommon. When it does occur, it may be associated with dehydration, insufficient water intake, primary aldosteronism, Cushing's disease, diabetes insipidus, and use of anabolic steroids or corticosteroids.[6]

Serum Fasting Blood Glucose

Glucose is formed from carbohydrate digestion and by conversion of glycogen to glucose in the liver. The two hormones that directly regulate blood glucose are glucagon and insulin. Glucagon accelerates glycogen breakdown in the liver, causing blood glucose to rise. Insulin increases cell membrane permeability to glucose, stimulates glycogen formation, and reduces blood glucose levels. Driving glucose into the cells requires insulin and insulin receptors. After a meal, the pancreas releases insulin, which binds to receptors on the surface of fat and muscle cells. This opens channels that allow glucose to pass into cells where it is metabolized, producing energy.

Patient preparation for fasting blood glucose (FBG) requires a 12-hour fast. Water is permitted. If possible, the diabetic patient should defer taking insulin or oral hypoglycemics until after the FBG has been drawn. Normal adult values for serum FBG are between 65 to 110 mg/dl.

Elevated blood sugar (hyperglycemia) occurs in diabetes mellitus. A fasting glucose greater than 140 mg/dl on more than one occasion is usually diagnostic for diabetes mellitus. An oral glucose tolerance test is not usually necessary in this instance. However, mild "borderline" patients may present with normal fasting glucose values. In such cases, if diabetes is suspected, a glucose tolerance test can help confirm the diagnosis.

Other conditions that produce elevated blood glucose levels include Cushing's disease (increased glucocorticoids produce elevated blood sugar levels), myocardial infarction, and, occasionally, severe infection. Hyperglycemia during pregnancy may signal potential for onset of diabetes later in life.

If a person with known or suspected diabetes experiences headaches, irritability, dizziness, weakness, fainting, or impaired cognition (all symptoms of hypoglycemia), a blood glucose test or fingerstick test must be done before giving insulin. Insulin administration in the face of the hypoglycemia could be lethal for the patient.

When blood glucose values are greater than 300 mg/dl, urine output increases as does the risk of dehydration.[6] The polyuria produced by this condition could contribute to incontinence in susceptible patients.

Blood Urea Nitrogen

Urea forms in the liver and, along with CO_2, constitutes the final product of protein metabolism.

The renalyte test for BUN is used as a gross index of glomerular filtration. However, the BUN is less sensitive than the creatinine clearance test and may not be abnormal until the creatinine clearance is moderately abnormal. Normal adult BUN is between 7 to 20 mg/dl.

Increased BUN levels (azotemia) occurs in impaired renal function, congestive heart failure (which results in poor renal perfusion), dehydration, shock, gastrointestinal tract bleeding, and excessive protein intake or protein catabolism (starvation). In patients with an elevated BUN, fluid and electrolyte regulation may be impaired.

Decreased BUN levels are associated with liver failure, malnutrition, anabolic steroid use, IV feedings with overhydration, nephrotic syndrome, SIADH, and a low-protein/high-carbohydrate diet. Last, BUN tends to be lower in children and women because of a smaller muscle mass than adult males.[6]

Serum Creatinine

Creatinine is a by-product in the breakdown of muscle. It is produced at a constant rate, depending on the muscle mass of the person, and is removed from the body by the kidneys. A disorder of kidney function reduces excretion of creatinine, resulting in increased blood levels. Normal adult serum creatinine values are between 0.6 to 1.3 mg/dl. Panic value is 10 mg/dl in nondialysis patients.

The serum creatinine test is used to diagnose impaired renal function. Increased blood creatinine levels occur in chronic renal failure. Other causes of elevated blood creatinine include muscle disease (acromegaly, myasthenia gravis, muscular dystrophy, poliomyelitis), rhabdomyolysis, congestive heart failure, shock, dehydration, and a diet high in meat content. Serum creatinine should always be checked before giving nephrotoxic chemotherapies (methotrexate, cisplatin, cyclophosphamide [Cytoxan], mithramycin, or semustine).[6]

Other Important Tests Pertaining to the Genitourinary System

Serum Calcium

Approximately 50% of blood serum calcium (Ca^{++}) is ionized; the rest is protein-bound. Only ionized Ca^{++} can be used by the body in such vital processes as muscular contraction, cardiac function, transmission of nerve impulses, and blood clotting.

The amount of protein in the blood affects Ca^{++} levels as 50% of the blood Ca^{++} is protein-bound. Thus, a decrease in serum albumin results in a profound decrease in total serum Ca^{++}. The decrease, however, does not alter the concentration of the ionized form. Measurement of ionized Ca^{++} is done to monitor patients with renal disease, renal transplantation, hemodialysis, hyperparathyroidism or hypoparathyroidism, pancreatitis, or malignancy.

Hyperparathyroidism and cancer (particularly metastatic bone cancers; Hodgkin's disease; lymphoma; leukemia; multiple myeloma; and primary squamous cell tumors of the lung, neck, and head) are the most common causes of hypercalcemia. Hypoalbuminemia is the most common cause of decreased total calcium. Hypocalcemia is also commonly associated with hyperphosphatemia caused by renal failure.

Normal values for total adult Ca^{++} are 8.6–10.0 mg/dl; normal adult ionized Ca^{++} is between 4.65 to 5.28 mg/dl. Panic values for total Ca^{++} are less than 6 mg/dl and greater than 13 mg/dl. Panic values for ionized Ca^{++} are less than 2 mg/dl and greater than 7 mg/dl. Severe hypocalcemia may produce tetany and convulsions, whereas hypercalcemia may cause cardiotoxicity, arrhythmias, and coma.[6]

Glucose Tolerance Test; Oral Glucose Tolerance Test

If the fasting serum glucose is greater than 140 mg/dl on two separate occasions, or a 2-hour postprandial blood glucose is greater than 200 mg/

dl on two separate occasions, an oral glucose tolerance test (OGTT) is not necessary to establish the diagnosis of diabetes mellitus.

If fasting and postprandial glucose test results are borderline, however, the OGTT can support or rule out diabetes mellitus. It can also be a part of a workup for unexplained renal disease. Before the OGTT, the patient should fast for 12 hours. Only water may be taken during the fasting time and test time. Use of tobacco products is not permitted during testing as smoking increases serum glucose levels. Certain drugs impair glucose tolerance levels, including insulin, oral hypoglycemics, large doses of salicylates, oral contraceptives, corticosteroids, and estrogens. If possible, these drugs should be withheld for at least 3 days before testing. A diet of 150 g of carbohydrates or greater should be eaten for 3 days pretest. A 5-ml sample of venous blood is drawn. After the blood is drawn, the patient drinks a specially formulated glucose solution containing 75–100 g of glucose. Blood and urine samples are then obtained at 30 minutes and 1, 2, 3, 4, and 5 hours after glucose ingestion. Normal values are as follows: fasting adult, 70–110 mg/dl; 30-minute adult, 110–170 mg/dl; 60-minute adult, 120–170 mg/dl; 2-hour adult, 70–120 mg/dl; and 3-hour adult, 70–120 mg/dl.

All blood values must fall within normal limits, and all urine samples should test negative for glucose to be considered a normal OGTT. Prescribed insulin or oral hypoglycemics should be administered once the test is done, and the patient should eat a short time later.

Next, the test results are interpreted: An impaired OGTT test result would include a 1-hour glucose level greater than 200 mg/dl and a 2-hour glucose greater than 140 mg/dl. The non–insulin-dependent (adult onset) diabetic patient has a 1-hour glucose greater than 200 mg/dl and a 2-hour glucose greater than 200 mg/dl. The insulin-dependent diabetic patient has a fasting glucose greater than 140 mg/dl, a 1-hour glucose greater than 200 mg/dl, and a 2-hour glucose greater than 200 mg/dl. In most cases of overt diabetes, no insulin is secreted, and abnormally high glucose levels persist throughout all stages of the test.

Patients with a new diagnosis of diabetes need diet, medication, and lifestyle-modification instructions.[6]

Uric Acid

Uric acid is formed from the breakdown of nucleic acids and is an end product of purine metabolism. The kidneys excrete two-thirds of the uric acid produced daily. Measurement of uric acid is used most commonly in the evaluation of renal failure, gout, and leukemia. Increased uric acid levels could ultimately lead to renal stones. Normal uric acid values are 3.5–7.2 mg/dl in men and 2.6–6.0 mg/dl in women.

Elevated uric acid levels (hyperuricemia) occur in starvation and gout (due to excessive catabolism of nucleic acids), chronic renal failure (due to inability to excrete uric acid), lymphoma and leukemia (due to excessive production and destruction of cells), alcoholism, dehydration, after chemotherapy or radiation treatment (which causes excessive cell destruction), and with a purine-rich diet (liver, kidney, sweetbreads).[6]

Acid Phosphatase

Acid phosphatases are enzymes that are widely distributed throughout the body. Their greatest diagnostic significance is in the prostate gland, however, where acid phosphatase activity is 100 times higher than in other tissues.

The acid phosphatase test helps to diagnose metastatic cancer of the prostate and monitors the effectiveness of treatment. Elevated levels of acid phosphatase are seen when prostate cancer has metastasized beyond the prostatic capsule. Once the carcinoma has spread, the cancerous prostate tissue starts to release acid phosphatase, resulting in an increased blood level. Normal acid phophatase values are 0.0–3.1 ng/ml.

A significantly elevated acid phosphatase value is almost always indicative of metastatic cancer of the prostate. If the tumor is successfully treated through surgery, chemotherapy, or radiation, enzyme levels drop within several weeks. Moderate elevations of acid phosphate values also occur in the absence of prostate cancer with any cancer that has metastasized to bone and with benign prostatic hypertrophy.

Palpation of the prostate gland before testing causes increases in the serum level of acid phosphatase. Therefore, rectal examination should not be performed within the 2–3 days before this test.[6]

Prostate-Specific Antigen

Prostate-specific antigen (PSA) is localized in both normal prostatic epithelial cells and prostatic carcinoma cells. It has proven to be the most reliable marker for monitoring recurrence of prostate cancer and effectiveness of treatment. Testing for both PSA and prostate acid phosphatase increases detection of early-stage prostate cancer. The greatest value of PSA is as a marker in the follow-up of patients at high risk for disease progression. PSA should be used in conjunction with the digital rectal examination. However, the serum specimen must be collected before palpation of the prostate is performed.

Normal PSA values in men are 0–4 ng/ml. Patients with benign prostatic hypertrophy (BPH) often demonstrate values between 4.0 and 8.0 ng/ml. Results between 4.0 and 8.0 ng/ml may represent either BPH or possible cancer of the prostate. Results above 8.0 ng/ml are highly suggestive (greater than 80% probability) of prostatic cancer. Increases above 4.0 ng/ml have been reported in approximately 8% of patients without prostate cancer or BPH. If a prostate tumor is completely and successfully removed, no antigen is detected.[6]

References

1. Williams RD. Urologic Laboratory Examination. In DR Smith (ed), General Urology (11th ed). Los Altos, CA: Lange Medical Publications, 1984;44–54.
2. Fischbach F. Urine Studies. In F Fischbach (ed), A Manual of Laboratory and Diagnostic Tests (5th ed). Philadelphia: Lippincott–Raven, 1996;147–252.

3. Fischbach F. Microbiologic Studies. In F Fischbach (ed), A Manual of Laboratory and Diagnostic Tests (5th ed). Philadelphia: Lippincott–Raven, 1996;441–511.
4. Fischbach F. Blood Studies. In F Fischbach (ed), A Manual of Laboratory and Diagnostic Tests (5th ed). Philadelphia: Lippincott–Raven, 1996;23–146.
5. Hoffbrand AV, Pettit JE. The White Cells. In AV Hoffbrand, JE Pettit (eds), Essential Hematology (2d ed). London: Blackwell Scientific, 1984;97–120.
6. Fischbach F. Chemistry Studies. In F Fischbach (ed), A Manual of Laboratory and Diagnostic Tests (5th ed). Philadelphia: Lippincott–Raven, 1996;302–440.

9   Common Disorders of the Urinary System

Jack L. Rook

Genitourinary Infections

Urinary tract infection (UTI) is one of the more common disorders seen by the clinician. Although most of these infections are uncomplicated and easily treated, some pose a threat to long-term kidney function. Infection in the bladder irritates the bladder wall, frequently resulting in unstable premature detrusor contraction. The premature contractions may produce incontinence in a person who is normally continent. Incontinence may recur in patients who had successfully gotten it under control, or the partially compensated incontinent patient may leak more frequently. The recurrence of incontinence or its increased frequency is known as *instability incontinence*.

The major cause of UTI in women is invasion of the urinary tract by bacteria, which have ascended the urethra from contamination of the introitus. Infection of the male urinary tract is unlikely with an anatomically normal tract. The much lower incidence of UTI in men has been attributed to the long male urethra and to a "prostatic antibacterial factor" present in prostatic fluid.

The bladder has its own defense mechanisms against infection, including the washout of bacteria by periodic voiding and removal of surface organisms, either by bladder mucosal phagocytosis or surface antibody production. These defenses are severely limited in the presence of residual urine.

UTIs occur more regularly in both men and women who have structural abnormalities (i.e., pelvic floor weakness in women or prostatic hypertrophy in men) of the urinary tract or who have been catheterized or instrumented. Vesicoureteral reflux may be associated with ascending infection.[1]

The gram-negative bacteria *Escherichia coli* accounts for approximately 80% of UTIs. More than 100 serotypes of *E. coli* exist. Other gram-negative bacteria, gram-positive bacteria, viruses, mycobacteria, fungi, and parasites account for the remainder of UTIs.

Clinical symptoms of UTI include persistent cloudy urine, the presence of blood or sediment in urine, or the development or recurrence of incontinence/leakage (instability incontinence).

Diagnosis

Microscopic Urinalysis

Microscopic urinalysis is the most important study when evaluating a patient suspected of having a UTI. Collection of the urine specimen requires special attention to prevent bacteria and cells on the skin near the external urethra from contaminating the specimen. A carefully instructed patient can usually obtain a clean-caught midstream specimen. However, some obese women or individuals with various disabilities require that their urine be obtained by bladder catheterization to prevent contamination. Catheterization of the urinary bladder requires careful preparation and cleansing of the urethral meatus to minimize the risk of introducing an infection.[1]

To perform this test, the urine sample is centrifuged, and a drop of the sediment is examined using the high-powered lens of a light microscope. The presence of white blood cells and bacteria suggests infection is likely. Quantitation of white blood cells after centrifugation is also used to determine UTI. It has been estimated that two to five leukocytes per high-powered field is abnormal. In men, the finding of any number of white cells should be considered abnormal. The identification of white cell casts is diagnostic of pyelonephritis. Red blood cells (RBCs) within the urine sediment are often associated with infection but may represent a number of other processes as well.[1,2]

Urine Dipstick

The urine may be analyzed by a multiple reagent dipstick; a pH greater than 7.0 suggests the presence of infection by a urea-splitting organism, usually a *Proteus* species. With UTIs, there may be a nonspecific positive test for blood or protein, or both. Bacteria in the bladder reduce nitrate to nitrite, and the latter can be measured colorimetrically using the urine nitrate test on the dipstick. This test is most sensitive when performed on the first-voided morning specimen.[1]

Urine Culture

When UTI is suspected and before therapy is given, a culture should always be obtained. Culture of the urine must be performed within a few minutes after collection. Culture of urine specimens contaminated by surface bacteria yields multiple species. When contamination occurs, a repeat clean-caught urine specimen should be obtained by catheterization, if necessary.[1]

Prostate Massage

Infection in the male patient may involve the prostate or bladder, or both. Suspected prostatic infection can be confirmed by comparison of quantitative bacterial counts on the first 10 ml of voided midstream urine specimen versus the first 5–10 ml of urine voided after prostatic massage. Prostatic massage is accomplished during rectal examination by firm rolling pressure working from the upper lateral margin of the prostate toward its midline and inferior margin. In the performance of this segmented collection technique, the patient must have some urine in the bladder at the time of prostatic massage.[1] Relatively higher bacterial counts obtained after massage suggest the prostate as the focus of infection.

Treatment

More than 80% of UTIs are cured with any of a number of antibiotic regimens. Oral sulfonamides, such as sulfisoxazole or trimethoprim-sulfamethoxazole are the agents of choice. Potential side effects of sulfa drugs include rash, urticaria, and gastrointestinal disturbances. Most of the failures or relapses occur in upper UTIs.[3]

Failure to improve after 3 or 4 days usually suggests either the presence of an organism resistant to the antibiotic or an upper UTI. Additional complications, including urinary tract obstruction and renal abscess formation, should also be suspected. Blood cultures should then be obtained and antibiotic sensitivities determined. If indicated, appropriate workup should be performed to help diagnose the additional complications.

Urinary Stones

Urinary stone disease is a common problem in the United States, usually encountered in one of five clinical settings involving patients with acute colic, persistent or recurrent UTI, isolated hematuria, a stone discovered incidentally on an x-ray taken for other purposes, or a history of having had a prior stone.[4]

Urinary stones may occur as a consequence of or contribute to urinary incontinence. The patient with frequent UTIs is prone to the development of struvite stones, a consequence of persistent bacteriuria. Frequent UTIs are associated with incontinence due to pelvic floor weakness (weakened barrier to infection), bladder outlet obstruction as in benign prostatic hypertrophy (urinary retention with increased postvoid residuals are associated with an increased incidence of infection), and spinal cord injury (due to introduction of organisms via straight catheterization).

The patient with stone disease due to hypercalcemia is prone to an osmotic diuresis that could contribute to incontinence in normally asymptomatic but susceptible patients. The spinal cord–injured patient is particularly prone to hypercalcemia post injury, predisposing him or her to calcium stone formation and possibly exacerbating the underlying neurogenic incontinence.

Acute Colic: Presentation

Most patients with urinary stones have an acute episode of colic, whereby the obstructing stone causes ureteral spasm, resulting in severe intermittent flank pain. As the stone moves distally, pain radiates in a characteristic pattern around the groin and into the testicle in the male or into the labia majora in the female. Nausea, vomiting, paralytic ileus, and other gastrointestinal symptoms may be associated with the colic pain. Examination reveals an uncomfortable, restless patient with costovertebral angle tenderness. No associated signs of peritoneal irritation are present (guarding, rebound, or rigidity). Fever is usually not present (unless UTI has developed in the obstructed urinary tract). Urinalysis almost always demonstrates microscopic or gross hematuria.[4]

Management

Management of a patient with colic should provide for relief of discomfort, surveillance for infection, determination of whether stones may pass spontaneously or require surgical removal, and measures to prevent future stone formation.

The abdominal x-ray is useful in monitoring the site and progression of radiodense stones. Approximately 90% of renal stones are radiodense and are seen on an abdominal x-ray.

In general, stones that are smaller than 5 mm in diameter pass spontaneously. Stones measuring 5–10 mm have a 50% chance of passing spontaneously, and those larger than 10 mm usually require surgical removal.

An intravenous pyelogram should also be obtained as soon as possible in the patient with colic to help establish a diagnosis (especially in patients with radiolucent stones) and to help determine if urgent urologic consultation should be obtained. Surgical intervention may be necessary if an intravenous pyelogram demonstrates a nonfunctioning kidney due to an obstructed ureter, a partially obstructed ureter from a solitary kidney, urine extravasation, or a stone larger than 10 mm in diameter (in which case spontaneous passage is unlikely).

Safe imaging techniques for the occasional colic patient allergic to intravenous radiologic dye are ultrasonic study of the renal collecting system or either an antegrade or retrograde pyelogram.

Most patients can be managed at home with the appropriate analgesics and forced hydration of 2–3 liters of fluid per 24 hours. This is necessary to maintain good urinary flow and to help in moving the stone along. All voided urine should be collected and strained through a fine screen or filter paper so that the passed stone may be saved and analyzed. Stones that pass from the ureter into the bladder generally pass with ease through the urethra, unless the bladder outlet obstruction prevents its passage, resulting in a retained bladder stone.

The physician will want to follow the patient by arranging for a weekly x-ray of the abdomen to determine progression of the stone. Urologic consultation or hospitalization may be necessary if by 6 weeks the stone has not passed or should fever, pain not easily controlled, or vomiting develop.

Several options for stone removal exist. Lower ureteral stones may be removed by using a basket inserted through a cystoscope. Stones located more proximally may require open removal by ureterolithotomy,

TABLE 9.1 Causes of hypercalciuria that may not be associated with hypercalcemia

Idiopathic hypercalciuria
Administration of loop diuretics (furosemide, ethacrynic acid, or bumetanide)
Excessive salt ingestion
Exogenous adrenal corticosteroids
Cushing's syndrome
Paget's disease of bone
Immobilization
Progressive bone disease
Malignant tumors
Hyperthyroidism
Sarcoidosis
Renal tubular acidosis
Other causes of metabolic acidosis
Medullary sponge kidney
Severe phosphate deprivation

---

pyelolithotomy, or, in the case of a staghorn calculus, nephrolithotomy.

The closed technique, extracorporeal shock-wave lithotripsy, has the distinct advantage of lower postprocedural morbidity. This procedure requires that a patient be positioned in a water bath. Then, by focusing shock waves on the calculus, the stone is fragmented into smaller particles that can then pass spontaneously.[4]

Types of Stones and Their Causes

Five main types of urinary calculi exist, including calcium, uric acid, oxalate, cystine, and struvite (infection) stones. Calcium stones are by far the most common.

Calcium Stones

Hypercalciuria can occur with or without hypercalcemia. Generally, the upper limits of calcium excretion for individuals eating a normal diet are 250 mg per 24 hours for women and 300 mg per 24 hours for men. Patients with hypercalciuria without hypercalcemia are commonly seen and tend to have variable pathogenesis of their stones. Table 9.1 lists the causes of hypercalciuria that may be unassociated with hypercalcemia.[4] Table 9.2 shows common metabolic and clinical disorders in calcium stone formers.

The most common cause of minimal, asymptomatic hypercalcemia is that associated with the use of thiazide diuretics. This problem is fully reversible on withdrawal of the drug.[5] Another common cause of benign hypercalcemia in patients is hyperparathyroidism, whereby small, indolent, and usually harmless parathyroid adenomas produce hypercalcemia in approximately 1 of 1,000 patients screened.[6]

A more ominous setting is the patient with hypercalcemia, anorexia, and weight loss. In this scenario, a calcium elevation is more likely attributable to a malignant process. In the event that malignancy is not apparent, primary hyperparathyroidism should be ruled out through determination of parathyroid hormone (PTH) concentration. However, elevations of PTH

TABLE 9.2   Metabolic and clinical disorders in calcium stone formers

Disorder	%
Idiopathic hypercalciuria	20
Marginal hypercalciuria	11
Hyperuricosuria	15
Hypercalciuria and hyperuricosuria	12
Hyperuricemia	6
Primary hyperparathyroidism	5
Renal tubular acidosis	4
Inflammatory bowel disease	5
Medullary sponge kidney	1
Sarcoidosis	1
No disorder found	20

are often due to ectopic PTH production by tumors, and although tumor-produced PTH is not identical to normal PTH, the testing used to quantitate PTH often fails to distinguish between these substances (Table 9.3).[5]

Diagnosis   The symptoms of hypercalcemia should alert the physician to its potential diagnosis (Table 9.4). However, most cases of hypercalcemia are detected by routine automated analysis of blood electrolytes.

Hypercalcemia is established as being present when serum calcium levels are found to be greater than 10.5 mg/dl on multiple determinations.

The next step is to determine the cause of the hypercalcemia. Assay of PTH in blood should be performed to rule out hyperparathyroidism. In cases of long-standing hyperparathyroidism, bone x-ray studies reveal a variety of changes, including demineralization (osteopenia), and subperiosteal resorption.[5]

Treatment   Calcium restriction in conjunction with thiazide diuretic administration has been shown to result in up to a 90% reduction in stone formation by causing a fall in urinary calcium excretion.[4]

Inorganic phosphate administration may result in the cessation of new urinary calculi formation in 90% of patients.[7] Cellulose phosphate (Calcibind) is an ion exchange resin powder that is mixed with water and taken within 30 minutes of each meal. Sodium phosphate salts given orally (K-Phos) can also be used but may produce diarrhea. Asymptomatic patients with mild hypercalcemia should probably not be treated with phosphate.

TABLE 9.3   Common causes of hypercalcemia

Condition	Comment
Thiazide drugs	Mild elevation (not >12.5 mg/dl; requires 2 or more weeks to subside)
Hyperparathyroidism	Frequently asymptomatic; commonly discovered on routine blood test
Malignancy	Most common among hospitalized patients; may lead to initial encounter in ambulatory patients
Spurious	Inappropriate technique while drawing blood (venous stasis produces hemoconcentration)

TABLE 9.4   Symptoms and signs of hypercalcemia

Short term (readily reversible)
   General: weakness, anorexia, weight loss, fatigue
   Gastrointestinal: nausea, vomiting, constipation
   Genitourinary: polyuria, azotemia
   Musculoskeletal: bone aches
   Neurologic: lethargy, sleepiness, difficulty concentrating, confusion, psychosis
   Cardiovascular: bradycardia, electrocardiographic abnormalities (short Q-T interval,
      arrhythmias, digitalis toxicity)
   Ophthalmologic: difficulty focusing
   Dermatologic: pruritus
Long term (irreversible or slowly reversible)
   Gastrointestinal: peptic ulcer, pancreatitis
   Genitourinary: renal calculi (colic, hematuria); nephrocalcinosis; polyuria
   Skeletal: bone loss (osteopenia); subperiosteal resorption, bone cysts, pseudogout
   Ophthalmologic: band keratopathy; conjunctival calcifications (usually requiring
      slit lamp examination)
   Neuromuscular: muscle atrophy

The patient should also be on a restricted calcium diet.[4,5]

When the diagnosis of hyperparathyroidism is well established, the main question becomes whether surgical intervention is warranted. The rate of development of complications (urolithiasis, emotional disorders, bone disease, decreased renal function, peptic ulcer, and pancreatitis) may determine the need for surgery. In experienced hands, an adenoma, if present, is located and easily removed. Failure to identify the adenoma may necessitate partial thyroidectomy.

The medical therapy of hyperparathyroidism with phosphate is ordinarily limited to those patients in whom surgery is not desirable but who require therapy.[5]

Uric Acid Stones

Uric acid stones are caused by the high insolubility of undissociated uric acid. Three factors associated with uric acid stone formation are hyperuricosuria, highly acid urine, and low urinary volume. The prevalence of uric acid stones in the general population is low. On the other hand, uric acid stones are prevalent in patients who have gout, asymptomatic hyperuricemia, hyperuricosuria, chronic diarrhea or excessive fluid loss from the skin (which causes highly concentrated urine), myeloproliferative disease, and those with solid tumors that are undergoing lysis (due to change or radiation therapy). Patients with gout also have more calcium stones than the general population.[4,8]

Treatment   Increasing urinary pH can reduce uric acid stone formation. Increasing the pH from 4.5 to 5.5 or 6.5 increases uric acid dissociation from 15% to 40% and 80%, respectively. The administration of sodium bicarbonate citrate salts or Diamox can accomplish alkalinization. Because sodium bicarbonate frequently causes gas and gastrointestinal discomfort, citrate salts are preferable. The metabolism of citrate results in the generation of bicarbonate. The dose should be adjusted as neces-

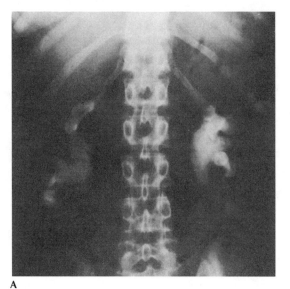

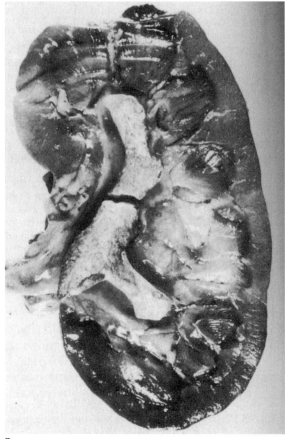

FIGURE 9.1 *(A) Plain abdominal radiograph shows a bilateral staghorn calculi. (B) Staghorn calculi in situ. (Reprinted with permission from A Cuschieri, GR Giles, AR Moosa [eds], Essential Surgical Practice [3d ed]. Oxford, UK: Butterworth–Heinemann, 1995;1484.)*

sary based on the results of regular urine pH testing. Proper alkalinization would be a urine pH greater than 6.5. If neither citrate nor bicarbonate is practical, urinary pH may be increased using Diamox, 250–500 g, four times a day.

Should these agents not be effective in controlling recurrence of uric acid stones, allopurinol (which decreases uric acid production) may be used and is effective in reducing stone recurrence.[4]

Struvite Infection Stones

Patients with frequent UTIs are prone to the development of struvite infection stones. Infection stones form as a consequence of the hydrolysis of urea and the production of ammonium by the bacterial enzyme urease. The majority of urea-splitting organisms are *Proteus* species. The production of ammonia alkalinizes the urine promoting the precipitation of magnesium, ammonium, and phosphate, the components of the infection-induced struvite stone.

Struvite stones are almost always a complication of another primary stone disease, in which the original stone becomes the focus for growth of the infection stone. Struvite stones are especially likely to grow into staghorn calculi, large stones that form a cast of all or a portion of the pelvocalyceal system (Figure 9.1). Staghorn calculi usually cannot pass out of the kidney.[1]

Treatment of struvite stones is essential, as infection stones are particularly virulent and make eradication of the infection nearly impossible. Untreated patients with infected staghorn calculi frequently develop sepsis and require urgent nephrectomy. Early urologic referral is suggested to determine the need for surgery. The goal of surgery in such patients is to remove the stone totally.[4] Lithotripsy may be an option for smaller infection stones.

Cystine Stones

Cystine stones are rare, forming because of crystallization of cystine when the urine is supersaturated with it. This disorder, an inherited autosomal recessive trait, occurs when there is a defect in renal tubular resorption of filtered cystine.[4]

Cystine stone formers have particularly virulent disease, best managed by raising the urinary pH in a manner similar to the method used in patients with uric acid stones. If stone activity continues, D-penicillamine is used. It forms complexes with cystine, thereby preventing its precipitation.[4]

Oxalate Stones

Patients with hyperoxaluria are prone to the development of oxalate stones. The aim of treatment in this group of patients is to lower oxalate excretion. The use of cholestyramine (8–16 g per day), increased calcium supplementation, and a low-oxalate diet are the hallmarks of treatment. In patients who have had ileal resection, pyridoxine (vitamin B_6) deficiency may develop, resulting in hyperoxaluria. In this situation, vitamin B_6 supplementation may provide benefit.[4]

Laboratory Assessment in Stone Formers

Laboratory assessment of patients who have formed urinary calculi should include urinalysis, microscopic urinalysis, and stone analysis. This evaluation should be accomplished without the patient modifying his or her diet so that an underlying process associated with urinary calculus disease is not masked.

The pH value of the urinalysis provides important information that may help determine the cause of the urinary calculus. The pH is usually acid in patients with uric acid or cystine stones and tends to be alkaline in patients with struvite stones.

The microscopic urinalysis may show crystals or evidence of infection. Crystals of cystine have the appearance of a benzine ring and are highly suggestive of cystinuria. Oxalate crystals normally appear in urine. Their identification may not be diagnostic of anything.[4] Monosodium urate is easily distinguished from calcium pyrophosphate dihydrate on the basis of crystal morphology and characteristics of the crystals under polarized light. Monosodium urate morphology includes rod- or needle-shaped crystals whose length approaches the diameter of polymorphonuclear leukocytes within the microscopic field. Under polarized light, they stand out brightly when the field is dark, and they have strong negative birefringence. Calcium pyrophosphate dihydrate crystals vary much more in size and shape, are never needlelike, and are usually shorter than monoso-

TABLE 9.5   Recommended tests for laboratory assessment of patients with urinary calculi

24-Hour urinary volume
24-Hour urinary calcium
24-Hour urinary uric acid
24-Hour urinary creatinine
Urinalysis
Urine cystine screen (cyanide-nitroprusside test)
Urine culture (if pyuria)
Urine pH (taken on first voided morning specimen)
Serum calcium
Serum phosphorus
Serum uric acid
Serum chloride
Serum bicarbonate
Serum creatinine
Serum urea nitrogen

dium urate crystals. Their length is often smaller than one lobe of a polymorphonuclear leukocyte nucleus. They are usually refractile without polarized light, do not increase appreciably in brilliance when the light is polarized, and are weakly positively birefringent.[9]

The presence of infection is suggested by the identification of white blood cells and bacteria through microscopic urinalysis.

In addition to the typical laboratory assessment of patients with urinary calculi (Table 9.5), parathyroid hormone should be measured if hypercalcemia and hypercalciuria are documented. Perform a 24-hour study for urinary oxalate when hyperoxaluria is expected clinically.[4] Twenty-four hour studies are also available for urinary uric acid, calcium, and cysteine.

If a stone is available, it should be analyzed. Stone analysis can be performed inexpensively at most commercial laboratories.

Diabetes Mellitus

Diabetes mellitus is a condition caused by an abnormality of glucose utilization, resulting in an elevation of blood glucose concentration. Long-standing diabetes mellitus leads to sequelae affecting the urinary system, including diabetic neuropathy and nephropathy. The peripheral neuropathy associated with long-standing diabetes affects both myelinated and unmyelinated fibers of the somatic and autonomic nervous systems. Somatic nervous system involvement may lead to pelvic floor denervation (damage to the pudendal nerve) causing weakness of the striated external sphincter, thereby contributing to stress incontinence. Autonomic nervous system involvement, particularly of the sacral parasympathetic fibers, weakens detrusor contraction, leading to a flaccid distended bladder prone to overflow incontinence.

The osmotic diuresis caused by hyperglycemia may precipitate urgency incontinence in normally continent individuals or may worsen incontinence in the formally incontinent patient who had been successfully treated.

Last, the same microangiopathy that leads to diabetic neuropathy also contributes to renal end-organ damage. This, known as *diabetic nephropathy*, over time contributes to chronic renal failure.

The insulin-dependent type (type 1) of diabetes usually has its onset in youth. Insulin deficiency requires exogenous insulin to prevent complications (ketosis-acidosis).

The non–insulin-dependent type (type 2) of diabetes generally has onset after age 40 years, particularly in overweight individuals. These patients are not insulin dependent or ketosis prone, but they may need insulin for control of persistent hyperglycemia. Weight control of the non–insulin-dependent subtype may ameliorate disease. Non–insulin-dependent type 2 represents 90% of all cases of diabetes.[10]

Clinical Presentation

Most diagnoses of diabetes mellitus are made at an asymptomatic stage of the disease as a result of routine blood tests that reveal hyperglycemia. Of those patients who are symptomatic at time of diagnosis, most complain of excessive thirst with increased fluid intake (polydipsia) and increased urination (polyuria). If the disease is severe, weight loss occurs despite increased appetite and increased food consumption (polyphagia). These symptoms are manifestations of excessive blood sugar with secondary glucosuria. Other symptoms associated with hyperglycemia include blurred vision, vaginitis, and skin infections.[10]

Diagnosis

Elevation of blood sugar concentration is the hallmark of diabetes mellitus. Criteria diagnostic for diabetes includes: elevation of plasma glucose concentration associated with classic symptoms of diabetes mellitus, multiple elevated fasting plasma glucose (FPG) determinations, or elevation of plasma glucose after an oral glucose challenge on more than one occasion. A single elevated FPG or abnormal oral glucose tolerance test never establishes the diagnosis (Table 9.6).

Elevation of FPG should be followed up by several repeat measurements of the FPG on different days.

The oral glucose tolerance test (OGTT) is not necessary if the FPG is elevated on more than one occasion or if there is unequivocal elevation of plasma glucose in a patient who has classic symptoms of diabetes.

A number of considerations impose limitations on the usefulness of the FPG and OGTT. Stress and illness may elevate FPG; abnormalities of the OGTT are produced by a variety of illnesses, both acute and chronic. Infection, trauma, certain drugs, physical inactivity, febrile illness, and myocardial infarction may produce a "diabetic" OGTT. Smoking before or during testing or the ingestion of caffeine-containing drinks (coffee, tea) in the period of fasting both can contribute to abnormal results. Therefore, a diagnosis of diabetes cannot be established on the basis of a single abnormal test.[10]

TABLE 9.6   Diagnosis of diabetes: diagnostic concentrations of glucose

Normal plasma glucose concentrations
    Fasting state (10–16 hrs postprandial)
        Venous plasma: <115 mg/dl
        Venous whole blood: <100 mg/dl
        Capillary whole blood: <100 mg/dl
    2-Hour oral glucose tolerance test (OGTT)
        Venous plasma: <140 mg/dl
        Venous whole blood: <120 mg/dl
        Capillary whole blood: <140 mg/dl
Diabetic glucose concentrations
    Fasting state (10–16 hrs postprandial)
        Venous plasma: >140 mg/dl
        Venous whole blood: >120 mg/dl
        Capillary whole blood: >140 mg/dl
    OGTT preparation: fasting 10–16 hrs during which no caffeine-containing drinks or
        smoking is permitted.
    75 g glucose (40 g/m^2)
    Use in nonpregnant adults: (1.75 g/kg for children. Up to 75 g maximum.)
        Dosage form: flavored water, 25 g of glucose/100 dl. Drink over 5 minutes.
        Obtain blood samples at 0, $\frac{1}{2}$, 1, $1\frac{1}{2}$, and 2 hours.
    Test positive for diabetes mellitus: both the 2-hour sample and at least one other
        sample must meet following criteria:
        Venous plasma: >200 mg/dl
        Venous whole blood: >180 mg/dl
        Capillary whole blood: >200 mg/dl

Treatment

Juvenile-onset diabetes (type 1 diabetes) is caused by the absence of insulin due to the destruction of insulin-producing cells. It most frequently occurs in persons younger than 40 years of age. These patients require lifelong insulin therapy. When beginning insulin therapy, the diabetic should initially be treated with an intermediate-acting insulin, either neutral protamine Hagedorn (NPH) or lente, given subcutaneously each morning. The intermediate insulins typically peak at 6–14 hours after injection, with 18–28 hours' duration of action. Patients should be started at low doses, approximately 10–20 U per day, and the dose can be increased appropriately to control hyperglycemia.

If hyperglycemia consistently occurs in the late morning or early afternoon, rapid-acting insulin (regular or semilente) should be given along with the morning NPH or lente. The activity of regular insulin peaks in 3–4 hours and lasts up to 7 hours; semilente peaks in 3–4 hours and lasts for 10–16 hours.

Adult-onset diabetes (type 2 diabetes) is commonly seen in obese persons. In contrast to the insulin-deficient type 1, insulin levels are frequently elevated at the onset of type 2 disease. Adult-onset diabetes may be caused by insensitivity to the effects of insulin. Because adult-onset diabetes can usually be alleviated or even cured by weight loss and diet, these patients are said to be insulin independent. However, insulin injections are often required in patients who find it impossible to maintain weight loss. Oral hypoglycemic agents are commonly used in the treatment of type 2 diabetes. The dosage must be properly tailored for each patient. The oral agents are appropriate only in the treatment of adult-onset, type 2 diabetes.

The principal aims of therapy for both types of diabetes are to ameliorate the symptoms of hyperglycemia (polydipsia, polyuria, and polyphagia), prevent ketoacidosis and hyperosmolar coma, and to prevent or delay long-term complications of the disease (neuropathy, retinopathy, nephropathy, and cardiovascular disease).

With newly diagnosed diabetes, patient education is necessary to help plan diet therapy including, if necessary, a practical weight reduction diet high in fibers. The diabetic patient should be instructed about this illness and how to provide self-care, including how to perform insulin injections. The benefits of regular exercise for type 2 diabetic patients should also be stressed. In addition to promoting overall cardiovascular fitness and weight loss, exercise may lead to increased end-organ insulin sensitivity.

Patients should be seen frequently after initiation of therapy to reassess the insulin dosage and reinforce diabetic teaching. Insulin requirements may change with alterations in the patient's diet and with intermittent illnesses (which may necessitate an increase in the insulin dose). Aggressive therapy to maintain as normal a blood sugar as possible (euglycemia) is called *tight control*.[11]

Perhaps the most significant complication of insulin-dependent diabetes is diabetic crisis or ketoacidosis, a disease of insulin deficiency. Circulating insulin normally inhibits peripheral lipolysis. When insulin levels are markedly reduced or absent, lipolysis is accelerated, and triglycerides are degraded into three fatty acids that are released into the circulation. On reaching the liver, the fatty acids are oxidized to ketone bodies, and ketone bodies accumulate. Infection ranks as the leading precipitant of ketoacidosis, as infection raises the body's insulin requirement. Other causes of ketoacidosis include pregnancy, failure to continue insulin therapy, and the stress of myocardial infarction.

The typical prodrome of diabetic ketoacidosis consists of 12–24 hours of weakness, polyuria, polydipsia, Kussmaul hyperventilation, visual disturbances, and abdominal pain with vomiting. As the syndrome progresses, all patients become significantly dehydrated. Stupor and coma may ensue.

Therapy for diabetic ketoacidosis consists of prompt administration of intravenous fluids, potassium, and insulin, and a thorough search for and treatment of the precipitating cause.[11]

Disorders of Water Metabolism

The combination of excessive thirst, increased water intake, and increased urine output (polyuria) is a common clinical presentation of a number of conditions (Table 9.7). These symptoms are related to some event, which results in an excessive loss of fluid via the kidneys. Excessive urinary out-

TABLE 9.7   Causes of polyuria

Disorder	Mechanism
Glucosuria	Osmotic diuresis
Excessive intake of water	Psychogenic
Various drugs	Often due to anticholinergic effects producing dryness of mouth; possible central effects
Decreased antidiuretic hormone (ADH) effect	Deficiency of ADH secretion (idiopathic diabetes insipidus or due to pituitary-hypothalamic disease: nephrogenic diabetes insipidus
Renal disease, plus renal effects of potassium depletion, hypercalcemia, and lithium therapy	In all of these disorders, impairment of renal concentrating ability is present
Hyperthyroidism	Impairment of urinary concentrating ability; decreased salivary flow

put may contribute to the development of incontinence in normally continent individuals, or it may worsen the degree of incontinence in a compromised individual.

Hyperglycemia causes a large solute load (glucose) to be presented to the renal tubules. Water loss ensues, known as an *osmotic diuresis*. Hypercalcemia produces renal tubular abnormalities resulting in impaired ability to concentrate urine. Lithium, used for treatment of manic depressive disorder, impairs the action of antidiuretic hormone, thereby producing water loss.

A rare disorder of water metabolism is diabetes insipidus, a deficiency of antidiuretic hormone. This condition, also known as the *syndrome of inappropriate antidiuretic hormone*, is either idiopathic, in which case it is not associated with any pituitary hypothalamic disease or, more commonly, is secondary to pituitary gland, hypothalamus, or pituitary stalk disease (tumor, craniopharyngioma, aneurysm). Other causes of the syndrome of inappropriate secretion of antidiuretic hormone include head trauma, neurosurgical procedures, and central nervous system infections.[5]

Management of Polydipsia and Polyuria

An initial laboratory workup should be performed to help determine the cause of polydipsia and polyuria. Testing should include a urine glucose, a 24-hour urine test, serum sodium, osmolality, potassium, calcium, blood urea nitrogen (BUN), and creatinine. The 24-hour urine samples should be examined to determine the total volume, osmolality, and creatinine excretion, the latter serving as a marker for completeness of the collection.

These tests provide insight into the diagnosis. Unless considerable glucosuria is present, the patient's problem is not due to uncontrolled diabetes mellitus. The presence of normal serum calcium and potassium concentrations excludes several metabolic problems, whereas abnormalities of calcium, potassium, or renal function suggest that the problem is not one of water metabolism.

Normal urine volume ranges up to 2,500 ml per 24 hours. In both diabetes insipidus and psychogenic water drinking, urine volume usually exceeds 4 liters per day. If the serum sodium and osmolality are low and the urine volume is large with low osmolality, a diagnosis of psychogenic water drinking is likely. If the serum sodium or osmolality is high and the urine volume is large with low osmolality, the diagnosis would be diabetes insipidus.[5]

Treatment

The treatment of psychogenic water drinking involves psychiatric counseling and perhaps psychotropic medications. Treatment of diabetes insipidus involves use of antidiuretic hormone in some form. Formerly, intramuscular Pitressin Synthetic in oil was the preferred agent. Antidiuretic hormone may also be administered as a nasal spray.[5]

Proteinuria

Proteinuria is frequently encountered in clinical practice. It may signify a serious underlying disorder or simply an abnormal laboratory finding in an asymptomatic individual with little or no effect on present or future health.

Normally, there is limited glomerular filtration of albumin and lower molecular weight proteins, with nearly complete tubular resorption of filtered proteins. The quantity of protein remaining in the urine is usually less than 150 mg per 24 hours.

Certain disease states that affect the glomeruli or the tubules, or both, result in increased amounts of protein in the urine. Screening for proteinuria is easily and inexpensively accomplished by using the urine dipstick. When moistened with urine, the stick becomes yellow when protein is absent and as protein concentration increases, it develops an increasingly green color. This technique is simple and inexpensive, but has limitations. It is important to quantitate proteinuria by examining a 24-hour urine sample or by determining the protein to creatinine ratio, as this helps to classify the disorder and assist in the development of a differential diagnosis.[12]

The 24-hour collection is best done on a day when the patient will be using one toilet. A container without preservatives is required. The first-voided morning specimen is discarded, and then all urine in the next 24 hours, including the next morning's first-voided specimen, is collected in the container.

When quantifying urine protein, any value greater than 200 mg per 24 hours is considered abnormal. Protein is classified as non-nephrotic if the excretion is between 200 and 3,500 mg in 24 hours and classified as nephrotic when the excretion is greater than 3,500 mg in 24 hours.

The simultaneous measurement of urinary creatinine when performing the 24-hour test is an index of the adequacy of the collection. Most individuals of average body mass produce between 800 and 1,500 mg of creatinine per day.

TABLE 9.8   Causes of proteinuria not due to a primary renal disease

Congestive heart failure
Epinephrine administration
Exercise
Fever
Stress resulting in catecholamine release

The protein to creatinine ratio is measured as milligrams per deciliter of protein divided by milligrams per deciliter of creatinine. This value may eliminate the need for 24-hour urine testing, as the ratio can be calculated with any volume of urine. A ratio of greater than 0.2 mg of protein per mg of creatinine is considered abnormal, and a ratio of greater than 3.5 mg of protein per mg of creatinine represents nephrotic range proteinuria. Determination of protein to creatinine ratio should be used whenever there is doubt regarding the adequacy of the 24-hour collection.[12]

Non-Nephrotic Proteinuria

A clinician considering the differential diagnosis of a patient with non-nephrotic proteinuria should first rule out problems that are not primarily renal (Table 9.8). These can be eliminated by brief questioning and repeat semiquantitative assessment for urine protein. A variety of primary renal and systemic diseases may be associated with non-nephrotic range proteinuria, and most, if not all, patients with nephrotic range proteinuria may have had, at some time, non-nephrotic range protein excretion.[12]

Nephrotic Proteinuria

When a 24-hour protein quantitation reveals greater than 3.5 g of protein, or the protein to creatinine ratio is greater than 3.5, nephrotic range proteinuria is established and is indicative of glomerular disease.[12] Many causes of nephrotic syndrome exist (Table 9.9), a condition characterized by albuminuria, hypoalbuminemia, hyperlipidemia, and edema. These abnormalities are consequences of excessive glomerular leakage of plasma proteins into the urine.

Damage to the glomerular capillary wall underlying the excessive filtration of plasma proteins can arise as a consequence of a wide variety of disease processes, including immunologic disorders, toxic injuries, metabolic abnormalities, biochemical defects, and vascular disorders. Thus,

---

TABLE 9.9   Most common causes of nephrotic syndrome in adults

Diabetes mellitus: most common
Idiopathic membranous glomerulopathy: second most common
Idiopathic lipoid nephrosis: third most common in adults (most common in children)
Drug toxicity (nonsteroidal anti-inflammatory agents, captopril, lithium, or gold)

---

the nephrotic syndrome may be viewed as a common end point of a variety of disease processes that damage the normal permeability properties of the glomerular capillary wall.

Heavy proteinuria is the hallmark of the nephrotic state. Sustained heavy proteinuria produces hypoalbuminemia, which results in decreased plasma oncotic pressure. This leads to a disturbance in the Starling forces acting across peripheral capillaries, and intravascular fluid migrates into the interstitial tissues, resulting in unrelenting edema. The diminished plasma oncotic pressure also appears to stimulate hepatic lipoprotein synthesis, causing the hyperlipidemia seen with nephrotic syndrome.[13]

Management of Patients with Proteinuria

Non-nephrotic proteinuria requires no special treatment. The physician's major effort is directed at diagnosis, education, surveillance, and at treatment of any underlying disease. When a drug is the suspected cause of the proteinuria, the drug should be discontinued. Proteinuria from drugs may take several months to resolve, and occasionally it is permanent.

Treatment of patients with nephrotic-range proteinuria includes adequate protein intake, accomplished with protein supplements. In the presence of edema, a salt restriction diet is appropriate. If the edema is more severe and is unresponsive to the no-added-salt diet, then the cautious use of diuretics may be helpful.[12]

Hematuria

Hematuria, especially microscopic, is a common finding, seen in nearly 3–4% of apparently healthy adults.[14]

Under certain conditions, the finding of red urine or RBCs in the urine may be considered normal, commonly seen just after pelvic or prostatic examination, bladder instrumentation, catheterization, after prostate or renal biopsy, or even after vigorous exercise. Therefore, in these situations, repeat urinalyses should be performed before other potential causes of the problem are investigated. Also, the menstruating female patient should not be evaluated for hematuria until after menstruation stops.[14,15]

On the other hand, hematuria may be a manifestation of a serious disease, which may be otherwise asymptomatic, such as tumor of the genitourinary tract. Table 9.10 lists causes of hematuria.[14]

Diagnostic Tests

Dipstick Screening Test
Most multipurpose reagent strips have a colorimetric test that detects both hemoglobin and myoglobin pigments. Therefore, it is not specific for blood in the urine, but it may be the first clue to the presence of hematuria. A positive reaction is produced by both hemoglobin from intravascular hemolysis and myoglobin released from injured muscles. Therefore, the dipstick

TABLE 9.10   Causes of hematuria

Hematuria alone
    Disorders anatomically adjacent to the urinary tract
        Aortic aneurysm
        Renal artery aneurysm
    Anticoagulant drugs
    Benign prostatic hypertrophy
    Calculi
    Neoplasia (benign or malignant)
    Trauma
    Urethritis
Hematuria and pyuria
    Infection (anywhere in the genitourinary tract)
Hematuria with casts and/or significant proteinuria (>1 g/24 hrs)
    Hypertension
    Arterial emboli
    Glomerulonephritis
    Nephrotoxins:
        Nonsteroidal anti-inflammatory drugs
        Lithium
        Penicillin and its derivatives

screening technique should never be taken as diagnostic, and hematuria should always be confirmed by microscopic urinalysis.[14]

Microscopic Urinalysis

Microscopic hematuria is identified by microscopic examination of centrifuged urine. Normally, 1–2 million RBCs are lost in the urine every 24 hours. However, when studied microscopically in centrifuged urine, this amounts to only one to two RBCs per high-powered field. Therefore, the finding of more than three or four RBCs per high-powered field should be considered abnormal and requires further assessment.[14]

Approach to the Patient with Hematuria

The source of hematuria must always be determined. This requires a progressively detailed examination of the urinary tract by cystoscopy, retrograde pyelography, arteriography, renal ultrasonography, and computed tomography and magnetic resonance imaging scanning to disclose tumor, stone, cysts, or other causes. Computed tomography and magnetic resonance imaging are particularly helpful in detecting and evaluating renal cysts and tumors and should precede cystoscopy and arteriography.

Hematuria with infection or overt renal disease usually requires no steps beyond intravenous pyelography.[16]

Chronic Renal Failure

Renal insufficiency, occurring either as a primary event or complicating another illness, is a common clinical problem.

The healthy kidney performs a wide variety of functions that contribute to maintenance of the internal environment of the body. In addition to its role in maintaining water and electrolyte balance, the kidney has important endocrine and metabolic functions. It produces hormones responsible for normal bone formation (1,25-dihydroxy vitamin D_3), RBC production (erythropoietin), and blood pressure control (renin, prostaglandins). The kidney is responsible for degrading a number of polypeptide hormones, including parathyroid hormone, insulin, gastrin, and prolactin, among others. Also, the kidney serves as a major excretory route for many toxic metabolic wastes and a wide variety of drugs or their breakdown products.[17]

The patient with incontinence due to pelvic floor or sphincter weakness or insufficiency is prone to frequent UTIs. This predisposes to upper tract infection and pyelonephritis. Chronic kidney infection and inflammation produce renal scarring, with the development of chronic renal failure (CRF).

Patients with overflow incontinence due to outlet obstruction as in benign prostatic hypertrophy or detrusor sphincter dyssynergia with spinal cord injury are prone to vesicoureteral reflux. Chronic reflux damages renal interstitial tissues, contributing to CRF.

Patients with longstanding nonhealing decubiti are prone to a condition known as *amyloidosis*. With amyloidosis, amyloid deposits settle in various organs, including the kidney. In time, this leads to CRF.

Last, patients with renal damage that contributes to polyuria (see Disorders of Water Metabolism, earlier) may develop chronic renal failure in association with the incontinence that may be caused by the increased urine load.

Pathophysiology of Chronic Renal Insufficiency

The course of CRF is characterized by the progressive loss of functioning nephrons. Even while nephrons are being destroyed, the kidney undergoes various adaptive changes that allow most patients with chronic renal failure to have few signs or symptoms until 80% of the original number of nephrons is lost. In conjunction with the progressive destruction of nephrons, patients pass through a sequence of clinical stages before reaching end-stage renal failure (the point at which dialysis is required).

During the initial stage of renal impairment, the BUN and serum creatinine concentrations are often within the normal range, despite a fall of the glomerular filtration rate (GFR) to as low as 50 ml per minute.

As renal function declines further (GFR 20–50 ml per minute), the BUN and serum creatinine levels begin to increase. During this stage of renal insufficiency, the patient begins to experience symptoms related to anemia (fatigue), loss of urine-concentrating ability (polyuria), or volume expansion (dyspnea or edema, or both).

When the GFR falls below 20 ml per minute, the serum creatinine concentration begins to rise greater than 5 mg/dl. This stage, known as *renal failure*, is associated with a deterioration of the kidney's ability to maintain homeostasis as the renal reserve capacity is overwhelmed. Multiple biochemical abnormalities ensue, including hypocalcemia, hyperphosphatemia, metabolic acidosis, and fluid overload. The term *uremia* is used

TABLE 9.11   Major physiologic and clinical abnormalities of uremia

Fluid and electrolyte abnormalities
  Volume expansion
  Hyperkalemia
  Hypocalcemia
  Hyperphosphatemia
  Metabolic acidosis
Endocrine-metabolic abnormalities
  Vitamin D deficiency
  Hyperparathyroidism
  Carbohydrate intolerance
  Impotence and infertility
  Hypertriglyceridemia
Hematologic-immunologic abnormalities
  Impaired platelet function
  Abnormal T- and B-cell function
  Anemia
Cardiovascular abnormalities
  Hypertension
  Accelerated atherosclerosis
  Pericarditis
Dermatologic abnormalities
  Pruritus
  Increased pigmentation
  Acne
Gastrointestinal abnormalities
  Nausea and vomiting
  Anorexia
  Pancreatitis
Neuromuscular abnormalities
  Peripheral neuropathy
  Seizures
  Coma
  Asterixis
  Myoclonus

to describe the entire set of signs, symptoms, and metabolic disturbances that occurs in advanced kidney failure (GFR less than 10 ml per minute, serum creatinine concentration usually greater than 8 mg/dl). Uremia results from failure of the kidney to fulfill its excretory, endocrine, and metabolic functions. In the uremic patient with end-stage renal disease, virtually every organ system is affected to some degree. Uremic manifestations include nausea, vomiting, anorexia, lassitude, sleep disturbance, heart failure, hypertension, pruritus, and infertility (Table 9.11).[17]

Laboratory Diagnosis of Chronic Renal Failure

Diagnostically, the urinalysis can often provide important information. RBCs can be seen with any renal disorder, whereas RBC casts are more indicative of a glomerular lesion. White blood cells, with or without casts, are found in the interstitial nephropathies, including bacterial pyelonephritis.

Measurements of the concentration of blood glucose, serum electrolytes (Na, K^+, Cl, CO_2, Ca, PO_4), uric acid, and liver tests (alkaline phosphatase, bilirubin, serum transaminases) are helpful in monitoring the patient with CRF.

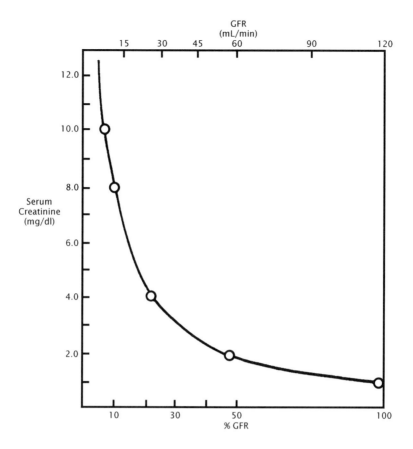

FIGURE 9.2 *The relationship of the serum creatinine concentration to the glomerular filtration rate (GFR) in patients with normal muscle mass (produces 1.0 g creatinine per day).*

A 24-hour urine specimen should be obtained to quantify proteinuria and to calculate the creatinine clearance. The finding of nephrotic range proteinuria (greater than 3 g per day) usually indicates a glomerular lesion, whereas lesser amounts are seen in some glomerular disorders and in most interstitial forms of nephritis.

Although the serum creatinine concentration is a better indicator of renal function than is the BUN, in the early stages of renal insufficiency, serum creatinine concentration is an insensitive indicator of functional impairment because it may remain in the normal range (less than 1.5 mg/dl) until GFR has decreased by as much as 50%. The general relationship between the serum creatinine concentration and the GFR is shown in Figure 9.2. It is not until the GFR falls from 50% to 25% of normal that the serum creatinine concentration begins to rise from 2 to 4 mg/dl. Therefore, most of the loss of functioning nephrons occurs at levels of serum creatinine that would be considered to be only modestly elevated. However, once the GFR is reduced to 20–30% of normal, the curve expressing the relationship between serum creatinine and the GFR rises steeply.

Calculation of the creatinine clearance provides a more accurate reflection of the severity of renal disease than does the serum creatinine concentration. The creatinine clearance is a close approximation of the GFR. The formula used for calculating clearance is UV over P divided by 1,440, where U is the urine creatine in mg/dl, V is the urine volume in ml per day, P is the plasma creatinine concentration in mg/dl, and 1,440 is the number of minutes in 24 hours. The result is expressed in milliliters per minute. The normal creatinine clearance is approximately 100–140 ml per minute in men and 85–125 ml per minute in women.

A normochromic, normocytic anemia develops in patients with chronic renal failure, its severity being proportional to the degree of renal insufficiency. Hematocrit values generally fall to between 15% and 25% in a patient with advanced CRF. The anemia of renal failure results from shortened RBC survival, and decreased RBC production due to lack of erythropoietin.[17]

Management of Renal Disease

Regardless of the etiology of renal damage, the patient with CRF requires therapeutic intervention to ameliorate symptoms and prevent further system deterioration. Initial therapy is conservative and directed toward the management of diet, fluid, electrolytes, and calcium/phosphate balance.

The availability of dialysis therapy in CRF has enabled patients to overcome the potentially fatal complications of uremia. Hemodialysis is a potent clinical tool with many indications, complications, and psychosocial consequences. Absolute indications for hemodialysis include uremic pericarditis, progressive motor neuropathy, intractable volume overload, and life-threatening acidosis or hyperkalemia.

Renal transplantation is a reasonable alternative to chronic hemodialysis. After transplantation, the mainstay of medical management is continuous immunosuppression to avoid allograft rejection by the patient's immune system.[18]

References

1. Burton JR, Smolev JK. Genitourinary Infections. In LR Barker, JR Burton, PD Zieve (eds), Principles of Ambulatory Medicine (2d ed). Baltimore: Williams & Wilkins, 1986;334–346.
2. Stamm WE, Wagner KF, Ansel RL, et al. Causes of the acute urethral syndrome in woman. N Engl J Med 1980;303:409.
3. Fishman MC, Hoffman AR, Klausner RD, et al. Urinary Tract Infections. In MC Fishman, AR Hoffman, RD Klausner, et al.(eds), Medicine. Philadelphia: Lippincott, 1981;410–412.
4. Burton JR, Smolev JK. Urinary Stones. In LR Barker, JR Burton, PD Zieve (eds), Principles of Ambulatory Medicine (2d ed). Baltimore: Williams & Wilkins, 1986;532–542.
5. Gregerman RI. Selected Endocrine Problems: Disorders of Pituitary, Adrenal, and Parathyroid Glands; Pharmacological Use of Steroids; Hypo and Hypercalcemia; Osteoporosis; Water Metabolism; Hypoglycemia. In LR Barker, JR Burton, PD Zieve (eds), Principles of Ambulatory Medicine (2d ed). Baltimore: Williams & Wilkins, 1986;1013–1040.

6. Heath H III, Hodgson SF, Kennedy MA. Primary hyperparathyroidism. Incidence, morbidity, and potential economic impact in a community. N Engl J Med 1980;302:189.
7. Thomas WC Jr. Use of phosphates in patients with calcereous renal calculi. Kidney Int 1978;13:390.
8. Yu T, Gutman AB. Uric acid nephrolithiasis in gout. Predisposing factors. Ann Int Med 1967;67:1133.
9. Townes AS. Crystal Induced Arthritis. In LR Barker, JR Burton, PD Zieve (eds), Principles of Ambulatory Medicine (2d ed). Baltimore: Williams & Wilkins, 1986;905–916.
10. Gregerman RI. Diabetes Mellitus. In LR Barker, JR Burton, PD Zieve (eds), Principles of Ambulatory Medicine (2d ed). Baltimore: Williams & Wilkins, 1986;951–986.
11. Fishman MC, Hoffman AR, Klausner RD, et al. Diabetes Mellitus. In MC Fishman, AR Hoffman, RD Klausner, et al. (eds), Medicine. Philadelphia: JB Lippincott, 1981;221–234.
12. Burton JR. Proteinuria. In LR Barker, JR Burton, PD Zieve (eds), Principles of Ambulatory Medicine (2d ed). Baltimore: Williams & Wilkins, 1986;511–516.
13. Glassock RJ, Brenner BM. The Major Glomerulopathies. In RG Petersdorf, RD Adams, E Braunwald, et al. (eds), Harrison's Principles of Internal Medicine (10th ed). New York: McGraw-Hill, 1983;1632–1641.
14. Smolev JK, Burton JR. Hematuria. In LR Barker, JR Burton, PD Zieve (eds), Principles of Ambulatory Medicine (2d ed). Baltimore: Williams & Wilkins, 1986;517–521.
15. Siegel AJ, Hennekins CH, Solomon HS, VanBoeckel E. Exercise related hematuria. JAMA 1979;241:391.
16. Coe FL, Glassock RJ, Brenner BM. Proteinuria, Hematuria, Azotemia, and Oliguria. The Major Glomerulopathies. In Petersdorf RG, Adams RD, Braunwald E, et al. (eds), Harrison's Principles of Internal Medicine (10th ed). New York: McGraw-Hill, 1983;211–216.
17. Briefel GR. Chronic Renal Failure. In LR Barker, JR Burton, PD Zieve (eds), Principles of Ambulatory Medicine (2d ed). Baltimore: Williams & Wilkins, 1986;543–568.
18. Fishman MC, Hoffman AR, Klausner RD, et al. Chronic Renal Failure. In MC Fishman, AR Hoffman, RD Klausner, et al. (eds), Medicine. Philadelphia: Lippincott, 1981;163–172.

10   Eight Types of Incontinence

Jack L. Rook

Background

Urinary incontinence is defined as "the uncontrolled loss of urine of sufficient amount and frequency to cause a social or hygienic problem for the
patient or his family."[1,2] Because of its social connotations, urinary incontinence is an underreported problem, and the absolute incidence of incontinence among individuals in the United States remains unknown. The
National Institutes of Health estimates that at least 10 million adults experience urinary incontinence, at an annual cost exceeding 10 billion dollars.[1,3] In
the elderly institutionalized adult population, as many as 50% are incontinent
and 70% experience at least occasional urinary leakage.[1,4] Among elderly in
the community, approximately 15–30% experience urinary incontinence.[1,3]
Many of these cases are transient, brought on by infection, immobility, or
acute disease. The remaining incontinent individuals have a chronic condition that persists until proper treatment and bladder management strategies
are initiated.[1]

Several classification systems for chronic urinary incontinence exist.
Gray and Dougherty[5] identified four types of incontinence:

1. Stress incontinence is the leakage of urine with physical exertion
   but without detrusor contraction.
2. Instability incontinence is the leakage of urine caused by unstable or
   hyperreflexic detrusor contractions: Urge incontinence is the presenting symptom with unstable detrusor contractions in the face of
   normal bladder sensation, whereas reflex incontinence is the presenting symptom when unstable contractions occur without normal
   bladder sensations.
3. Overflow incontinence occurs with urinary retention, the inability to
   completely empty the bladder by voiding.
4. Extraurethral incontinence occurs when ectopia, fistula, or surgical
   diversion procedures produce leakage through some route that
   bypasses the normal sphincter mechanism.

The North American Nursing Diagnosis Association uses a system of six diagnoses for incontinence: *Altered patterns of urinary elimination* is a broad diagnosis intended to describe any dysfunctional voiding state. *Stress incontinence* describes milder cases of sphincter dysfunction, whereas a more vague diagnosis, *total incontinence* is used for both severe stress incontinence caused by sphincter incompetence and extraurethral leakage. The North American Nursing Diagnosis Association labels instability leakage by its presenting symptoms, *urge incontinence* or *reflex incontinence*. Leakage that results from urinary retention corresponds to the diagnosis *overflow incontinence*, and *functional incontinence* refers to urinary leakage associated with altered mobility, dexterity, or cognition.[1,6]

This text describes incontinence based on eight different types of pathophysiologic abnormalities, including (1) stress incontinence due to pelvic descent, (2) stress incontinence due to sphincter incompetence, (3) instability incontinence, (4) incontinence due to involuntary detrusor contractions, (5) overflow incontinence secondary to urinary retention caused by impaired detrusor contraction, (6) overflow incontinence secondary to urinary retention due to obstruction (in males, this condition is usually due to benign prostatic hypertrophy; however, enlargement of the prostate due to prostate cancer can also cause this type of incontinence, and a separate chapter is devoted to its discussion), (7) total or extraurethral incontinence, and (8) functional incontinence.

The identification and successful treatment of incontinence are critical to prevent potential complications, including psychosocial sequelae (shame, humiliation, and social isolation), skin irritation and breakdown, and painful pressure ulcers in bedridden individuals.

Spinal cord–injured patients can develop a whole host of physical problems as a result of urinary dysfunction. Detrusor sphincter dyssynergia (uncontrolled bladder contraction against a closed sphincter) can occur with upper motor neuron spinal cord injury. This condition can lead to upper urinary tract damage, contribute to autonomic dysreflexia, and worsen spasticity. Uncontrolled incontinence can contribute to skin breakdown and pressure ulcers in this population. Frequent catheterization of the urinary tract of spinal cord–injured patients can predispose to urinary infections.

Stress Urinary Incontinence

Stress urinary incontinence refers to leakage in response to physical exertion (jumping, exercise, and change of position), or increases in intra-abdominal pressure (coughing, sneezing). With this condition, the amount of urine lost varies from a few drops to gushes of urine that necessitate containment products. Stress incontinence is associated with either loss of structural support of the bladder neck and proximal urethra or intrinsic sphincter dysfunction.[1,7]

The pelvic floor muscles and ligaments support the lower urinary tract and reproductive organs. Pelvic descent results from weakness of the pelvic floor support structures. Factors that contribute to their weakening in women include childbearing (particularly with multiple or difficult deliveries), loss of circulating estrogen, and pelvic floor denervation. Distortion of the urethrovesical anatomy adversely affects sphincter muscle tone and efficient closure of the urethral sphincter.[1]

Stress incontinence caused by pelvic floor relaxation is classified as type I or II, according to the degree of pelvic descent. Intrinsic sphincter dysfunction in women is classified as type III stress incontinence. For these patients, the incontinence is not due to pelvic descent, but, rather, to actual loss of sphincter function. With type III incontinence, the vesicle neck and proximal urethra remain open during filling, allowing for incontinence with little provocation. Active leakage may be noted when the patient is only standing, without coughing or straining. When the urethral sphincter mechanism is damaged and fails to close completely, urethral pressure is low, leakage occurs with only minimal activity, and the incontinence is often severe. Correct identification of sphincter damage in women is important, because the management differs from the maneuvers used to treat pelvic descent.[1]

Urine leakage in men is referred to as *sphincteric incontinence*. Iatrogenic sphincter incompetence is a rare complication of transurethral resection of the prostate and an uncommon complication of radical prostatectomy procedures.[1,7,8]

Instability (Reflex) Incontinence

Instability (reflex) incontinence, leakage without warning signals of sensory urgency, can be caused by disease or trauma affecting the spinal cord above the sacral micturition center (S2 through S4), which results in detrusor muscle instability with loss of normal bladder sensations.[1]

Suprasacral spinal cord lesions result in loss of voluntary control of micturition, as well as a loss of bladder-sphincter coordination due to interruption of the pontine sacral axis. This condition is known as *detrusor external sphincter dyssynergia* or *detrusor sphincter dyssynergia*. *Detrusor sphincter dyssynergia* refers to the loss of coordination between the striated sphincter mechanism and the detrusor muscle. The "dyssynergic" sphincter fails to relax during micturition, causing bladder outlet obstruction, increased intravesical pressure, and urinary retention. During this uncoordinated voiding, the intravesical pressure may rise to extremely high levels. When high-pressure voiding remains untreated, upper urinary tract deterioration ensues secondary to the development of vesicoureteral reflux.[1,7]

Incontinence Caused by Involuntary Detrusor Contractions

Involuntary detrusor contractions due to detrusor instability or uninhibited contraction are the most common cause of storage problems. In this condition, the bladder contracts involuntarily during filling.[7]

Patients with involuntary detrusor contractions may perceive each contraction as an urge to void (urgency). Once aware of the contraction, some patients are able to maintain continence by contracting the external urinary sphincter. Those without sufficient external sphincter closure are incontinent (urge incontinence). Still others are completely unaware of the contraction and simply void uncontrollably. These patients typically have cerebral dysfunction and are said to have uninhibited contractions.[7]

Bladder instability may be caused by bladder outlet obstruction, bladder inflammation, cerebral neurologic conditions, or unknown factors.

Incontinence Associated with Obstructive Uropathy

Chronic urinary retention is the inability to evacuate the bladder completely. Micturition occurs, but some urine remains in the bladder, resulting in more frequent attempts to empty the bladder and predisposing the individual to complications, including urinary tract infection, vesicoureteral reflux, and upper tract damage. Dribbling, overflow incontinence, frequent urination, compromised force of stream, and nocturia are presenting symptoms of urinary retention. Two pathophysiologic conditions cause urinary retention— obstruction and deficient detrusor contractility.[1]

Bladder outlet obstruction principally affects men as a result of prostatitis, benign prostate glandular hypertrophy, or prostate cancer. Bladder outlet obstruction is relatively uncommon in women but can occur due to urethral distortion from pelvic descent or trauma or as an uncommon complication of urethropexy or periurethral injection.[1]

Bladder outlet obstruction predisposes the urinary system to the adverse effects of increased intravesical pressure and urinary stasis. The deleterious effects of obstruction are described by the concept obstructive uropathy, with complications including urinary tract infection, pyelonephritis, vesicoureteral reflux, compromised renal function, and lithiasis.[1]

Obstructive uropathy results from the complete or partial obstruction of urinary flow.[9] Obstruction of the bladder outlet adversely affects the detrusor muscle, which undergoes hypertrophy in an attempt to sustain more powerful contractions. As the smooth muscle bundles undergo hypertrophy, collagen is deposited. Over time, there is general disruption of the bladder wall, and trabeculation is noted. Neurologic and histologic changes in the detrusor muscle increase the intravesical pressure during the filling and storage phases. As this condition of "compromised compliance" worsens, pressure levels above normal ureteral peristalsis ensues, resulting in vesicoureteral reflux.[10] Vesicoureteral reflux ultimately causes dilation of the ureters and kidneys (hydronephrosis). Therefore, with long-standing obstruction, there is dilatation of urinary tract proximal to the site of obstruction, and hydronephrosis (dilatation of the pyelocalyceal system with renal enlargement) may occur.

Because the kidney is encased within a fairly inflexible capsule, it has a limited capacity for expansion. The increased urinary tract pressure is transmitted to the renal tubules, gradually damaging them. The inability to form concentrated or acid urine is among the earliest signs of obstructive uropathy. Intrarenal pressures eventually become so high that renal blood flow and glomerular filtration rate decline.[11] The reduction in glomerular filtration rate is due to loss of functioning renal parenchyma, resulting from pressure atrophy, ischemia, and any associated infection (which hastens nephron destruction). Rapid parenchymal atrophy and shrunken "end-stage" kidney may be the end result. Uremia with progressive azotemia (increased blood urea nitrogen or creatinine) may become manifest. Therefore, obstruction should be sought in all cases of unexplained renal failure. The term *obstructive nephropathy* refers to these functional and histopathologic changes in the kidney that result from obstruction of urine flow.[9]

Obstruction of the lower urinary tract also predisposes to infection. Spontaneous infection with benign prostatic hypertrophy occurs in 8.6% of cases. Residual urine is a good culture medium for bacterial replication. Decreased blood flow to the distended bladder may impair local defense mechanisms.[9] The risk of infection is markedly increased in those patients undergoing invasive diagnostic tests. Ascending infection with pyelonephritis may complicate lower urinary tract infection.

Lithiasis may also complicate urinary obstruction. Bladder calculi may occur because stasis and infection seem to predispose to stone formation.[9]

The potential for recovery of renal function after relief of obstruction depends on the completeness and duration of the obstruction and the presence or absence of infection. The level of function 3 months after relief of obstruction probably is permanent.[9]

Overflow Incontinence Due to Impaired Detrusor Contractions

In contrast to obstruction, deficient detrusor contractility affects both women and men equally. Detrusor deficiency can occasionally be traced to a reversible, transient cause, including medications (antispasmodics, antidepressants, narcotics, psychotropic medications, antiparkinsonian drugs, recreational hallucinogens or cannabis, or calcium channel blockers), constipation or fecal impaction, hysterical retention, immobility due to illness, or after acute bladder overdistension.[1]

Chronic deficient contractility is usually traced to a neurologic condition that may or may not be reversible, including lower motor neuron spinal injury due to trauma, herniated disk, or spinal stenosis, cauda equina syndrome, or peripheral neuropathy secondary to diabetes mellitus, chronic ethanol abuse, and so forth.[1]

Urinary retention caused by deficient detrusor contractility predisposes the individual to overflow incontinence, and adversely affects the urinary system. Incomplete bladder evacuation causes urinary stasis and contributes to bladder ischemia, increasing the risk of urinary tract infection.[1]

Extraurethral Incontinence

Extraurethral incontinence refers to the uncontrolled leakage of urine through some fistulous or ectopic communication that bypasses the normal urethral sphincter mechanism. The urinary leakage is continuous and relatively unaffected by physical exertion. In some cases, extraurethral leakage manifests as a continuous dribble coexisting with a relatively normal voiding pattern, whereas in other instances, the leakage is severe and replaces normal voiding.[1]

Functional Incontinence

Functional incontinence refers to urinary leakage due to a functional deficit (impaired physical mobility, dexterity, or cognition), rather than due to organic dysfunction of the urinary system.[1,12–14] Functional incontinence is relatively unusual as an isolated finding. More commonly, stress, instability, overflow, and continuous incontinence are complicated or exacerbated by functional deficits. A comprehensive management plan must include measures to alleviate both the primary voiding dysfunction problem and any associated functional aspects of urinary leakage.[14]

The population of patients who could be afflicted with functional incontinence includes those with orthopedic, musculoskeletal, and/or neurologic deficits.

Conclusion

Previous chapters described the normal anatomy and physiology of the urinary tract, assessment of the patient with urinary tract dysfunction, and pathologic conditions associated with urinary tract dysfunction. Those chapters serve as a necessary foundation for the following chapters. One must understand normal anatomy and pathophysiology to appreciate how various pathologic conditions can produce different types of incontinence. Proper assessment helps define the underlying pathologic condition, necessary to initiate an appropriate treatment program. Appreciation of potential complications, particularly with regards to kidney function, helps the clinician understand the urgency of the situation—to correct or control the underlying condition. The following chapters review the eight types of incontinence, each chapter including a discussion of pathophysiology, assessment, diagnostic workup, conservative treatment, and, if appropriate, surgical correction of the underlying problem.

References

1. Gray M. Urinary Incontinence/Voiding Dysfunction. In M Gray (ed), Genitourinary Disorders. St. Louis: Mosby, 1992;90–159.
2. Bates CP, Rowen D, Bradley WE, et al. Standardization of terminology of lower urinary tract function. Urology 1977;9:237.
3. National Institutes of Health. Consensus Development Conference Statement: Urinary Incontinence in Adults (vol 7, no 5). Bethesda, MD: U.S. Department of Health and Human Services, 1988.
4. Cella M. The nursing costs of urinary incontinence in a nursing home population. Nurs Clin North Am 1988;23:159.

5. Gray ML, Dougherty MC. Urinary incontinence: pathophysiology and treatment. J Enterost Ther 1987;14:152.
6. Kim MJ, McFarlane GH, McLane AM. Pocket Guide to Nursing Diagnosis. St. Louis: Mosby–Year Book, 1991.
7. Blaivas JG, Oliver L. Pathophysiology of Urinary Incontinence. In DB Doughty (ed), Urinary and Fecal Incontinence: Nursing Management. St. Louis: Mosby, 1991;23–46.
8. Wheatley JK. Causes and treatment of bladder incontinence. Comp Ther 1983;9:27.
9. Phelps KR, Lieberman RL. Nephrology. In EA Friedman, RM Stillman (eds), Internal Medicine Review and Assessment. New York: Appleton-Century-Crofts, 1982;184–229.
10. Gray M. Obstructive Uropathies. In M Gray (ed), Genitourinary Disorders. St. Louis: Mosby, 1992;160–199.
11. Fishman MC, Hoffman AR, Klausner RD, et al. Obstructive Uropathy and Nephrolithiasis. In MC Fishman, AR Hoffman, RD Klausner, et al. (eds), Medicine. Philadelphia: Lippincott, 1981;173–180.
12. Gray ML. Functional Incontinence. In JM Thompson (ed), Clinical Nursing (2d ed). St. Louis: Mosby–Year Book, 1989.
13. Kim MJ, McFarland GH, McLane AM. Pocket Guide to Nursing Diagnoses (3d ed). St. Louis: Mosby–Year Book, 1989.
14. Gray M, Siegel SW, Troy R, et al. Management of Urinary Incontinence. In DB Doughty (ed), Urinary and Fecal Incontinence: Nursing Management. St. Louis: Mosby, 1991;95–150.

11 Stress Incontinence Due to Pelvic Descent

Jack L. Rook

Stress urinary incontinence refers to leakage in response to physical exertion (jumping, exercise, and change of position), or increases in intra-abdominal pressure (coughing, sneezing). With this condition, the amount of urine lost varies from a few drops to gushes of urine that necessitate containment products. Stress incontinence is associated with either loss of structural support of the bladder neck and proximal urethra, or intrinsic sphincter dysfunction.[1,2] This chapter is devoted to a discussion of the former.

The pelvic floor muscles and ligaments support the lower urinary tract and reproductive organs. Pelvic descent results from weakness of the pelvic floor support structures. Factors that contribute to their weakening in women include childbearing (particularly with multiple or difficult deliveries), loss of circulating estrogen, and pelvic floor denervation. In both men and women, pelvic floor denervation due to peripheral neuropathy, pudendal nerve damage, sacral spine lesions, and cauda equina syndrome lead to decreased tone of the pelvic floor musculature. In addition, alpha-blocking medications (phenoxybenzamine, prazosin) may further aggravate pelvic descent by causing relaxation of the striated sphincter.[1]

The hypoestrogenic state of menopause or after total abdominal hysterectomy with oophorectomy can contribute to pelvic floor changes and pelvic descent. Estrogen benefits pelvic muscle tone and the compressive abilities of the sphincter mechanism. Loss of circulating estrogen also causes vaginal and urethral atrophic changes.[1]

Pathophysiology

Stress incontinence with pelvic descent occurs due to distortion of urethrovesical anatomy that causes loss of normal pressure transmission

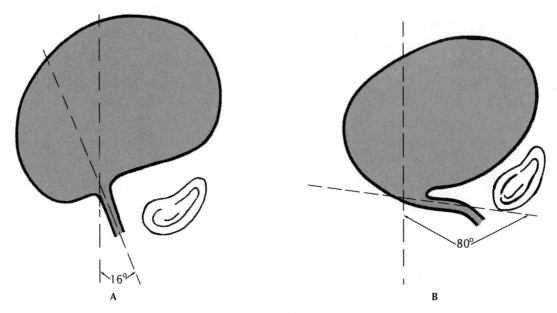

FIGURE 11.1 **(A)** *The normal female urethra exits the bladder at a 16-degree angle and follows a straight course to its meatus within the vaginal introitus.* **(B)** *Pelvic descent causes urethral excursion with loss of the normal 16-degree angle. This results in less efficient bladder outlet closure.*

from the abdomen to pelvis. The distorted urethrovesical anatomy adversely affects efficient closure of the urethral sphincter. Normally, the urethra exits the bladder at a 16-degree angle from the base of the bladder and follows a straight course to its meatus within the vaginal introitus. This anatomic course provides for optimal positioning of the circular and longitudinal urethral muscles, which during contraction, can effectively seal the urethra and prevent leakage (particularly when the bladder is stressed by physical exertion). Pelvic descent causes urethral excursion, loss of the 16-degree angle, and less efficient closure (Figure 11.1).[1]

With a healthy pelvic floor, the base of the bladder is flat and situated above the superior margin of the pubic symphysis (Figure 11.2).[3] The blad-

FIGURE 11.2 *With a healthy pelvic floor, the base of the bladder is situated above the superior margin of the pubic symphysis. The bladder neck and proximal urethra are well supported in this intra-abdominal position. This positioning helps to maintain continence as any increase in intra-abdominal pressure is transmitted equally to both the bladder* (large arrows), *and the bladder neck and proximal urethra* (small arrows).

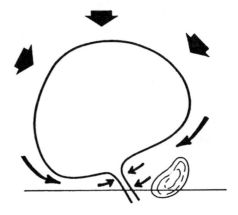

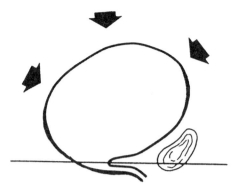

FIGURE 11.3   *With loss of support of the pelvic floor, the bladder positions itself outside of the abdominal cavity. When this occurs, increases in abdominal pressure are transmitted to the bladder (arrows), but not to the bladder neck and proximal urethra. This results in a sharp increase in intravesical pressure without a concomitant increase in urethral pressure, and leakage may ensue.*

der neck and proximal urethra are well supported in this intra-abdominal position. This positioning is important for continence because any increase in intra-abdominal pressure is transmitted equally to both the bladder and the bladder neck and proximal urethra. With loss of support, the pelvic floor descends and repositions the bladder neck and proximal urethra outside the abdominal cavity (Figure 11.3). When this occurs, increases in abdominal pressure (as occur with coughing, laughing, lifting, etc.) are transmitted to the bladder, but not to the bladder neck and proximal urethra. This results in a sharp increase in intravesical pressure without a concomitant increase in urethral pressure. Leakage may ensue.[2]

Stress incontinence caused by pelvic floor relaxation is classified as type I or II, according to the degree of pelvic descent demonstrated by video urodynamic studies. With type I stress incontinence, the bladder neck is closed at rest and situated at or above the inferior margin of the pubic symphysis. During stress, the bladder neck and proximal urethra descend less than 2 cm, open, and leakage occurs. In type II stress incontinence, the bladder neck is closed at rest and situated at or above the inferior margin of the pubic symphysis. During stress, however, it descends more than 2 cm, opens, and leakage occurs. A cystourethrocele occurs in this situation.[2]

History

The woman with type I or type II stress incontinence reports urinary leakage provoked by physical exertion, coughing, laughing, and sneezing. The leakage occurs without urgency to void. There may be symptoms of suprapubic pressure and low back pain aggravated by standing and walking and alleviated when lying down. This represents a referred pain from stretched sensory receptors within the pelvic floor musculature.

Patients with stress incontinence may report that their collection devices do not adequately contain the urinary leakage. Poor hygiene, impaired activities of daily living, and avoiding others (isolation) often occur with advanced incontinence.[1]

Physical Examination

In women with pelvic descent, physical examination of the pelvic floor reveals either a cystocele (bulging of bladder into the anterior vaginal vault), rectocele (bulging of rectum into the posterior vaginal vault), or uterine prolapse (migration of cervix and uterus into vagina). In addition, the postmenopausal, hypoestrogenic woman has dry, tender, nonrugated vaginal mucosa.[1]

Women with chronic incontinence may have moist, odorous perineal skin. A red, maculopapular rash with satellite lesions is characteristic of *Candida*, whereas pale, papillary lesions are seen with ammonia contact dermatitis. Collection devices and clothing may be noted to be moist or saturated.[1]

Diagnostic Studies

Urodynamics (Cystometrogram, Urine Flow Studies)

Urodynamic studies in patients with type I or II stress incontinence demonstrate characteristic features: The filling cystometrogram usually demonstrates normal capacity, compliance, and filling sensation. The detrusor appears stable. With long-standing disease, capacity and compliance may decrease; the voiding pressure study shows a normal but low-pressure contraction, a result of reduced bladder outlet resistance (Figure 11.4). Simultaneous uroflowmetry demonstrates an explosive flow pattern occurring concurrently with the filling cystometrogram low-pressure contraction. The pelvic floor electromyogram response is normal.[1]

Urethral Pressure Profile

Urethral pressure study may demonstrate reduced maximum closure pressure (less than 50 cm H_2O) and reduced functional length (less than 3 cm).[4]

Video Urodynamics

Video urodynamic studies of stress incontinence due to pelvic descent demonstrate urethral excursion (movement) with or without leakage on provocation. For example, coughing or increasing intra-abdominal pressure by bearing down provokes urethral excursion. Occasionally, the bladder descends below the inferior margin of the symphysis pubis even at rest, when the patient is upright. In contrast to the upright studies, the bladder contour appears normal when the patient is supine (Figures 11.5 and 11.6).[1]

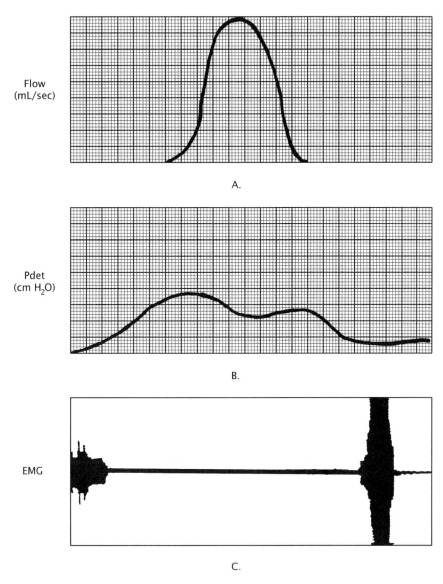

Flow
(mL/sec)

A.

Pdet
(cm H$_2$O)

B.

EMG

C.

FIGURE 11.4   *Urodynamic study in the patient with type I or type II stress urinary incontinence. (A) Uroflowmetry demonstrates an explosive flow pattern occurring concurrently with a (B) cystometrogram low-pressure contraction. (C) The simultaneous electromyogram (EMG) response is normal. (Pdet = detrusor muscle pressure.)*

Treatment

The goals of treatment for patients with stress urinary incontinence include prevention of urinary leakage if at all possible, urinary containment with proper skin care when continence is unobtainable, and preventing complications of uncontrolled stress urinary incontinences (cystitis, urinary tract infection, altered skin integrity, renal dysfunction, odor, shame, humiliation, and social isolation).[5]

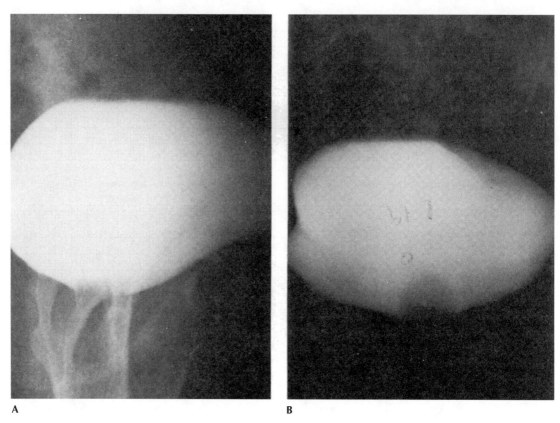

A   B

FIGURE 11.5   *Supine (A) and lateral (B) cystogram of a woman with normal pelvic support. (Reprinted with permission from MB Chancellor, JG Blaivas [eds]. Practical Neurology: Genitourinary Complications and Neurologic Disease. Boston: Butterworth–Heinemann, 1995;252.)*

Treatment for the patient with stress urinary incontinence (type I, type II) includes containment and skin care, pharmacologic management, pelvic muscle exercises, electrostimulation, pessary devices, and definitive surgical repair procedures.[1]

Containment and Skin Care

The patient should be prescribed an appropriate urinary containment device. The ideal containment product protects skin and clothing by completely absorbing leakage, minimizes odor, is not detectable under clothing, and is affordable. Initially, the collection device provides temporary relief for the patient, while more definitive management techniques are attempted to alleviate the incontinence.[1]

The patient with stress incontinence should try to void on a timed schedule. This helps to prevent leakage by preventing the bladder from reaching high urine volumes. In addition, the patient should avoid excessive fluid consumption with meals, which would likely produce unstable detrusor contractions and intensify frequency.[1]

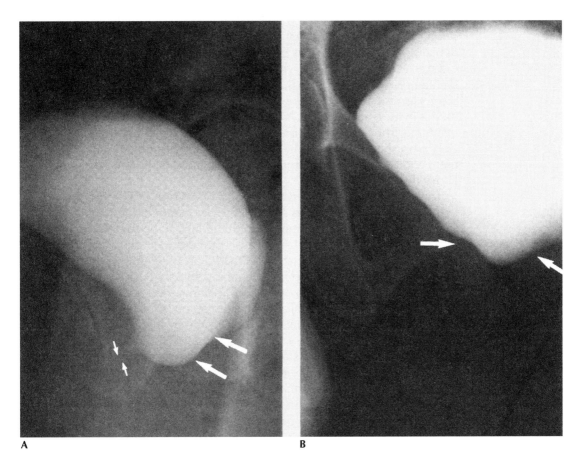

A   B

FIGURE 11.6   *Supine (A) and lateral (B) voiding cystourethrogram of a woman with a cystocele, urethrohypermobility, and genuine stress urinary incontinence (type II). Note the descent of the bladder neck (large arrows) on both A and B with Valsalva maneuver. The cystocele is noticeable on A (large arrows). The urethra is delineated with small arrows on B. (Reprinted with permission from MB Chancellor, JG Blaivas [eds]. Practical Neurology: Genitourinary Complications and Neurologic Disease. Boston: Butterworth–Heinemann, 1995;253.)*

All patients with incontinence should be instructed in the principles of skin care, including regular washing, complete drying, protecting skin with a moisture barrier, and use of a collection device. Candidal rashes are managed by routine skin care in conjunction with application of an antifungal cream or powder. Ammonia contact dermatitis (which occurs with prolonged exposure of the skin to urine) should be treated with regular cleansing of the skin with soap and water.[1]

Pharmacologic Management

Stress incontinence may also respond to pharmacologic manipulation. Alpha sympathomimetic agents, available over the counter and by prescription, palliate or eradicate leakage. These medications increase tone of the internal (smooth muscle) and rhabdosphincter. They should be taken only during daytime hours, as they have a stimulant effect, and before physically demanding activities such as exercise or walking.[1,5]

Over-the-counter alpha sympathomimetic preparations available include pseudoephedrine (Sudafed) and phenylpropanolamine (Dexatrim). Generic substitutes are available. Side effects of alpha sympathomimetics include tachycardia, hypertension, anxiety, nervousness, and insomnia. They should be used with caution in patients with hypertension, who should monitor their blood pressure after initiation of treatment and discontinue the drug promptly should their blood pressure rise above desired levels.[1,5,6]

These drugs are marketed as diet pills or decongestants, but they also help to increase urethral resistance and thus can benefit the patient with stress incontinence. The patient should be instructed to take the medication only during waking hours because of the drugs, stimulant effects, and because stress incontinence is rarely a problem during sleep.[5]

In some patients, exertion triggers an involuntary detrusor contraction, which in conjunction with pelvic floor incompetence causes the patient to void suddenly and uncontrollably. This condition is known as *stress-urge incontinence*. Stress incontinence complicated by this urge instability may be treated with imipramine, a tricyclic antidepressant. Imipramine relieves the symptoms of bladder instability (urgency, frequency, urge incontinence, and nocturia), and exerts a mild alpha-adrenergic effect that helps promote urethral closure. Imipramine is administered at 10–25 mg orally three to four times per day. Its side effects include drowsiness, urinary retention, dry mouth, constipation, hypertension, and mydriasis.[1,5]

Postmenopausal women with estrogen deficiency may be treated with topical or systemic estrogens. Long-term therapy is necessary for palliation of symptoms. Exogenous estrogens may alleviate stress urinary incontinence by promoting compression of urethral tissue and vascular cushion growth. This leads to more effective sphincter closure and greater integrity of the pelvic floor.[1,5,7]

Local (intravaginal) estrogen therapy can be administered as a cream (estradiol vaginal cream 0.01%) with an intravaginal dispenser. Dosage is 2–4 g per day for 1–2 weeks, followed by 1–2 g per day for the next 2 weeks. A maintenance dose of 1 g, one to three times per week, may be used after restoration of vaginal mucosa has been achieved.

Oral systemic estrogen therapy using estradiol, estradiol cypionate, and estradiol valerate can be administered orally at 1–2 mg per day with a cyclic regimen. Estrogen therapy is also available as a transdermal patch. Side effects include nausea, abdominal cramps and discomfort, constipation, headache, migraine, risk of thromboembolic disorders, and hypertension.[1,8,9]

Pelvic Muscle Exercise Program

Pelvic muscle exercises may alleviate or even cure stress incontinence by strengthening periurethral striated muscles of the sphincter mechanism.[10] The patient with stress incontinence due to pelvic floor weakness should be taught the Kegel pelvic muscle exercise program. When performing Kegel exercises, the patient should avoid contraction and relaxation of distant muscle groups. Several methods may be used to help the patient isolate the proper muscles while performing Kegel exercises, including the use of an intravaginal balloon, electrodes, or a nurse's gloved finger. A custom-designed intravaginal balloon that acts as a pressure transducer can be used to evaluate the efficiency and magnitude of circum-vaginal muscle contraction.[1,5,10,11] Likewise, a percutaneous needle electrode, needle, or patch electrodes placed at the anal sphincter or perineum can be used to assess contraction of pelvic floor and periurethral muscles. Last, a nurse may gently place a gloved finger in the anterior vaginal vault to assess contraction of the pelvic floor muscles, which causes opposition of the posterior and anterior vaginal walls.[5]

The patient should be provided with a schedule for a regular home Kegel exercise program, emphasizing both maximum strength and endurance. Pelvic muscle exercises produce long-term results only when maintenance programs are continued indefinitely.[1]

Electrostimulation

Electrostimulation can be used along with pelvic muscle exercises, using a transvaginal or transrectal route. It is particularly useful for women with markedly weak pelvic muscles. Stimulation and rest period duration, pulse frequency, pulse width, and duration of each session can be adjusted over time, as appropriate. The device should be used daily and the patient followed up regularly to evaluate progress.[1]

Pessary

Stress incontinence due to pelvic descent may also be managed by placement of an appropriate pessary, a ring-shaped, doughnut-shaped, spheric, or oblong device manufactured of rubber or some inert material, which can be placed within the vaginal vault to lend support to the pelvic floor.

A pessary may be used for those women with significant pelvic floor weakness and uterine prolapse who do not benefit from exercise regimens and are not candidates for surgery. When inserted correctly, it can be worn comfortably and may relieve symptoms of stress urinary incontinence without obstructing urinary flow. It does this by mechanically restoring a more normal urethrovesical position.

The pessary is successful only when cared for meticulously. It should be replaced as necessary. The principal complications of pessary use are erosion and local infection resulting from infrequent changes. Proper hygiene, regular replacement, and regular follow-up by experienced clinicians help prevent these complications.[1,5,12]

Surgery for Management of Urinary Incontinence

The role of surgery in the management of urinary incontinence may be considered when less-invasive forms of management have failed. Surgical treatment of types I or II stress incontinence is designed to relocate the bladder neck to a relatively fixed intra-abdominal position. Many surgical procedures that have evolved since the 1940s can accomplish this goal. The most commonly performed procedures for stress urinary incontinence are suprapubic repairs or combined suprapubic-transvaginal repairs. Suprapubic procedures include the Marshall-Marchetti-Krantz procedure, Burch colposuspension, and anterior urethropexy. Combined suprapubic-transvaginal procedures include the modified Pereyra bladder neck suspension, Stamey procedure, and Gittes procedure.[5]

With suprapubic procedures, a low abdominal transverse incision is made to gain access to the retropubic space, the bladder neck and urethra are identified, and the surgeon approximates and anchors the periurethral fascia of the vesicourethral junction to the cartilage of the posterior symphysis pubis (Marshall-Marchetti-Krantz procedure), to Cooper's ligament (retropubic colposuspension or Burch procedure), or to the periosteum of the symphysis pubis bone (anterior urethropexy).[1,5,13]

To perform the combined suprapubic/vaginal approach procedure, a vaginal incision is made, the vagina and urethra are carefully separated, and the urethra is mobilized to an intra-abdominal position by ligature carriers that are passed through a small abdominal incision made above the symphysis pubis. Next, the sutures are anchored to the abdominal rectus fascia. This procedure elevates the bladder neck to an intra-abdominal position.[1,5,14]

In general, the suprapubic and combined suprapubic-transvaginal repair procedures are equally effective, with both producing cures in approximately 90% of patients with stress incontinence. Complications of these procedures include urinary retention, wound infection, and urinary tract infection.[1,5,15]

References

1. Gray M. Urinary Incontinence/Voiding Dysfunction. In M Gray (ed), Genitourinary Disorders. St. Louis: Mosby, 1992;90–159.
2. Blaivas JG, Oliver L. Pathophysiology of Urinary Incontinence. In DB Doughty (ed), Urinary and Fecal Incontinence: Nursing Management. St. Louis: Mosby, 1991;23–46.
3. Blavias JG, Olsson CA. Stress incontinence: classification and surgical approach. J Urol 1988;139:727.
4. Webster GD. Urodynamic Studies. In MI Resnick, RA Older (eds), Diagnosis of Genitourinary Disease. New York: Thieme-Stratton, 1982;173–206.
5. Gray M, Siegel SW, Troy R, et al. Management of Urinary Incontinence. In DB Doughty (ed), Urinary and Fecal Incontinence: Nursing Management. St. Louis: Mosby, 1991;95–150.
6. Govoni LE, Hayes JE. Drugs and Nursing Implications. Norwalk, CT: Appleton-Century-Crofts, 1982.
7. Staskin DR, Zimmern PE, Hadley HR, Raz S. Pathophysiology of stress incontinence. Clin Obst Gynecol 1985;12:357.

8. Govoni LE, Hayes JE. Drugs and Nursing Implications. Norwalk, CT: Appleton-Century-Crofts, 1988.

9. Benness C, Abbott D, Cardozo L, et al. Lower urinary tract dysfunction in postmenopausal women: the role of estrogen deficiency. Neurol Urodyn 1991;10:315.

10. Dougherty MC, Bishop KR, Abrams RM, et al. The effect of exercise on the circum-vaginal muscles in postpartum women. J Nurse Midwifery 1989;34:8.

11. Dougherty MC, Abrams RA, McKey PA. An instrument to assess the dynamic characteristics of the circum-vaginal musculature. Nurs Res 1985;35:202.

12. Stanton SL. Vaginal Prolapse. In S Raz (ed), Female Urology. Philadelphia: Saunders, 1983.

13. Siegel SW, Montague DK. Surgery for Stress Urinary Incontinence. In BH Steward, AC Novick, SB Streem, JE Pontes (eds), Stewart's Operative Urology (2d ed, vol 2). Baltimore: Williams & Wilkins, 1989.

14. Barrett DM, Wein AJ. Voiding Dysfunction: Diagnosis, Classification and Management. In JY Gillenwater, JT Grayhack, SS Howards, et al. (eds), Adult and Pediatric Urology (2d ed). Chicago: Mosby–Year Book, 1991.

15. Spencer JR, O'Conor VJ, Schaeffer A. A comparison of endoscopic suspension of the vesical neck with suprapubic vesicourethropexy for treatment of stress urinary incontinence. J Urol 1987;137:411.

12   Stress Incontinence Due to Sphincter Incompetence

Jack L. Rook

The sphincter mechanism can be adversely affected by anatomic distortion caused by pelvic descent in women, directly damaged by surgical trauma in men, or by denervation of its muscular elements in both sexes.[1]

Intrinsic sphincter dysfunction in women is classified as type III stress incontinence. For these patients, the incontinence is not due to pelvic descent, but rather due to actual loss of sphincter function. With type III incontinence, the vesicle neck and proximal urethra remain open during filling, allowing for incontinence with little provocation. Active leakage may be noted when the patient is only standing, without coughing or straining. When the urethral sphincter mechanism is damaged and fails to close completely, urethral pressure is low, leakage occurs with only minimal activity, and the incontinence is often severe. Correct identification of sphincter damage in women is important because the management differs from the maneuvers used to treat pelvic descent.[1]

Urine leakage in men is referred to as *sphincteric incontinence*. Sphincteric incontinence may be caused by surgical procedures that damage the urethral sphincter, sphincter denervation, or both.[2]

Iatrogenic sphincter incompetence is a rare complication of transurethral resection of the prostate and an uncommon complication of radical prostatectomy procedures.[1,3] Transurethral resection of the prostate requires endoscopic incision and resection of obstructive prostatic tissue. In rare cases, inadvertent incision of the sphincter causes its incompetence, which contributes to stress urinary incontinence. Radical prostatectomy involves the surgical resection of the entire prostate and its capsule for treatment of cancer. Because this is a lifesaving procedure, partial resection of sphincter tissue may be necessary. It is the proximal urethral sphincter that is removed during this procedure. Therefore, continence after radical prostatectomy depends on preservation of the distal ureteral (striated) sphincter.[1,2,4–6]

Denervation of the pudendal nerve or lesions of the sacral micturition center (sacral cord levels 1 through 3) increase the risk of sphincter

TABLE 12.1   Causes of type III (sphincter incompetence) stress incontinence

Sphincter insufficiency (men)
    Rare complication of transurethral resection of the prostate
    Uncommon complication of radical prostatectomy
Pudendal nerve damage
    Anteroposterior resection of the rectum
    Radical prostatectomy
    Radical hysterectomy
    Pelvic radiation therapy
Lesions of the sacral spinal cord or its nerve roots (S1–S3)
    Spina bifida
    Low back injuries with cauda equina damage
    Spinal stenosis
    Herniated disk

incompetence and stress urinary leakage. Procedures that may potentially damage the pudendal nerve include abdominal-perineal resection of the rectum, prostatectomy, radical hysterectomy, and pelvic radiation therapy. Spina bifida defects often damage lumbosacral nerve segments, producing denervation of pelvic floor muscles with intrinsic sphincter dysfunction. Cauda equina abnormalities due to low back injuries (affecting bony segments T12 or lower) may also denervate muscular components of the sphincter mechanism (Table 12.1).[1,2]

History

Patients with incontinence due to sphincter incompetence complain of leakage caused by minimal physical exertion (walking, lifting, position changes), a frequent need to urinate, or a complete absence of voiding with continuous leakage into a containment device. Continuous leakage may cause perineal skin problems, including redness, rash, itching, and odor. Social isolation may occur due to the incontinence, odor, or reluctance or inability to participate in exertional activities that require interaction with others.[1]

Men with sphincter incompetence may have a history of prior prostatectomy (transurethral resection of the prostate). Surgical procedures that can lead to sphincter incompetence due to pudendal nerve injury include abdominal-perineal resection of the rectum and radical hysterectomy. Pelvic irradiation for prostate, rectal, gynecologic, or pelvic tumors could cause the sphincter to become fibrotic and rigid with associated incompetence. Low back trauma, lumbar disk herniation, or spina bifida defects could cause lumbosacral nerve root injury and denervation of the sphincter.

Physical Examination

Stress incontinence may be provoked by minimal exertion. The skin may be moist and odorous. Pelvic descent, cystocele, rectocele, or uterine prolapse may be seen on gynecologic examination, but is usually more commonly associated with type I or type II incontinence. With patients

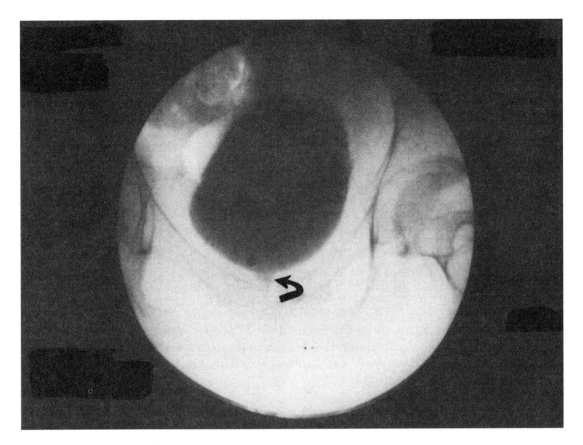

FIGURE 12.1   *Type III stress urinary incontinence of intrinsic sphincter deficiency. Note the open bladder neck during filling* (curved arrow). *(Reprinted with permission from MB Chancellor, JG Blaivas [eds]. Practical Neurology: Genitourinary Complications and Neurologic Disease. Boston: Butterworth–Heinemann, 1995;254.)*

who have impaired skin integrity, red, maculopapular rashes with satellite lesions represent candidal infection, whereas pale papillary lesions represent ammonia contact dermatitis.[1]

Urodynamic Studies and Videourodynamics

Urodynamic studies of sphincter incompetence demonstrate reduced cystometric capacity with stable detrusor activity. Stress urinary incontinence occurs with minimal exertion. The voiding-pressure study shows an explosive flow pattern (on uroflowmetry), with a low-pressure detrusor contraction characteristic of reduced bladder outlet resistance.

The urethral pressure profile study shows a profoundly low, maximum urethral closure pressure (20 cm H_2O or less).

Video urodynamics demonstrate a funneled (open) bladder outlet on upright cystogram during filling, with stress urinary incontinence provoked by minimal exertion. Pelvic descent and urethral hypermobility are absent with type III incontinence (Figure 12.1).[1]

TABLE 12.2   Treatment of stress incontinence due to sphincter incompetence

Appropriate containment device
Skin care
    Regular wash and dry
    Skin sealant
    Appropriate collection device
    Antimonilial cream or powder
Alpha sympathomimetic pharmacologic agents
Physical therapy
    Pelvic muscle exercises
    Electrostimulation
Surgical procedures
    Pubovaginal sling
    Artificial urinary sphincter
    Periurethral injection therapy

Treatment

The treatment of stress incontinence due to sphincter incompetence includes containment, skin care, pharmacologic management with alpha sympathomimetic drugs, physical therapy, electrical stimulation, and, if necessary, surgery (Table 12.2).

Containment

The patient with type III incontinence should use an appropriate containment device. After containment is achieved, the patient should be encouraged to seek a more definitive management program for urinary leakage. The ideal urinary collection device protects skin and clothing by completely absorbing leakage.[1]

Skin Care

The patient should be taught proper procedures to maintain skin integrity, including regular cleansing with complete drying. Moisture barriers, skin sealants, and collection devices offer some protection from exposure to urinary leakage.

Routine skin care and local application of an antimonilial cream or powder manage candidal rashes. Ammonia contact dermatitis occurs as a result of prolonged exposure of the skin to urine. Regular washing and drying, a moisture barrier or skin sealant, and a collection device help to minimize exposure.[1]

Pharmacologic Management

The patient with type III incontinence may require alpha sympathomimetic medications to stop or minimize urinary leakage. The alpha sympathomimetic agents increase sphincter closure by stimulating urethral smooth muscle and the rhabdosphincter, ablating urinary leakage in mild cases, but, more commonly, reducing the severity of leakage.[1]

Physical Therapy and Electrical Stimulation

Physical therapy and electrical stimulation are noninvasive interventions used to strengthen the pelvic floor musculature. Their effect on stress incontinence related to sphincter incompetence remains unclear. However, a trial of such therapy may be appropriate for the patient who does not wish to undergo surgical repair or pharmacologic management. Pelvic muscle exercises alleviate stress incontinence through active strengthening of pelvic floor muscles, whereas electrical stimulation passively exercises the periurethral muscles.[1]

Surgical Procedures

A number of surgical procedures are available to help restore normal support for the bladder neck and proximal urethra in women with type I and type II stress incontinence. The goal of these procedures is to allow the bladder neck to maintain an intra-abdominal position during stress maneuvers.

For women with type III stress incontinence, simple restoration of pelvic floor support is usually ineffective. Surgical procedures that provide urethral compression become necessary, the most common being the pubovaginal sling, in which a small fascial "sling" is created to provide urethral compression. Surgical treatment options for the male patient with sphincteric incontinence include artificial urinary sphincter implantation and periurethral injection therapy.[7]

Pubovaginal Sling Procedure

For the pubovaginal sling procedure, a strip of anterior rectus fascia is harvested through a transverse abdominal incision. The fascial defect is then closed. The rectus fascia is used to create a fascial sling that is positioned around the bladder neck through a midline vaginal incision. The limbs of the sling are then pulled through the retropubic space and anchored to the anterior rectus fascia above the pubic bone.

Postoperatively, the sling tension should be sufficient to obstruct the urethral outlet during rest, yet allow voiding when appropriate. Typically, when the patient performs a stress maneuver, the abdominal muscles tighten, thus, tightening the sling and preventing stress incontinence. During voiding, the abdominal muscles relax, alleviating tension on the sling, and voiding commences.[7,8]

Complications of the pubovaginal sling procedure include urinary retention, wound infection, and urinary tract infection.[1]

Artificial Urinary Sphincter Implantation

A second alternative for management of intrinsic sphincteric incompetence in women, and the principal procedure available for men, is implantation of an artificial urinary sphincter.[9,10] The artificial urinary sphincter

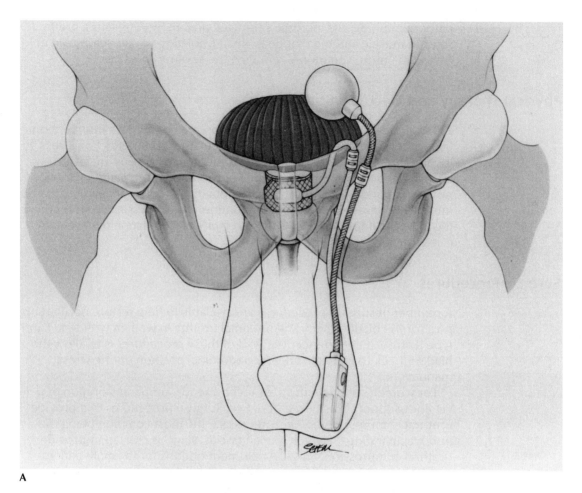

A

FIGURE 12.2 *The American Medical Systems, Inc., Sphincter 800 urinary prosthesis has three principal components, including an abdominal balloon reservoir, a periurethral cuff, and a pump mechanism. The cuff is placed near the bladder neck or bulbus urethra in men (**A** and **B**), and near the bladder neck in woman (**C**). (Courtesy of American Medical Systems, Inc., Minnetonka, MN. Medical Illustrations by Michael Schenk.)*

(AUS) is a urologic prosthetic device with three principle components: an abdominal balloon reservoir, a periurethral cuff, and a pump mechanism (Figure 12.2). The cuff is placed near the bladder neck or bulbous urethra in men and near the bladder neck in women. The device works by directing fluid through a silicone-tubing network from the cuff to the abdominal reservoir and back again. Candidates for the AUS procedure must have appropriate mobility to toilet, dexterity to manipulate the device, and motivation to proceed with surgery and lifelong follow-up.[1,7]

The pump mechanism of the AUS is placed in the scrotum in men or underneath the labia in women. The balloon reservoir is placed in the prevesical space and the cuff around the bladder neck. The pump mechanism is capable of transferring fluid between the balloon reservoir and the cuff. To establish continence, the cuff self-inflates over a period of 3–5

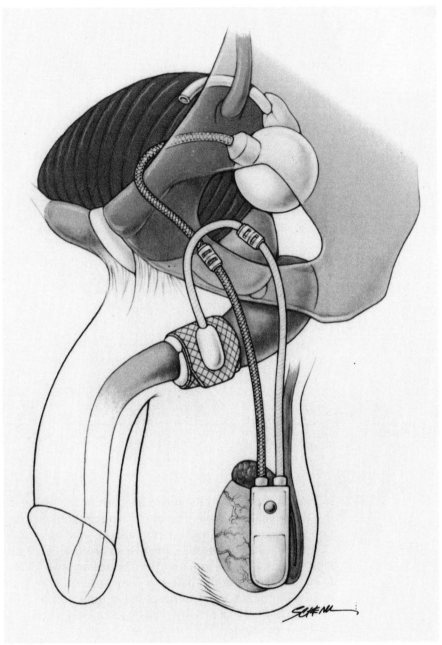

B

FIGURE 12.2 *Continued*

minutes. The cuff, placed at the bladder neck, is designed to occlude the urethra when inflated. Appropriate fit of the cuff, is critical to the effectiveness of the device. Several cuff sizes are available, allowing custom fitting for each patient during surgery.[1,7,11,12]

The AUS operates by mechanical compression of the urethra, which substitutes for the damaged muscular elements. Before bladder evacuation, the

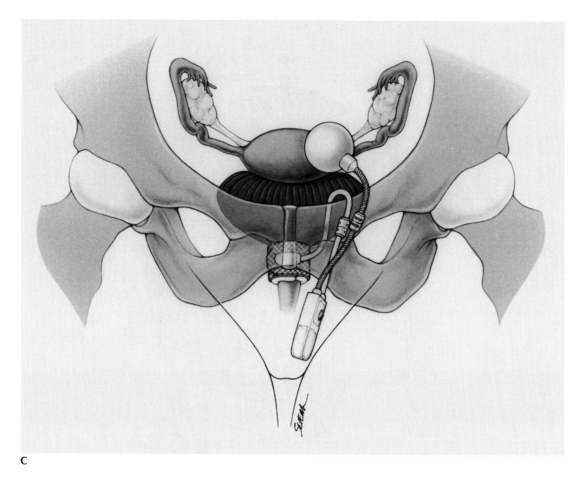

C

FIGURE 12.2 *Continued*

individual compresses the pump mechanism, diverting fluid from the cuff to the abdominal reservoir, thus decreasing urethral pressure. Bladder evacuation is then accomplished by spontaneous voiding or via catheter.[1]

Implantation of the AUS improves continence for most patients. Even with successful AUS implantation, however, stress leakage may result from excessive bladder filling or vigorous exertion. Removal is most often necessitated by complications such as infection or erosion, or both. Modifications of normal activity may be necessary, such as modified seating for bicycle riding.[1,7,11,13]

Contraindications to the AUS procedure include patients who lack the dexterity required to operate the pump mechanism, uncontrolled detrusor hyperreflexia, compromised bladder wall compliance, and vesicoureteral reflux. Preoperative workup is directed toward identification of these contraindications. It should include a history and physical, intravenous pyelogram, cystoscopy, voiding cystourethrogram, cystometrogram with electromyography, urinary flow studies, assessment of postvoid residual volume, and a psychological evaluation. If such testing confirms the patient's candidacy, AUS implantation may proceed.[1,7]

Periurethral Injection Therapy

Periurethral injection therapy uses bulking agents (collagen or Teflon) to reduce urethral caliber and prevent leakage. The indication for this procedure is stress incontinence due to sphincter incompetence. The agents are injected transurethrally or transperitoneally using local anesthesia with or without systemic sedation. Because of potential for a hypersensitivity response to semisynthetic collagen, a skin test is given before periurethral injection. The urologist uses a cystoscope to visualize the urethral lumen while the material is injected circumferentially beneath the urethral wall. The injections continue until the urethral lumen appears to be obstructed through the cystoscope.[1,7,14-16]

The major advantages of periurethral injection therapy over surgical procedures are that it is less invasive; the balking agents are injected, and no incision is required; the procedure is completed on an outpatient basis; and repeat injection can be done within the next 30 days if the initial treatment does not restore continence.[1]

Complications of periurethral injection therapy include persistent or recurrent stress incontinence and transient urinary retention. Occasionally, the urinary retention may be long term, requiring chronic intermittent catheterization. Stress urinary incontinence may recur several years post procedure as collagen is reabsorbed. Reinjection may be required.

Contraindications to periurethral injection include type I or II stress incontinence, detrusor hyperreflexia, and hypersensitivity to the injection substance.[1]

References

1. Gray M. Urinary Incontinence/Voiding Dysfunction. In M Gray (ed), Genitourinary Disorders. St. Louis: Mosby, 1992;90–159.
2. Blaivas JG, Oliver L. Pathophysiology of Urinary Incontinence. In DB Doughty (ed), Urinary and Fecal Incontinence: Nursing Management. St. Louis: Mosby, 1991;23–46.
3. Wheatley JK. Causes and treatment of bladder incontinence. Comp Ther 1983;9:27.
4. Chilton CP. The Distal Urethral Sphincter Mechanism and the Pelvic Floor. In AR Mundy, TP Stephenson, AJ Wein (eds), Urodynamics: Principles, Practice, and Application. Edinburgh: Churchill Livingstone, 1984.
5. Worth PHL. Postprostatectomy Incontinence. In AR Mundy, TP Stephen, AJ Wein. Urodynamics: Principles, Practice, and Application. Edinburgh: Churchill Livingstone, 1984.
6. Hadley R, Zimmern P, Raz S. Surgical Treatment of Urinary Incontinence. In S Yalla, E McGuire, A Elbadawi, J Blaivas (eds), Neurology and Urodynamics: Principles and Practice. New York: MacMillan, 1988.
7. Gray M, Siegel SW, Troy R, et al. Management of Urinary Incontinence. In DB Doughty (ed), Urinary and Fecal Incontinence: Nursing Management. St. Louis: Mosby, 1991;95–150.

8. McGuire EJ, B Lytton. Pubovaginal sling procedure for stress incontinence. J Urol 1978;199:82.
9. Fishman IJ, Shabsigh R, Scott FB. Experience with the artificial urinary sphincter model AS800 in 148 patients. J Urol 1989;141:307.
10. Scott FB. The use of the artificial sphincter in the treatment of urinary incontinence in the female patient. Urol Clin North Am 1985;12:305.
11. Faller NA, Vinson RK. The artificial urinary sphincter. J Enterost Ther 1985;12:7.
12. Goldwasser B, Furlow WL, Barrett D. The model AMS800 artificial urinary sphincter: Mayo Clinic experience. J Urol 1987;137:668.
13. Scott FB. The artificial urinary sphincter: experience in adults. Urol Clin North Am 1989;16:105.
14. Shortliffe LMD, Freiha FS, Kessler R, Stamey TA, et al. Treatment of urinary incontinence by the periurethral implantation of the glutaraldehyde lined collagen. J Urol 1989;141:538.
15. Politano VA. Periurethral polytetrafluoroethylene injection for urinary incontinence. J Urol 1982;127:439.
16. Kaufman M, Lockhart JL, Silverstein MJ, Politano VA. Transurethral polytetrafluoroethylene injection for post prostatectomy urinary incontinence. J Urol 1984;132:463.

13   Instability Incontinence

Jack L. Rook

Disease or trauma affecting the spinal cord above the sacral micturition center (S2–S4) results in detrusor muscle instability with loss of normal bladder sensations. This can cause instability (reflex) incontinence, with leakage without warning signals of sensory urgency.[1]

Suprasacral spinal cord lesions result in loss of voluntary control of micturition, as well as a loss of bladder-sphincter coordination due to interruption of the pontine-sacral axis. However, the parasympathetic and somatic reflex arcs between the bladder and sacral cord are maintained. Thus, the bladder may contract spontaneously, via the sacral parasympathetic reflex arc, at low volumes or in response to stimuli such as exposure to cold or stroking perineal skin. Simultaneously, the external sphincter may contract, because the somatic reflex arc innervating the pelvic floor remains intact, whereas the neural pathways that control sphincter relaxation (from the brain and pons to the sacral cord and external sphincter) have been lost (Figure 13.1). This condition is known as *detrusor external sphincter dyssynergia* or *detrusor sphincter dyssynergia* (DSD).[1,2]

DSD refers to the loss of coordination between the striated sphincter mechanism and the detrusor muscle. The "dyssynergic" sphincter fails to relax during micturition, causing bladder outlet obstruction, increased intravesical pressure, and urinary retention. During this uncoordinated voiding, the intravesical pressure may rise to extremely high levels. When high pressure voiding remains untreated, upper urinary tract deterioration ensues secondary to the development of vesicoureteral reflux.[1,2]

The etiology of suprasacral spinal cord injury (SCI) includes trauma, multiple sclerosis, atherosclerotic vascular disease with spinal cord infarction, cervical or thoracic spondylosis, spina bifida defects, transverse myelitis, and other related conditions. Suprasacral SCI due to these various disorders can result in detrusor instability without sensations of bladder filling and DSD.[1]

Upper urinary tract distress may occur as a complication of instability incontinence when it is associated with DSD. Specifically, pyelone-

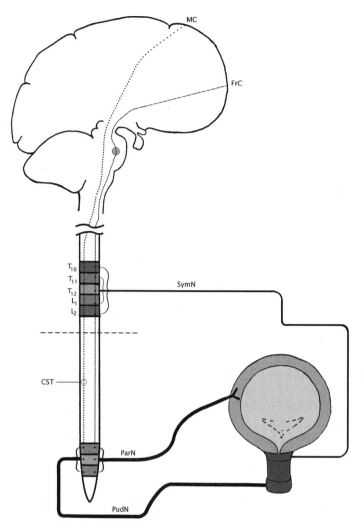

FIGURE 13.1   *Suprasacral spinal cord lesions* (dashed line) *result in loss of voluntary control of micturition, as well as a loss of bladder sphincter coordination. The bladder may contract spontaneously, via the sacral parasympathetic reflex arc (ParN), even at low volumes. The external sphincter may contract simultaneously, as the somatic reflex arc (PudN) innervating the pelvic floor musculature remains intact. Neural pathways to inhibit micturition and sphincter relaxation have been lost (SymN) as a result of the suprasacral spinal cord lesion. This condition is known as* detrusor sphincter dyssynergia. *(MC = motor cortex; FrC = frontal cortex; CST = corticospinal tract.)*

phritis, vesicoureteral reflux, upper urinary tract dilatation, hydronephrosis, and compromised renal function may result from dyssynergia and instability incontinence.[1] Compromised renal function occurs when chronic infection or hydronephrosis causes permanent renal parenchymal scarring.

Autonomic dysreflexia may also occur in association with instability incontinence.[3] *Autonomic dysreflexia* refers to the sudden, massive sympathetic nervous system firing that occurs with high thoracic or cervical SCI in response to noxious stimuli occurring below the spinal lesion.

Bladder distension and high-pressure detrusor contractions are the most common cause of dysreflexia. Signs and symptoms occurring with this massive neural sympathetic discharge include elevated blood pressure (to potentially dangerous levels), a pounding headache, tachycardia with palpitations, pupillary dilatation, and anxiety.[1]

Other complications of reflex incontinence include altered skin integrity, shame, humiliation, and social isolation.[1]

History

The patient with instability incontinence reports frequent, uncontrolled bladder evacuation without sensations of urgency. Voiding stream may be intermittent. Because of the SCI, mobility is affected, and some quadriplegic patients may have difficulty manipulating clothing. Signs and symptoms of a current urinary tract infection may be reported, including foul-smelling urine and fever.[1]

The incontinent patient may report social isolation. Some high-level (upper thoracic) paraplegic and quadriplegic patients may report symptoms of autonomic dysreflexia, including sudden onset of diaphoresis, a pounding headache, palpitations, and anxiety. Last, the patient may report rashes and perineal skin lesions, which are related to chronic urine exposure.[1]

Physical Examination

Physical examination of the patient with an upper motor neuron SCI reveals hyperreflexia, paraparesis or quadriparesis, sensory loss, mobility problems, and, with quadriplegic patients, varying degrees of upper extremity weakness.

The perineal skin may be moist and odorous, with compromised integrity. If the patient is seen during an episode of autonomic dysreflexia, there is severe hypertension, diaphoresis (above the level of the injury), and tachycardia.[1]

Diagnostic Studies

Urodynamics, cystometrogram and electromyogram, in reflex incontinence demonstrates small cystometric capacity, high detrusor pressure during contraction, unstable detrusor contractions, and dyssynergia on sphincter electromyogram (Figure 13.2).[1]

Fluoroscopy during a dysreflexia contraction demonstrates funneling of the bladder neck with narrowing of the membranous urethra in men and mid urethra in women. Bladder trabeculations, diverticula (herniation of bladder mucosa through muscular wall), and vesicoureteral reflux (retrograde movement of contrast from bladder to ureters and kidney) may be present (Figures 13.3 and 13.4).[1,4]

Imaging studies of the upper urinary tract, including the intravenous pyelogram or intravenous urogram, may demonstrate ureteral dilatation

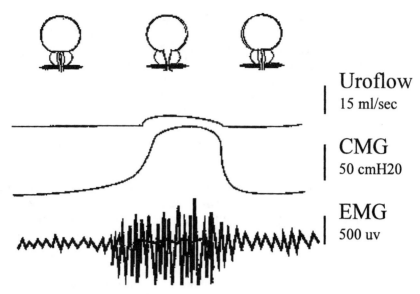

FIGURE 13.2   *Urodynamics in reflex incontinence demonstrate high detrusor pressure during contractions on cystometry, dyssynergia on sphincter electromyogram (EMG), and poor urine flow. (CMG = cystometrogram.) (Reprinted with permission from MB Chancellor, JG Blaivas [eds]. Practical Neurology: Genitourinary Complications and Neurologic Disease. Boston: Butterworth–Heinemann, 1995;79.)*

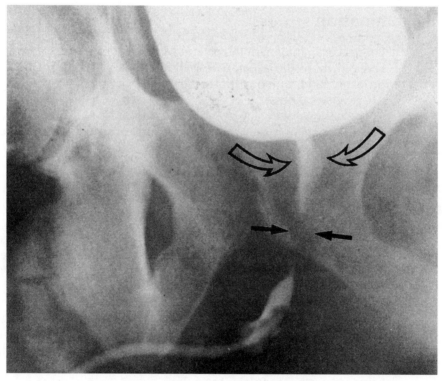

FIGURE 13.3   *Combined voiding cystourethrogram and retrograde urethrogram in a C7 quadriplegic patient demonstrate detrusor sphincter dyssynergia without bladder neck obstruction. The straight arrows denote the narrowed external sphincter; the curved arrows point to the open bladder neck. (Reprinted with permission from Chancellor MB, Blaivas JG [eds]. Practical Neurology: Genitourinary Complications and Neurologic Disease. Boston: Butterworth–Heinemann, 1995;314.)*

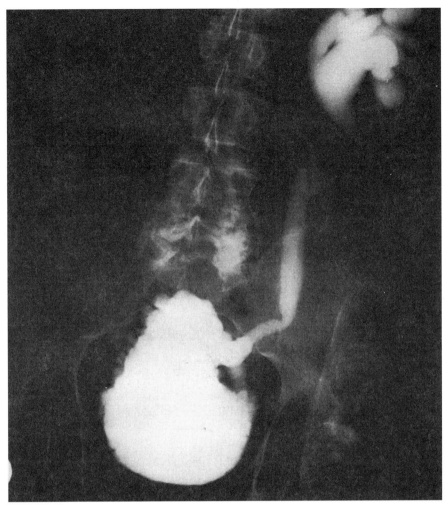

FIGURE 13.4   *A 19-year-old paraplegic patient managed with a condom catheter and admitted with left pyelonephritis. Urodynamic evaluation revealed detrusor hyperreflexia with detrusor external sphincter dyssynergia. On this voiding cystourethrogram, a classic "Christmas tree" neurogenic bladder with trabeculation and diverticula formation was found. In addition, high-grade left vesicoureteral reflux was apparent. The patient was started on anticholinergic agents and switched to intermittent catheterization. He was noncompliant with the medication and frequency of catheterization and developed recurrent pyelonephritis; he subsequently underwent intestinal bladder augmentation and left ureteral reimplantation. (Reprinted with permission from MB Chancellor, JG Blaivas [eds]. Practical Neurology: Genitourinary Complications and Neurologic Disease. Boston: Butterworth–Heinemann, 1995;305.)*

of one or both collecting systems; hydronephrosis and parenchymal damage is suggested by delayed accumulation of contrast within the kidney(s) during the nephrogram phase of the urogram.[1]

Radionuclide studies may demonstrate focal renal scarring, and serum laboratory studies demonstrate abnormal blood urea nitrogen and creatinine in untreated late-stage disease.[1]

TABLE 13.1 Treatment of instability (reflex) incontinence

Administer antispasmodic agents in conjunction with an intermittent catheterization program.

In men, condom catheter drainage with pharmacologic sphincterotomy using alpha blockers.

Routine evaluation of upper urinary tract function.

Prevention and management of complications (urinary tract infection, altered skin integrity, and autonomic dysreflexia).

If necessary, indwelling suprapubic or urethral urinary catheter.

When conservative treatment fails, or the medications cannot be tolerated, surgical management is an alternative. Surgical techniques available for management of this condition include

    Sphincterotomy with condom catheter containment in men

    Augmentation enterocystoplasty and an intermittent catheterization program

    Urinary diversion with a pouch containment device[1]

SOURCE: Adapted from Gray M. Instability (Reflex) Incontinence. In M Gray (ed), Genitourinary Disorders. St. Louis: Mosby, 1992;90–159.

Treatment

Treatment goals for the patient with the reflex incontinence should include[1,2]

1. Protection of the upper urinary tract by eliminating the high-pressure obstructed voiding caused by DSD
2. Prevention of instability incontinence by teaching the patient how to regularly evacuate his or her bladder
3. Prompt management of urinary tract infections
4. Maintaining skin integrity
5. Prompt management of autonomic dysreflexia
6. Prevention of social isolation

General management of patients with instability incontinence is summarized in Table 13.1.

Antispasmodic Medication and Intermittent Catheterization

Initial treatment of instability incontinence should include an intermittent catheterization program with pharmacotherapy using either a calcium channel blocking drug or tricyclic antidepressant in combination with an antispasmodic agent. Calcium channel blockers and tricyclic antidepressants both act synergistically with antispasmodics to inhibit unstable detrusor contractions.[1]

Clean intermittent catheterization is usually the best bladder management program for patients with reflex incontinence and dyssynergia. This technique ensures complete, regular bladder emptying. It is associated with an acceptably low rate of urinary tract infection, particularly when compared to indwelling catheter drainage. A clean intermittent catheterization schedule of four times during waking hours is considered ideal, although more frequent catheterization may be required. Antispasmodic pharmacotherapy helps ablate unstable contractions and leakage between catheterizations. The antispasmodics also help prevent unstable, high-pressure bladder contractions that can stress the upper urinary system.[1,5,6]

Alpha Blockers and Condom Drainage

Males whose incontinence cannot be controlled by clean, intermittent catheterization and antispasmodic agents, or who cannot catheterize themselves because of physical disability (i.e., the quadriplegic patient with decreased dexterity), may manage their bladders with a program of reflex voiding with condom drainage. Such a program is feasible only for patients who do not have DSD, or for those with DSD that can be controlled by medications or surgical sphincterotomy.[5]

Alpha-adrenergic blocking agents may be used to reduce urethral sphincter resistance. These medications reduce obstruction caused by vesicosphincteric dyssynergia by decreasing muscle tone in the bladder neck, proximal urethra, and rhabdosphincter.[1,5]

Alpha-blocking drugs include phenoxybenzamine (Dibenzyline), prazosin (Minipress), and terazosin (Hytrin). These medications selectively block $alpha_1$-adrenergic receptors of bladder neck, prostatic urethra, and rhabdosphincter, thus preventing the muscle contraction that would be induced by receptor binding of the adrenergic neurotransmitter, norepinephrine. Alpha blockers are used to reduce the obstruction produced during DSD. Medication titration may be required and nighttime (hs) administration is recommended to avert side effects, which include fatigue, postural hypotension, and rhinitis.

Dosage for phenoxybenzamine is 10–20 mg at hs; prazosin, 1–10 mg at hs; and terazosin, 1–10 mg at hs.[1,7]

Routine Evaluation of the Urinary Tract

All patients with reflex incontinence should have an annual upper urinary tract evaluation. These patients are at high risk for complications such as infection (caused by bacteria introduced into the bladder during intermittent catheterization), bladder stones (which can occur with immobility), and vesicoureteral reflex, all of which may contribute to upper urinary tract decompensation. An intravenous pyelogram, urinalysis, and serum renal electrolytes should be performed annually as part of this evaluation.[2,8]

Prevention and Management of Complications

The patient with reflex incontinence must be instructed how to monitor for and respond to complications associated with his or her bladder dysfunction and bladder management program, including cystitis, pyelonephritis, impaired skin integrity, and autonomic dysreflexia.

The patient must be taught to recognize symptoms of urinary tract infection, including cloudy, concentrated urine, the presence of blood or sediment in urine, or recurrent leakage in the face of a previously stable bladder program. Signs of serious infection involving the kidneys include a temperature greater than 100°F, nausea and vomiting, and flank or back discomfort. A lower urinary infection may lead to pyelonephritis and sepsis if left untreated. However, the presence of asymptomatic bacteriuria is the rule among individuals with instability incontinence managed by intermittent catheterization. Attempts to maintain continuously sterile urine in these patients only leads to colonization of the bladder with resistant organisms. Therefore, asymptomatic bacteriuria should be tolerated among these patients and suppressive or prophylactic anti-infective drug therapy used sparingly.[1,5]

Ascending infection from the urethra is the most common cause of a symptomatic lower urinary tract infection. The use of clean catheters and collection bags along with good perineal hygiene helps reduce the number of bacteria available to invade the reflex neurogenic bladder. Adequate fluid intake helps flush the urinary system, promoting mechanical movement of bacteria away from the kidneys.[1]

Impaired skin integrity related to chronic exposure to urine may be treated with an appropriate urinary collection device, which protects skin by absorbing leakage and minimizing urine contact. Maintenance of skin integrity relies on regular cleansing, complete drying, and the frequent use of moisture barriers or skin sealants, which offer some protection from exposure to urinary leakage.[1]

Collection Devices

Condom Drainage Device

The male patient who is not a candidate for intermittent catheterization should obtain and use an appropriate condom drainage device (assuming appropriate drainage has been achieved pharmacologically or through surgical sphincterotomy). The ideal condom device is easy to put on, forms a watertight seal, and readily drains without kinking or twisting at its distal end. This drainage device should remain in place continuously. A temporary indwelling catheter is indicated for these patients when skin integrity is compromised.[1]

Routine skin care and local application of an antifungal cream or powder manage candidal rashes. Ammonia contact dermatitis, resulting from prolonged exposure of the skin to urine, requires regular, complete drying; use of a moisture barrier or skin sealant; and a collection device to minimize exposure.[1]

The high thoracic paraplegic or quadriplegic patient should be able to recognize the signs and symptoms of autonomic dysreflexia, including a pounding headache, diaphoresis, palpitations, and a rapid pulse. When this occurs, the patient or caretaker must quickly move the patient to an upright position, which may temporarily reduce blood pressure. Antihypertensive drugs are required to relieve the severe hypertension associated with this disorder.[1] Sublingual preparations (nifedipine [Procardia]) have a faster onset of action than oral agents.

Autonomic dysreflexia can be triggered by noxious stimuli emanating from the bladder. Bladder distention with frequent unstable contractions is a common, readily reversible cause of dysreflexia. Other noxious stimuli resulting from chronic incontinence, such as pressure sores, may precipitate dysreflexia.[1]

Indwelling Catheter

Women with instability incontinence may require indwelling catheters, as currently there are no suitable external collection devices for women. Indwelling catheters seem to cause fewer problems in women as compared to men with a chronic indwelling catheter. In men, a temporary indwelling catheter is indicated when skin integrity is compromised.[1,2,9]

Transurethral Sphincterotomy

Transurethral sphincterotomy is indicated for men with instability incontinence and vesicosphincteric dyssynergia that does not respond to conservative management. Sphincterotomy is the surgical incision of the urethral sphincter using a transurethral approach. The membranous urethra is visualized endoscopically, and an incision is made. After the procedure, a three-way catheter with bladder irrigation is left in place temporarily to provide hemostasis and to prevent or evacuate clots from the bladder. After healing, the patient receives instruction on the use of, and is provided with, an appropriate condom catheter and leg bag.[1,2]

Bladder Augmentation

Surgical enlargement or augmentation of a small capacity, hyperreflexic bladder is an alternative to urinary diversion.[10] Patients having bladder augmentation are hospitalized preoperatively for bowel preparation and antibiotic prophylaxis. After the patient has been given a general anesthetic, a midline incision is made and a segment of intestine, such as the ascending colon, is isolated on its vascular pedicle. The intestinal segment is then fashioned as a pouch that is sutured to the bladder to increase its storage capacity (Figures 13.5–13.7).[5,11]

Postoperatively, prolonged use of a suprapubic or Foley catheter is usually necessary to prevent bladder distension until healing is complete. Because the intestinal pouch produces mucus, intermittent bladder irrigation may be necessary to prevent obstruction from a mucous plug. Other possible complications include anastomotic breakdown and urinary fistulae. Many patients who have had a bladder augmentation procedure require long-term intermittent catheterization to empty the bladder efficiently.[5]

Urinary Diversion

Construction of an ileal conduit is a major abdominal surgical procedure. Preoperatively, the patient must be hospitalized for a bowel preparation and

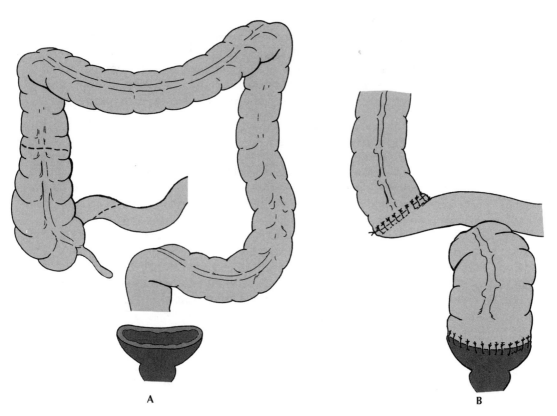

FIGURE 13.5   *With the bladder augmentation procedure, a segment of intestine, such as the ascending colon (A), is isolated on its vascular pedicle and the intestinal segment is fashioned as a pouch (B) that is sutured to the bladder to increase its storage capacity. (Modified from AC Novick. Augmentation Cystoplasty. In AC Novick, SB Streem, JE Pontes [eds]. Stewart's Operative Urology [2d ed]. Baltimore: Williams & Wilkins, 1989.)*

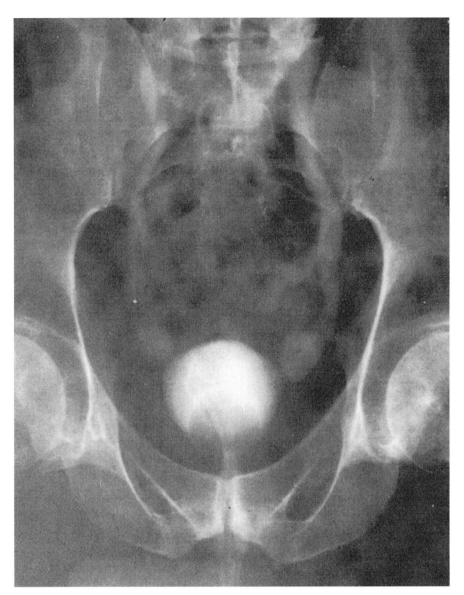

FIGURE 13.6   *End-stage neurogenic bladder in a paraplegic man managed with a long-term indwelling urethral catheter. Bilateral vesicoureteral reflux was seen on the cystometrogram. The bladder capacity was only 75 ml. The patient underwent a bladder augmentation cystoplasty procedure. (Reprinted with permission from MB Chancellor, JG Blaivas [eds]. Practical Neurology: Genitourinary Complications and Neurologic Disease. Boston: Butterworth–Heinemann, 1995;329.)*

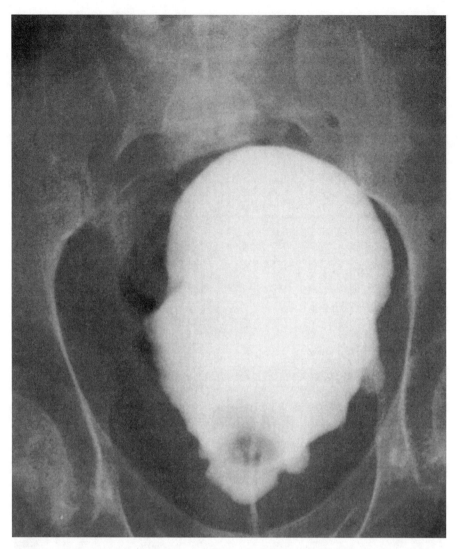

FIGURE 13.7 *Cystogram after the bladder augmentation procedure of the same patient as in Figure 13.6. Bladder capacity 1 month postoperatively was 350 ml, and bilateral ureteral reflux spontaneously resolved. The bladder capacity after 6 months was 600 ml. (Reprinted with permission from MB Chancellor, JG Blaivas [eds]. Practical Neurology: Genitourinary Complications and Neurologic Disease. Boston: Butterworth–Heinemann, 1995;330.)*

intravenous antibiotics. During the procedure, a segment of terminal ileum is isolated through a midline abdominal incision. The proximal end of the ileal segment is sutured closed, and the ureters, which are removed from the bladder, are anastomosed to it. Antirefluxing anastomoses of the ureters are included to protect the upper urinary tracts. The distal end of the ileal segment is brought to the abdominal wall to form a stoma (Figure 13.8).[5,12]

Disadvantages of an ileal conduit include deterioration of the upper tracts, which is known to occur over time, and the need to wear an external urine collection appliance, which some patients find undesirable.[5]

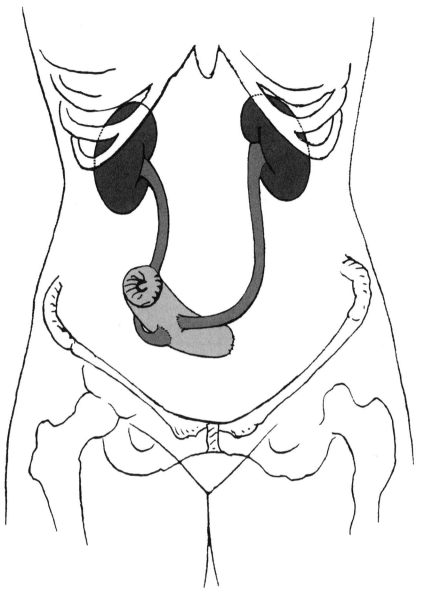

FIGURE 13.8 *For construction of an ileal conduit, a segment of terminal ilium is isolated, the proximal end of the ileal segment is sutured closed, and the ureters, which are removed from the bladder, are anastomosed to it. The distal end of the ileal segment is brought to the abdominal wall to form a stoma.*

References

1. Gray M. Instability (Reflex) Incontinence. In M Gray (ed), Genitourinary Disorders. St. Louis: Mosby, 1992;90–159.
2. Blaivas JG, Oliver L. Pathophysiology of Urinary Incontinence. In DB Doughty (ed), Urinary and Fecal Incontinence: Nursing Management. St. Louis: Mosby, 1991;23–46.

3. McGuire TJ, Kramer VN. Autonomic dysreflexia in the injured spinal cord: What the physician should know about this medical emergency. Postgrad Med 1986;80:81.

4. Blaivas JG, Chancellor MB. Catheterization Management. In MB Chancellor, JG Blaivas (eds), Practical Neurourology: Genitourinary Complications in Neurologic Disease. Boston: Butterworth–Heinemann, 1995;299–308.

5. Gray M, Siegel SW, Troy R, et al. Management of Urinary Incontinence. In DB Dougherty (ed), Urinary and Fecal Incontinence: Nursing Management. St. Louis: Mosby, 1991;95–150.

6. Lapides J, et al. Further observations on self-catheterization. Trans Am Assoc Genitourinary Surg 1975;67:15.

7. Govoni LE, Hayes JE. Drugs and Nursing Implications. Norwalk, CT: Appleton-Century-Crofts, 1988.

8. Amis ES, Blaivas JG. Neurogenic bladder simplified. Radiol Clin North Am 1991;29:571.

9. Lloyd LK. New trends in urologic management of spinal cord injured patients: Voiding dysfunction in patients with neurological disease. AUA Home Study Course, American Urological Association, 1988;Series XI[1]:27.

10. Linder A, Leach GE, Raz S. Augmentation cystoplasty in the treatment of neurogenic bladder dysfunction. J Urol 1983;129:491.

11. Novick A. Augmentation Cystoplasty. In A Novick, S Streem, J Pontes (eds), Stewart's Operative Urology (2d ed, vol 2). Baltimore: Williams & Wilkins, 1989.

12. Broadwell D. Principles of Ostomy Care. St. Louis: Mosby–Year Book 1982.

| 14 | **Storage Problems Caused by Involuntary Detrusor Contractions** |

Jack L. Rook

Involuntary detrusor contractions (detrusor instability, uninhibited contraction) are the most common cause of storage problems. In this condition the bladder contracts involuntarily during filling. Normally, the bladder does not contract unless the patient is trying to void, usually occurring when its volume nears capacity. Involuntary detrusor contractions are not volume dependent—that is, they may occur with any amount of urine in the bladder. Such contractions are not under voluntary control. They may occur spontaneously or may be provoked by rapid bladder filling, alterations in posture, and coughing.[1]

The symptoms that occur with involuntary contractions include urinary frequency, urgency, and urge incontinence. Patients with involuntary detrusor contractions may perceive each contraction as an urge to void (urgency). Once aware of the contraction, some patients are able to maintain continence by contracting the external urinary sphincter. Those without sufficient external sphincter closure are incontinent (urge incontinence). Still others are completely unaware of the contraction and simply void uncontrollably. These patients typically have cerebral dysfunction and are said to have uninhibited contractions.[1]

Causes

Bladder instability may be caused by bladder outlet obstruction, bladder inflammation, cerebral neurologic conditions, or unknown factors.

Bladder Outlet Obstruction

Uninhibited contractions may occur in association with bladder outlet obstruction. Urodynamic studies of patients with symptomatic benign prostatic hypertrophy (BPH) frequently reveal involuntary detrusor contractions. These patients commonly have symptoms of frequency, urgency, and urge incontinence typical of bladder instability.[1]

Inflammatory Bladder Conditions

Uninhibited contractions may also occur due to inflammation of the bladder wall. Urinary tract infection, bladder calculi, environmental or chemical irritants (i.e., some chemotherapeutic agents), and tumors are possible causes of inflammation. Inflammation increases irritability of the detrusor, precipitating involuntary contractions.[1]

Neurologic Conditions That Cause Loss of Inhibition

Normal voiding is voluntarily controlled by the cerebral cortex. With normal cerebrocortical function, voiding can be delayed, thus enabling the patient to maintain continence until he or she reaches a bathroom. The frontal cortex sends inhibitory messages to the pontine micturition center.[1,2] Neurologic lesions that damage the cortex (stroke, multiple sclerosis, Alzheimer's disease, and Parkinson's disease) may cause the loss of this ability to inhibit, resulting in involuntary contractions in conjunction with coordinated relaxation of the sphincters and pelvic floor, and incontinence.[1] Involuntary contractions caused by neurologic lesions are termed *uninhibited bladder*.

Idiopathic Bladder Instability

Some patients have bladder instability with no discernible cause. In these situations, the detrusor instability and involuntary contractions are termed *idiopathic*.[1]

History

The history of a patient suspected of having instability incontinence should include questions geared toward finding the etiology and contributing factors of the condition. The clinician should delineate whether the patient has urgency with continence, incontinence after urgency, or incontinence without urgency (as in stroke patients).

The patient should be questioned concerning conditions associated with bladder irritation. Patient responses may be consistent with a history of BPH, stones, or urinary tract infection (see Chapters 16 and 9, respectively, for details).

Patients with uninhibited bladder contractions have a history of some neurologic condition with cerebrocortical involvement, such as stroke, multiple sclerosis, or a neurodegenerative disorder (Parkinson's or Alzheimer's disease).

The patient may be taking medications that could worsen underlying urge incontinence. For example, alpha-blocking agents weaken urinary sphincters, contributing to incontinence due to involuntary contractions. Diuretics may provoke urge incontinence in susceptible patients due to rapid bladder filling.

The patient's food and fluid intake should be discussed. A history of bolus or excessive fluids, caffeinated beverages, and alcohol consumption, all could contribute to or worsen instability or urge incontinence. Alcohol can cause polyuria, frequency, urgency, sedation, immobility, and delirium.

Physical Examination

In men with BPH, rectal examination reveals the enlarged prostate.

Neurologic examination may reveal findings characteristically seen with cerebrovascular accident, Parkinson's disease, or Alzheimer's disease, all of which can be associated with uninhibited bladder contractions. The stroke patient's examination may demonstrate hemiparesis, cognitive impairment, hyperreflexia, and spasticity. Mobility or dexterity problems may be identified that can further aggravate the incontinence caused by uninhibited bladder contractions. Parkinsonian patients demonstrate tremor, mobility problems, and cognitive impairment (30% of these patients progress to an Alzheimer-like dementia). Skin evaluation may demonstrate candidal rashes or ammonia contact dermatitis.

Urodynamics

The filling cystometrogram usually demonstrates the presence of involuntary contractions for patients with detrusor instability or an uninhibited bladder. In particular, rapid bladder filling tends to precipitate a premature involuntary contraction in patients with detrusor irritability. The patient with an uninhibited bladder disorder also demonstrates premature detrusor contractions. However, uninhibited contractions are not associated with detrusor muscle irritability.

On cystometrogram, voluntary and involuntary (detrusor instability, uninhibited) contractions appear similar. Both contractions demonstrate similar pressure curves, and both produce urine flow. The only way to distinguish between a voluntary and involuntary contraction is to ask the patient during the study to indicate when he or she is trying to void.[1]

Treatment

Treatment options for patients with incontinence caused by involuntary detrusor contractions are conservative in nature. The goals of management of urge incontinence are to reduce bladder instability and improve bladder control. Treatment options include elimination of bladder irritants, prompted voiding programs, controlling fluid intake, electrostimulation, biofeedback, and exercises to strengthen the pelvic floor, and pharmacologic management.[3]

Elimination of Bladder Irritants

Bladder irritants can contribute to urinary frequency and incontinence. They should be eliminated as part of the bladder control program. Common irritant factors include urinary tract infections, bladder calculi, caffeinated or citrus beverages, and bubble bath preparations. The patient should be assessed for evidence of potential bladder irritants, and appropriate measures should be taken to eliminate them.[3]

Prompted Voiding Programs

Patients with urge incontinence should have an appropriate prompted voiding regimen in which he or she is asked to void "by the clock." After the clinician determines how long the patient can realistically postpone voiding, the individual is taught to void volitionally, at predetermined intervals, before leakage occurs.[3]

Fluid Control

Controlling fluid intake complements bladder-voiding regimens. With an appropriate fluid control regimen, beverages are consumed throughout waking hours, so that the patient prone to involuntary contractions is not forced to cope with large fluid volume over brief time periods. The patient is advised to maintain a fluid intake of 1.0–2.5 liters per day, to abstain from drinking more than 8 oz of fluids with meals, to sip liquids between meals, and to discontinue fluid consumption 2 hours before bedtime to alleviate nocturia.[3]

Electrostimulation, Biofeedback, and Pelvic Floor Exercises

Biofeedback therapy is sometimes used in conjunction with a pelvic floor exercise program. The strength of a pelvic muscle contraction is measured (through the use of patch electrodes on the perineum, or an intravaginal electrode in women), and the information is displayed so the patient can "visualize" the strength of his or her pelvic musculature contraction.[3] By continually attempting to increase the biofeedback response, a progressive strengthening of the pelvic floor ensues.

Electrical stimulation of the sphincter muscle is also used to strengthen the pelvic floor musculature and to help control unstable contractions. Electrostimulation is performed by placing a rectal or intravaginal probe that generates electrical pulses that act to contract and relax the pelvic floor and sphincter muscles. Sessions can be performed in the clinic or at home, last approximately 20 minutes, and can be repeated daily.[3,4]

Exercises that strengthen the pelvic floor (with or without biofeedback therapy) and electrical stimulation are effective in reducing leakage caused by involuntary detrusor contractions for a variety of reasons. Repeated contractions of the pelvic floor muscles strengthen their tone and contractility. Additionally, contraction of pelvic floor muscles reflexively inhibits detrusor muscle contractility. Electrostimulation also causes inhibition of the unstable detrusor contractions. Biofeedback therapy facilitates teaching the patient to suppress unstable bladder contractions by contracting the pelvic floor muscles.[3,5]

Pharmacologic Management

Antispasmodic or anticholinergic medications may be used in the management of patients who do not respond adequately to electro-stimulation, biofeedback, or pelvic floor exercises. These agents act by decreasing contractility and irritability of the bladder, thereby reducing symptoms of frequency, urgency, and urge incontinence, and increasing bladder capacity through reduction of bladder contractility. Various drugs may be used alone or in combination. Some patients are unable to tolerate the side effects of a particular drug and must discontinue its use before an effective dosage is reached. Pharmacologic management is most effective when used in conjunction with prompted voiding, controlled fluid intake, and a pelvic floor strengthening program.[3]

Anticholinergic Drugs

Stimulation of cholinergic receptors mediates bladder contractility. Anticholinergic agents inhibit detrusor contractility and may delay or reduce the amplitude of involuntary contractions, thus increasing functional bladder capacity.[2,3]

Propantheline (Pro-Banthine) is the most commonly used anticholinergic agent in the treatment of urge incontinence with detrusor instability. The usual dosage is 15–30 mg by mouth three times per day. It should be used with caution in patients with glaucoma, heart disease, hiatal hernia, high blood pressure, intestinal blockage, kidney disease, liver disease, lung disease, myasthenia gravis, prostatic hypertrophy, thyroid disease, ulcerative colitis, or urinary retention.

Common side effects of all anticholinergic agents include dry mouth, dry eyes, blurred vision, increased intraocular pressure, and constipation. With higher dosages, or in elderly patients receiving other drugs with anticholinergic effects (e.g., antidepressants or antipsychotics), propantheline can cause delirium, mental confusion, orthostatic hypotension, and tachycardia. Elderly patients usually require a lower therapeutic dose. The side effects of propantheline tend to decrease as the patient becomes accustomed to the medication.[3,5]

Direct Smooth Muscle Relaxants

Smooth muscle relaxants act directly on detrusor musculature, thereby reducing its contractility. They also have mild anticholinergic effects.

Oxybutynin (Ditropan) Oxybutynin (Ditropan) has a pronounced direct muscle relaxant effect. However, its level of anticholinergic action is also considered to be moderate to high. Oxybutynin is indicated in the management of patients with instability (urge or reflex) incontinence. The recommended dosage is 2.5–5.0 mg by mouth two to three times a day. Side effects profile and patient precautions are the same as those for propantheline.[3,6–8]

Dicyclomine (Bentyl) Dicyclomine (Bentyl) has both anticholinergic actions and direct smooth muscle relaxant effects. Oral dosage is 10–20 mg three times per day. The anticholinergic side effects most commonly seen are blurred vision, dry mucosa, headache, increased sensitivity to light, insomnia, and confusion. Contraindications and patient precautions are the same as those for propantheline.[3,6–8]

Flavoxate (Urispas) Flavoxate (Urispas) counteracts detrusor muscle contractility by cholinergic blockade and by a direct smooth muscle relaxant effect. In addition, it provides some local anesthesia and analgesia. The recommended adult dosage is 100–200 mg orally three to four times daily. This drug is contraindicated in patients with gastrointestinal obstructive lesions, ileus, or hemorrhage, or obstructive uropathies of the lower urinary tract. Flavoxate should be used with caution in patients with glaucoma. Its side effects include nausea and vomiting, dry mouth, nervousness, vertigo, headache, mental confusion (especially in elderly patients), blurred vision, and tachycardia. Driving and hazardous activities should be avoided if dizziness or drowsiness do occur.[3,6–8]

Imipramine (Tofranil) Imipramine (Tofranil) is a tricyclic antidepressant that produces systemic anticholinergic actions. Imipramine exerts a direct inhibitory effect on detrusor muscle. Imipramine is the only tricyclic antidepressant that has been used in the treatment of bladder instability. The usual dosage is 25–50 mg orally, three times daily. Contraindications include convulsive disorders, prostate hypertrophy, and the recovery phase of myocardial infarction. Side effects are the same as those for other anticholinergic agents. In addition, the patient must be observed for postural hypotension, sedation, and ventricular arrhythmias.[3,6–8]

References

1. Blaivas JG, Oliver L. Pathophysiology of Urinary Incontinence. In DB Doughty (ed), Urinary and Fecal Incontinence: Nursing Management. St. Louis: Mosby, 1991;23–46.
2. Amis ES, Blaivas JG. Neurogenic bladder simplified. Radiol Clin North Am 1991;29:571.
3. Gray M, Siegel SW, Troy R, et al. Management of Urinary Incontinence. In DB Doughty (ed), Urinary and Fecal Incontinence: Nursing Management. St. Louis: Mosby, 1991;95–150.
4. Eriksen BC, Bergmann S, Eik-Nes SH. Maximal electrostimulation of the pelvic floor in female idiopathic detrusor instability and urge incontinence. Neurourol Urodyn 1989;8:219.
5. Lindstrom S, Fall M, Carlsson CA, Erlandson BE. The neurophysiological basis of bladder inhibition in response to intravaginal electrical stimulation. J Urol 1983;129:405.
6. Romanowski GL, Shimp LA, Balson AB, Cahn MI. Urinary incontinence in the elderly: etiology and treatment. Drug Intel Clin Pharm 1988;22:525.

7. Olin BR. Professional's Guide to Patient Drug Facts. Philadelphia: Lippincott, 1990.
8. Skidmore-Roth RL. Mosby's 1990 Nursing Drug Reference. St. Louis: Mosby–Year Book, 1990.

15   Overflow Incontinence Due to Impaired Detrusor Contractility

Jack L. Rook

Incontinence may result from conditions that cause urinary retention, occurring when the bladder becomes so overfilled that urine leaks out. The primary causes of urinary retention are urethral obstruction with increased outflow resistance and insufficient detrusor contractility.[1] Chronic urinary retention is the inability to evacuate the bladder completely. Micturition occurs, but some urine remains in the bladder, resulting in more frequent attempts to empty the bladder and predisposing the individual to complications including urinary tract infection (UTI), pyelonephritis, vesicoureteral reflux, compromised renal function, and lithiasis.[2] Dribbling, overflow incontinence with frequent urination, compromised force of stream, and nocturia are the presenting symptoms of urinary retention.

Bladder outlet obstruction principally affects men. Prostatic outlet obstruction in men manifests as prostatitis, benign glandular hypertrophy, or prostate cancer. The outlet obstruction caused by benign prostatic hypertrophy and prostate cancer are discussed in detail Chapters 16 and 19. Bladder outlet obstruction is relatively uncommon in women. Women may experience obstruction because of urethral distortion from pelvic descent.[2]

In contrast to obstruction, deficient detrusor contractility affects both women and men. Transient detrusor deficiency can be traced to a reversible cause. Transient causes of urinary retention due to deficient contractility include medications (antispasmodic drugs, antidepressant drugs, opioids, psychotropic drugs, antiparkinsonian drugs, recreational drugs including hallucinogens and cannabis, and calcium channel blockers), constipation or fecal impaction, hysterical retention, or urinary retention associated with immobility or acute illness or acute overdistention injury.

Chronically deficient contractility is usually traced to a neurological condition that may or may not be reversible. Chronic causes of urinary retention include spinal injury of the sacral nerve roots (due to trauma, herniated disk, or spinal stenosis), peripheral neuropathies (diabetes mellitus, chronic ethanol abuse), or cauda equina syndrome. Urinary retention caused by deficient detrusor contractility adversely affects the urinary system. Incomplete bladder evacuation causes urinary stasis and contributes to bladder ischemia, increasing the risk of UTI.[2]

This chapter discusses loss of detrusor contractility due to a neurologic lesion. This condition is also known as *detrusor areflexia*. The patient with impaired detrusor contractility is unable to effectively empty his or her bladder, has a weak urinary stream, and experiences a feeling of incomplete emptying.[2]

Detrusor areflexia is most commonly caused by a neurologic process or injury that affects the lumbar or sacral nerve roots. The nerve fibers that innervate the bladder and sphincter mechanism exit the spinal cord at the lumbosacral level. Interruption of these pathways results in a denervated, acontractile bladder with loss of voluntary sphincter control. However, in most cases of detrusor areflexia, the bladder neck and sphincter remain closed. Conditions that may result in detrusor areflexia include:

- Herniated intervertebral disks in the lumbosacral spine
- Diabetic neuropathy
- Lesions or tumors of the lumbosacral cord with associated spinal cord injury (SCI)
- Pelvic surgery such as radical hysterectomy or abdominal perineal resection of the rectum (which on rare occasions may be associated with pelvic or pudendal nerve damage)

Damage to the pelvic plexus impairs bladder contractility, whereas damage to the pudendal nerve compromises voluntary control of the external sphincter.[1,3]

Neurogenic bladder dysfunction should be suspected when other symptoms of neurological disease are present, when disorders of bowel or sexual function coexist with urinary retention, or when a systemic disease exists that may be associated with neurological dysfunction (such as diabetes mellitus).

History

History of Lower Motor Neuron Bladder Dysfunction

Patients with urinary retention due to deficient detrusor contractility report poor or intermittent force of urinary stream, with a combination of urgency to void, yet hesitancy to initiate stream. All patients experience sensations of incomplete bladder evacuation. Irritative symptoms including urgency, diurnal urinary frequency (more often than q2h), and nocturia (more often than one episode per night) may occur.

Patients with retention have increased potential for UTI. Signs and symptoms of UTI include dysuria, foul-smelling urine, pyuria, fever, and chills.[2]

History of Peripheral Neuropathic Process

Patients with advanced peripheral neuropathy may also have bladder symptoms, including poor force of stream, difficulty initiating voiding, and overflow incontinence. Chronic constipation may occur concomitantly due to autonomic nerve involvement, and pudendal nerve damage may result in decreased sphincter tone with soiling of underwear. Sexual dysfunction may also occur due to the autonomic neuropathic process.

The history should include questions to help delineate the etiology of the peripheral neuropathic process. Diabetes mellitus, tabes dorsalis, chronic alcoholism, or exposure to toxic substances can all contribute to chronic nerve damage.

Typically, patients with peripheral neuropathy complain of sensory dysesthesias including numbness and tingling or burning paresthesias in the distal extremities. Extremity weaknesses such as foot dragging, unsteady gait, and decreased grip are motor manifestations.

History of Cauda Equina Syndrome

The patient's history may reveal a traumatic event that compromised the integrity of the spinal column, resulting in SCI. For example, a large traumatically induced herniated disk may cause a cauda equina injury. Such patients complain of radicular symptomatology involving one or both legs; bowel, bladder, or sexual dysfunction; and leg weakness, numbness, and paresthesias.

Patients with severe spinal stenosis may also develop a polyradiculopathy that resembles a cauda equina syndrome. These patients are described as having neurogenic claudication, with lower extremity pain on standing or walking that tends to decrease when they sit down. This problem should be differentiated from vascular claudication due to peripheral vascular disease. Patients with lumbar spinal stenosis complain of numbness in their feet or paresthesias. They tend to have weakness and atrophy of the lower extremity musculature. In contrast, the upper extremities are not involved. There may or may not be a history of low back pain.

Physical Examination

A brief neurological examination including evaluation of anal sphincter tone; genital and perineal sensation; and motor, sensory, and reflex activity of the lower extremities may disclose abnormalities that suggest an areflexic neurogenic bladder as the cause of the patient's urological symptoms. The neurological examination may help further differentiate the underlying cause of detrusor areflexia (i.e., lower motor neuron bladder secondary to peripheral neuropathy versus secondary to cauda equina injury).

Physical Examination for Peripheral Neuropathy

The motor examination in advanced peripheral neuropathy demonstrates atrophy of distal musculature, usually in all four extremities. In the upper extremities, it involves the hand intrinsic musculature, and in the lower extremities, foot intrinsic and calf musculature appear wasted. An associated decrease in motor strength occurs in the distal extremities. Sensory examination demonstrates decreased sensation in a stocking or glove distribution. Other sensations, including proprioception and temperature, are decreased.

Reflexes in early neuropathy tend to be diminished distally, affecting the lower extremities before the upper extremities. Over time, as the condition worsens, a global decrease in reflexes occurs.

With respect to gait, patients may develop a sensory ataxia. They can ambulate with their eyes open, but they cannot walk safely with their eyes closed because of lost proprioception.

Rectal examination may demonstrate decreased sphincter tone and a decreased anal wink reflex.

Patients may demonstrate difficulty initiating urinary stream and straining during urination with contraction of abdominal musculature. Poor force of stream may be due to weak detrusor contractions. Postvoid urinary residual volume often exceeds 25% of total bladder capacity (sum of voided volume and residual urinary volume).

Patients who have a urinary infection have foul-smelling urine, fever, and systemic illness. With ascending infection (pyelonephritis), flank pain may be elicited.

Physical Examination of the Patient with Cauda Equina Spinal Cord Injury

Sensory examination reveals a complete or incomplete sensory level in patients who have cauda equina syndrome.

On motor examination, the cauda equina injured patient has profound muscle atrophy and weakness that ranges from mild to complete paralysis below the level of the lesion. Tone is decreased, with no spasticity.

Reflexes are either decreased or absent. Plantar reflexes are equivocal.

Gait occurs with great difficulty with incomplete SCI. With complete lumbar-sacral SCI involvement, gait is only possible with long leg braces and crutches. Otherwise, mobility requires a wheelchair.

Rectal examination reveals decreased anal tone and strength on contraction. Bulbocavernosus reflex and anal wink are also decreased or absent.

On bladder evaluation, these patients have difficulty initiating urination, and they may require abdominal muscle contraction (Credé's maneuver) to void. The postvoid urinary residual volume exceeds 25% of total bladder capacity. Foul-smelling urine, fever, and signs of systemic illness may accompany urinary infections. With ascending infection, fever and flank pain occur.

Urodynamics

The normal bladder contracts strongly enough and long enough to empty its contents with a normal pattern of urinary flow. When detrusor contractility is impaired, the cystometrogram pattern demonstrates a low magnitude detrusor contraction, and the accompanying flow rate is low. Although diagnostic criteria have not been clearly established for this condition, a maximum detrusor pressure of 30 cm H_2O or less associated with a urinary flow rate less than 12 ml per second suggests a diagnosis of impaired detrusor contractility. The preceding discussion has dealt with impaired contractility caused by a neuropathic injury. A similar pattern of impaired contractility can also result from chronic distension.[1,4]

Electrodiagnostic Studies

Peripheral Neuropathy

The electrodiagnostic evaluation is important in the evaluation of suspected peripheral neuropathy. Early disease findings include prolongation of distal motor and sensory latencies in all four extremities, prolongation of F-waves, and prolongation of H-reflexes in the lower extremities. The lower extremities tend to be involved before the upper extremities, as the lower extremity distal-most peripheral nerves are further from the trunk.

With advanced peripheral neuropathy, slowing of all nerve conduction velocities (NCVs), absence of sensory nerve action potentials, absence of H-reflexes in the lower extremities, and decreased amplitude and temporal dispersion of the motor unit action potentials (MUAPs) and sensory nerve action potentials occur.

The electromyogram in late-stage disease demonstrates decreased insertional activity, an incomplete interference pattern on volitional testing, and possibly denervation potentials.

Lumbar Radiculopathy

Significant electrodiagnostic findings in lumbar radiculopathy include electromyographic evidence of lower extremity denervation potentials in a particular nerve root distribution(s) corresponding to the nerve rootlet(s) involved. In addition to the extremity denervation, the finding of ipsilateral paraspinal musculature denervation potentials confirms that nerve root irritation or damage is occurring at the spinal level.

Most motor NCVs and MUAPs are within normal limits. With an L5 radiculopathy, the peroneal NCV may be below normal and the extensor digitorum brevis MUAP may be diminished. In contrast, lower extremity sensory NCVs and SNAP amplitudes are normal as the sensory ganglion lies within the neural foramen, a distance from the site of compression. Last, with an S1 radiculopathy, there is prolongation or absence of the ipsilateral H-reflex.

Spinal Stenosis

The electrodiagnostic studies for spinal stenosis are fairly characteristic for this disorder. NCVs tend to demonstrate slowing of lower extremity conduction velocities with normal upper extremity NCVs. This suggests a polyradiculopathy involving only the lumbosacral nerve roots. The electromyogram may show diffuse and scattered denervation potentials involving both lower extremity and the paraspinal musculature.

Back Imaging Workup

Lumbar x-rays are useful in demonstrating degenerative changes that may contribute to radiculopathy or spinal stenosis. Instability may be seen with flexion and extension x-ray views of the lumbar spine. Such movement may cause entrapment of lumbosacral (cauda equina) nerve roots.

Computed tomography is useful in demonstrating spinal stenosis, both lateral recess and central. It also shows bony degenerative changes and herniated disks, which may be compromising nerve roots.

Magnetic resonance imaging is also useful in demonstrating spinal stenosis, degenerative changes, herniated disk(s), or tumor with nerve impingement or cauda equina involvement.

Myelography is useful to demonstrate impingement of nerve roots. Myelograms are performed with the patient upright as opposed to magnetic resonance imaging and computed axial tomography, which require the patient to be studied while supine. Therefore, myelography is a more physiological test, as it maximizes the effect of gravity on the intervertebral disks. Myelography is useful in demonstrating nerve impingement at a particular level(s). Knowing the appropriate level of involvement is critical in preparing for surgical intervention.

Laboratory Data

The complete blood cell count, urinalysis, and urine culture and sensitivity are laboratory tests useful in determining the presence of a UTI. Microscopic inspection of the urinary sediment may help delineate whether the infection involves the upper urinary tract (i.e., the presence of white blood count casts indicate renal involvement).

Treatment

Treatment options for patients with overflow incontinence due to impaired detrusor contractility include conservative toileting and fluid control programs, administration of medications, and clean intermittent catheterization (Table 15.1).[5]

Conservative Measures

The patient with urinary retention should be taught the technique of double voiding: The patient voids, then waits three to five minutes before voiding again. Double voiding improves the voided volume by allowing the detrusor to contract, relax, and rest, and then contract again. This

TABLE 15.1 Treatment of overflow incontinence due to impaired detrusor contractility

Conservative measures used in treating urinary retention
    Double voiding
    Recognize and treat urinary tract infection
    Timed schedule of voiding
    Fluid control program
Pharmacologic treatment of deficient detrusor contractility
    Cholinergic medication (bethanechol)
    Alpha-adrenergic blocking agents
Catheterization
    Clean intermittent catheterization
    Indwelling catheter (last resort)

technique may significantly reduce urinary retention in patients with deficient contractility.[2]

The patient must be able to recognize signs and symptoms of a UTI (foul-smelling urine, suprapubic or lower back pain, hematuria, dysuria, fever, or chills) and should seek prompt treatment if these symptoms occur. A UTI may worsen existing mild to moderate retention, causing a more severe acute urinary retention. Local UTI leads to systemic disease unless appropriately managed.[2]

The patient with deficient detrusor contractility and diminished sensations of filling should void on a timed schedule, every 3–4 hours. Timed voiding prevents bladder overdistension that further exacerbates the already deficient detrusor contractility among individuals with peripheral neuropathies.[2]

A fluid control program should also be instituted. Spacing fluids throughout the day helps to avoid bladder overdistension that may exacerbate symptoms of retention and reduces the risk of UTI.[2]

Pharmacologic Treatment of Deficient Detrusor Contractility

Patients with deficient detrusor contractility may benefit from a cholinergic medication. Detrusor contractility is mediated by stimulation of cholinergic (parasympathetic) receptors. Drugs that are agonists of these receptors can enhance bladder contraction and facilitate bladder emptying.[5]

Bethanechol chloride is a cholinergic analog that may improve bladder evacuation among some patients with deficient contractility. However, it is contraindicated when retention is caused by obstruction. The dosage is 10–30 mg by mouth three times daily. Side effects include bradycardia, postural hypotension, bronchoconstriction, increased secretion of gastric acid, and gastrointestinal discomfort. The patient should promptly notify the physician concerning any serious side effects such as severe dizziness or difficulty breathing.[2,5,6]

Alpha-adrenergic blocking agents may also help the patient with deficient detrusor contractility by relaxing the smooth muscles of the bladder neck, prostatic urethra, and rhabdosphincter. These drugs may be used as an adjunct with bethanechol chloride to help relieve urinary retention in patients with deficient contractility.[2]

Catheterization

In some patients, clean intermittent catheterization is the only viable treatment for detrusor areflexia. Intermittent catheterization provides regular, complete evacuation of the bladder with less risk for symptomatic bacteriuria than an indwelling catheter. The ideal intermittent catheter should be relatively small to minimize discomfort with insertion (approximately 12–14 French for adults) and should be constructed of a material that allows for washing and multiple uses. Occasionally, an indwelling catheter may be the only alternative for urinary retention. Its use is reserved for patients who are unable or unwilling to manage retention by other means.[2,5]

References

1. Blaivas JG, Oliver L. Pathophysiology of Urinary Incontinence. In DB Doughty (ed), Urinary and Fecal Incontinence: Nursing Management. St. Louis: Mosby, 1991;23–46.
2. Gray M. Urinary Incontinence/Voiding Dysfunction. In M Gray (ed), Genitourinary Disorders. St. Louis: Mosby, 1992;90–159.
3. Amis ES, JG Blaivas. Neurogenic bladder simplified. Radiol Clin North Am 1990;29:571.
4. Axelrod SA, Blaivas JG. The distinction between poor detrusor contractility and bladder outlet obstruction. Boston: Proceedings of the International Continence Society, 1986.
5. Gray M, Siegel SW, Troy R, et al. Management of Urinary Incontinence. In DB Doughty (ed), Urinary and Fecal Incontinence: Nursing Management. St. Louis: Mosby, 1991;95–150.
6. Romanowski GL, Shimp LA, Balson AB, Cahn MI. Urinary incontinence in the elderly: Etiology and treatment. Drug Intel Clin Pharm 1988;22:525.

16   Benign Prostatic Hypertrophy

Jack L. Rook

Benign prostatic hypertrophy (BPH) refers to enlargement of the prostate gland during the later decades of life. BPH is the most common cause of bladder outlet obstruction in middle-aged and older men, and the prevalence increases with age. By age 60 years, the incidence of BPH is 50%, and it increases to 80% by the age of 80 years.[1–3]

BPH begins in the mid-40s and becomes clinically significant when the gland extrinsically obstructs the bladder outlet, including the bladder neck and prostatic portion of the proximal urethra.[1,4] The causes of BPH are not clearly understood. The two factors necessary for its development are aging and functioning testes.[5,6] Testosterone, the principal hormonal product of the testes, serves as a precursor for dihydrotestosterone within the prostate. Dihydrotestosterone is a prominent androgen that influences interstitial prostatic growth. The exact role of dihydrotestosterone in the development of BPH remains unclear.[1,5]

The prostate is small at birth, but rapidly enlarges during puberty, reaching maturity at around the age of 20. A steady state lasts until age 45–50 years, when another gradual increase in prostate size and weight occurs in most males.[1,4–6]

Although the development of BPH itself is not harmful, the sequelae produced by this condition can cause significant morbidity and may prove fatal if left untreated. The signs and symptoms of BPH result from gradual encroachment of the hypertrophied prostatic tissue into the bladder outlet and proximal urethra.[1] As the enlarged prostate projects into the urinary bladder, it further impedes urinary flow by elevating the internal urethral orifice above the floor of the bladder, lengthening and distorting the prostatic urethra.[4]

Early obstructive symptoms include hesitancy, decreased force of urinary stream, diurnal frequency, and nocturia. Over time, the detrusor muscle, which is forced to contract against a closed outlet, develops compensatory hypertrophy, which may produce a reduction in symptoms. However, it should not be construed as an objective improvement in bladder outlet obstruction.[1,5,6] In untreated BPH, myogenic decompensation occurs when compensatory detrusor hypertrophy is no longer effective. The bladder wall then becomes increasingly distended, noncompliant, and hypotonic. This results in increased postvoid residuals and a greater chance of infection. Increased resistance at the ureterovesical junction combined with increased voiding pressure may contribute to vesicoureteral reflux, ureteral dilatation, progressive hydronephrosis, and an increased likelihood of pyelonephritis. Renal function is ultimately impaired.[1]

The three primary complications of BPH are urinary tract infection (UTI), acute urinary retention, and obstructive uropathy. UTI results from the increased postvoid residuals of advanced disease. The chronic presence of urine within the bladder decreases oxygenation of the bladder wall, which decreases resistance to bacterial invasion.[1,5] Acute urinary retention is a common complication due to overgrowth of the prostate's median lobe which forms a valvelike mechanism at the internal urethral orifice. Consequently, obstruction of the bladder outlet increases as the patient strains to void.[4]

Obstructive uropathy refers to the anatomic and physiologic changes that occur with long-standing disease. The chronically increased intravesical pressure with impaired urine flow results in detrusor trabeculation, diverticula, hypertrophy, and eventually decompensation. These anatomic changes are complicated by the presence of residual urine, infection, hematuria, vesicoureteral reflux, ureteral dilatation, hydronephrosis, and ultimately compromised renal function.

History

Bladder outlet obstruction is characterized by both obstructive and irritative symptoms. Early in the course of BPH, detrusor hypertrophy produces increased intravesical pressure during voiding, thereby maintaining urinary stream and ability to empty the bladder. In time, however, the bladder decompensates and symptoms of obstruction occur. Obstructive symptoms include difficulty starting urinary stream (hesitancy), diminished force and caliber of stream, prolonged voiding time, a feeling of incomplete emptying on completion of voiding, and postvoid dribbling. Other obstructive symptoms include diurnal frequency (greater than every two hours), and nocturia (with two or more visits to the bathroom per night). Urinary frequency and nocturia result from diminished bladder capacity due to bladder muscle hypertrophy in the early stages of BPH.[1,2,7]

With chronic urinary retention, patients report sensations of incomplete bladder emptying. With acute urinary retention, the patient suddenly reports a total inability to urinate with the acute onset of suprapubic discomfort that intensifies as the bladder fills.[1]

The classic symptoms of bladder instability (frequency, urgency, urge incontinence, and nocturia) also occur in conjunction with the obstructive symptoms.[2]

TABLE 16.1 Pharmacologic agents that aggravate symptoms of benign prostatic hypertrophy

Drugs that decrease bladder contractility
    Anticholinergic drugs (e.g., propantheline bromide [Pro-Banthine] or Donnatal)
    Tricyclic antidepressant drugs
Drugs that increase bladder outlet resistance
    Antiparkinsonian drugs (e.g., L-dopa [Sinemet])
    Sympathomimetic drugs (e.g., pseudoephedrine [Actifed, Sudafed], terbutaline
    [Brethine], dextroamphetamine [Dexedrine], isoproterenol [Isuprel], phenylpro-
    panolamine and guifenasin [Triaminic])
Drugs that increase urinary volume
    Diuretics

UTI may occur with BPH and urinary stasis. Patients with UTIs complain of irritative voiding symptoms and dysuria. Hematuria and fever occasionally occur.[1]

The patient's current medications may contribute to symptoms of bladder outlet obstruction. Anticholinergic agents (antispasmodic and antiparkinsonian drugs) and many antidepressant drugs depress bladder muscle contractility. Sympathomimetic agents (such as ephedrine) increase bladder outlet resistance. Diuresis, due to a diuretic agent may overstretch a partially compensated detrusor muscle and cause acute urinary retention (Table 16.1).[7]

Physical Examination

The physical examination of the patient with symptoms of bladder outlet obstruction should include observation of voided urinary stream, an abdominal examination, a rectal examination, and catheterization for postvoid residuals.

Observation

Observation of voided urinary stream reveals hesitancy to initiate the stream, diminished caliber, and prolonged voiding time. The stream may demonstrate intermittent flow with straining required enhancing evacuation.[1]

Abdominal Examination

Abdominal examination of the patient with advanced BPH may reveal several findings including

- A distended bladder from retention;
- Renal tenderness due to infection or hydronephrosis;
- Renal enlargement due to hydronephrosis; or
- An inguinal hernia from straining during urination in the face of outlet obstruction.[7]

Rectal Examination

A careful rectal examination of the prostate is important in evaluating the patient with suspected BPH or prostate carcinoma. However, there are certain limits to this evaluation as rectal palpation permits examination only of the posterior lobes of the prostate, and BPH most commonly involves the nonpalpable lateral and median lobes. Therefore, the size of the prostate gland, as estimated by rectal examination, is not necessarily directly related to the degree of urinary obstruction.[7]

The most important information obtained during the rectal examination is the consistency of the prostate gland. In patients with prostate enlargement, differences in consistency of the gland can be used to help differentiate from prostatic carcinoma with over 75% certainty. The prostate examination also permits determination of shape of the prostate, the presence of tenderness, and the adequacy of sphincter tone.[7]

Normal Prostate

The patient should void before rectal examination because a full bladder distorts the size of the prostate. The normal prostate is palpable through the anterior rectal wall, 2–5 cm from the anal verge. Normally, the examining finger can reach over the top of the prostate, as well as over each lateral border. A median sulcus is appreciated in the midline.[7]

With BPH, there is usually obliteration of the median sulcus, and also the examining finger may not reach the top of the gland. The consistency of the gland in BPH is smooth and rubbery, the gland is not tender, and the glandular enlargement tends to be symmetrical. Asymmetrical enlargement with palpation of distinct nodules (spheroids) is occasionally appreciated. The clinical differentiation between carcinoma and asymmetric or nodular BPH is based on the degree of hardness of the gland.[7]

Prostate Carcinoma

Classically, a rock-hard nodule or mass involving one or both posterior lobes characterizes prostate carcinoma. However, not all hard nodules turn out to be cancerous. In approximately 30–40%, biopsy of the tissue demonstrates either granulomatous prostatitis, prostatic calculi, spheroids of BPH, or nodularity resulting from transurethral prostatic resection.[7]

Catheterization

Catheterization may reveal a large urinary volume despite an inability to urinate. A urinary postvoid residual greater than 100 ml or 25% of total bladder capacity is consistent with urinary retention.[1]

Assessment

Assessment tools available to help evaluate the patient with urinary retention and suspected BPH include

1. Analysis of the voiding diary
2. Laboratory assessment
3. Catheterization for postvoid residual
4. Urodynamic studies (cystometrogram, urinary flow study, and urethral pressure profile)
5. Videourodynamic studies
6. Intravenous pyelogram
7. Renal ultrasound
8. Renal scan
9. Retrograde pyelogram
10. Prostatic ultrasound
11. Cystoscopy

Voiding Diary

The typical voiding diary of the patient with BPH and obstruction describes diurnal urinary frequency more often than every 2 hours and two or more episodes of nocturia per night. Urgency and urge incontinence may coexist.[1]

Laboratory Assessment

Preliminary laboratory assessment should include a urinalysis, urine culture (if infection is suspected), and measurement of serum creatinine and blood urea nitrogen or creatinine clearance. Bacteriuria and pyuria may be noted on urinalysis, and urine culture reveals the bacteria responsible for the UTI. The serum creatinine and blood urea nitrogen are elevated in advanced cases with compromised renal function.

Postvoid Residual Urine

Inserting a urethral catheter immediately after a patient has voided determines the amount of postvoid residual urine. A volume greater than 100 ml or more than 25% of the voided volume is considered abnormal. Catheter insertion can also help to determine if a urethral stricture is present.[7]

Urodynamic Studies

Most urodynamic studies are easily performed in a urologist's office, including the filling and voiding cystometrogram, urinary flow studies, and the urethral pressure profile.

Urodynamic abnormalities occur in BPH because the hyperplastic prostate gland impinges on and narrows the lumen of the urethra. As the prostate grows, its increasing size obstructs outflow.[2] Early on, the detrusor muscle compensates through hypertrophy, but over time it decompensates.

Early BPH voiding pressure studies demonstrate high-pressure contractions with normal to poor flow pattern, indicating outlet obstruction in the face of normal to hypertrophied detrusor musculature. With prolonged disease, decompensation of the detrusor occurs, with low pressure, poorly sustained contractions, large cystometric capacity, sensory urgency or detrusor instability, and compromised bladder wall compliance.[1,2] Early outflow obstruction pressure-flow analysis demonstrates a strong detrusor contraction (120 cm H_2O) of adequate duration occurring in conjunction with a poor flow rate (maximum of 4 ml per second) on uroflowmetry. With advanced disease, the cystometrogram demonstrates a low-pressure poorly sustained contraction with large cystometric capacity, and urinary flow studies demonstrate a poor flow pattern with low-maximum and average flow rates, and prolonged voiding time.

Urethral Pressure Profile

With BPH, the urethral pressure profile study demonstrates an increase in functional profile length, and the presence of prostatic peak (signifying increased intraluminal pressure) has been shown to correlate with obstruction.[8–10]

Videourodynamics

Videourodynamics (cystogram, voiding cystogram) visualize the narrowed prostatic urethra characteristic of BPH, trabeculation and diverticula of the bladder in advanced cases, and occasionally, vesicoureteral reflux. Deficient contractility is noted as a poorly contracting, smooth walled bladder with large capacity.[1]

Intravenous Pyelogram and Intravenous Urogram

The intravenous pyelogram and the intravenous urogram are reserved for cases in which upper urinary tract damage due to obstructive uropathy is suspected. Dilatation of the ureters, hydronephrosis, delayed excretion of contrast medium, and parenchymal thinning are seen in advanced cases.[1] Besides assessing the upper tract, the intravenous urogram may demonstrate bladder trabeculations and significant postvoid residual urine. The pelvic and vertebral bones can also be evaluated and may provide clues as to the presence of metastatic prostate cancer or advanced lumbar degenerative changes.[7]

Renal Ultrasound

If a patient has an allergy to intravenous contrast material, there are several alternative methods for studying the urinary tract:

- Renal ultrasound is useful in the detection of significant obstruction.
- Hydronephrosis is easily detected with this technique.

Renal Scan

A renal scan may be used to evaluate renal blood flow or delayed excretion suggesting obstruction.[7]

Retrograde Pyelogram

A retrograde pyelogram done in conjunction with cystoscopy provides visualization of dilated ureters. The dye used during this procedure is not absorbed and can be safely administered to patients allergic to intravenous contrast.[7]

Prostatic Ultrasound

Prostatic ultrasound in BPH demonstrates symmetrical enlargement of the gland without areas suspicious for malignant tumor. Prostatic calculi appear bright on ultrasound examination.[1]

Cystoscopy

The urologist may learn a great deal from a cystoscopic examination:

- The entire urethra is seen.
- The size of the prostate and degree of lumen occlusives can be assessed.
- Bladder trabeculation or diverticula can be directly visualized.

This information is important in helping the urologist decide the need for surgery.[7]

Treatment

Overflow incontinence, a dribbling leakage of urine accompanied by inability to empty the bladder, occurs as a consequence of BPH and is a symptom of urinary retention. The management program of urinary retention due to outlet obstruction is designed to correct and manage incontinence while promoting urinary elimination until surgical correction of the obstruction can be performed. Treatment options include[11]

- Double voiding
- Fluid control programs
- Avoidance of medications and conditions that promote urinary retention
- Pharmacologic manipulation
- Clean intermittent catheterization
- Indwelling catheter placement
- Ultimately, surgical correction of the underlying obstruction

Double Voiding Program

A program of double voiding may be effective in cases of mild to moderate BPH with outlet obstruction. The patient is taught to void twice during each trip to the bathroom. The patient voids, remains on the toilet, and voids again after a few minutes. Double voiding reduces residual urine volumes through more complete bladder evacuation in patients with mild to moderate obstructive symptoms.[1,11]

In addition to double voiding, the patient with mild to moderate obstructive symptoms should void on a timed schedule, every 2–3 hours. Regular bladder emptying prevents overdistension.[1]

Fluid Management Program

A fluid control program may benefit the patient with urinary retention. Adequate fluid intake must be maintained daily, but fluids should be distributed throughout waking hours. Curtailing fluid intake for 2 hours before sleep may help control symptoms of nocturia. Beverages during meals should be limited to about 8 oz. A fluid management program ensures adequate daily fluid intake while avoiding bolus fluids which increase the risk of acute urinary retention, detrusor instability, and infection.[1,11]

Avoiding Factors That Precipitate Urinary Retention

The patient with prostatic outlet obstruction should avoid factors that may precipitate an episode of acute urinary retention, including exposure to cold, consumption of large amounts of alcohol, use of over-the-counter cold medicines or diet pills, and avoidance of prescribed anticholinergic drugs or certain antidepressants with anticholinergic side effects.[11,12]

The patient should avoid over-the-counter decongestants or combination decongestant and antihistamine medications. Decongestant medications are alpha sympathomimetics. Besides relieving congestion in the upper airways, they increase tone at the bladder neck and prostatic urethra, thereby causing a predisposition to acute urinary retention. Likewise, over-the-counter diet pills rely on alpha sympathomimetics for their appetite suppressant actions and should be avoided.[1]

The patient with BPH should avoid excessive intake of alcohol. Alcohol has a diuretic effect, which can rather quickly cause bladder overdistension. This predisposes the patient to acute urinary retention.[1]

After prolonged exposure to cold temperatures, the patient with BPH should avoid trying to urinate until he warms his body. Exposure to cold causes increased urethral tone, indirectly related to shivering, and the shunting of blood away from the detrusor as the body works to prevent hypothermia and maintain core body temperature. This predisposes the patient to urinary retention. Rewarming the body before urination reverses this effect.[1]

Management of Acute Urinary Retention

The patient with BPH should be instructed on measures for the management of acute urinary retention. Acute urinary retention is characterized by the abrupt cessation of micturition followed by increasing feelings of suprapubic discomfort as the bladder fills without relief. This condition is particularly common in men with BPH and prostatic outlet obstruction.[11,12]

When acute retention occurs, the patient should be advised to relax, and attempt to void while sitting in a tub of warm water or standing in a warm shower. The warm water helps in relaxing the pelvic floor muscles, thus encouraging micturition. Drinking warm tea may also help stimulate micturition.[1,11]

The patient should seek urgent medical care if acute urinary retention persists or if suprapubic pain and urgency become unmanageable. Acute urinary retention is a medical emergency, with potential complications including infection, bladder rupture, and upper tract damage. Catheterization is required to prevent this complication.[1]

Intermittent Catheterization
Intermittent catheterization may be used to manage urinary retention. Catheterization provides for regular, complete bladder evacuation, helps to prevent urinary tract infection, and prevents the adverse effects of high-pressure voiding in the patient with outlet obstruction.[11]

Indwelling Catheter
An indwelling catheter is sometimes necessary for the management of urinary retention. It should be used only until a more definitive management program can be established. Occasionally, long-term catheter drainage is necessary. The individual with an indwelling catheter also needs an effective system for drainage. At night, the drainage reservoir should be large enough to store the urinary output for an 8-hour period.[11]

Pharmacologic Management of Obstruction

Medications for treatment of urinary retention secondary to BPH include alpha-adrenergic blockers, hormonal agents, and in cases with detrusor instability, anticholinergic and antispasmodic agents.

Alpha-Adrenergic Blocking Agents
Alpha-adrenergic receptors in the bladder neck and urethra cause an increase in urethral resistance when bound to by alpha agonists. Alpha agonists include norepinephrine (the sympathetic neurotransmitter) and pharmacologic sympathomimetics. Alpha-adrenergic blocking agents can be used to reduce urethral resistance and improve bladder emptying. Alpha-adrenergic blocking drugs work by causing relaxation of the smooth muscle bundles in the bladder neck, prostatic urethra, and prostatic capsule, which diminishes resistance to outflow during urination. These medications also help promote proximal urethral funneling during micturition, thus reducing retention. Alpha-adrenergic blockers include phenoxybenzamine (5–10 mg PO b.i.d.), prazosin (1–5 mg b.i.d.), terazosin (1–10 mg qhs), and doxazosin (1–16 mg qhs).[1,11]

Phenoxybenzamine produces alpha$_1$- and alpha$_2$-adrenergic blockade. All other agents provide selective alpha$_1$-adrenergic blockade. Common side effects of alpha blockers include

- Postural hypotension with dizziness
- Tachycardia
- Drowsiness
- Fatigue
- Rhinitis
- Nasal congestion
- Miosis
- Nausea
- Vomiting
- Depression
- Hallucinations
- Palpitations
- Rapid or irregular pulse
- Rash

Less common side effects include

- Weakness
- Lassitude
- Malaise
- Confusion
- Inhibition of ejaculation[1,11,13–15]

Hormonal Agents

Hormonal agents reduce prostatic enlargement by antagonizing testosterone and related androgens at the prostatic tissue receptors. The most widely used drug for the treatment of symptomatic BPH is finasteride (Proscar). There is a rapid regression of enlarged prostate glandular tissue in most treated patients. Approximately 60% of patients treated with finasteride experience an increase of urinary flow and improvement in symptoms of BPH. Although some patients may respond sooner, a minimum of six months, treatment may be necessary to determine whether an individual is responsive to the drug.

Finasteride is a specific inhibitor of the 5-alpha-reductase enzyme that converts testosterone to dihydrotestosterone. Side effects include headaches and loss of libido.[1,16]

Anticholinergic and Antispasmodic Agents

Detrusor instability may coexist with bladder outlet obstruction. Anticholinergic or antispasmodic medications may help to control unstable detrusor contractions.

Anticholinergic medications (i.e., imipramine) diminish the occurrence of unstable detrusor contractions while antispasmodic medications reduce bladder contractility. Reducing contractility may produce complete urinary retention in a patient with pre-existing retention. This situa-

TABLE 16.2   Detrusor antispasmodic agents

Hyoscyamine (Cystospaz)
Oxybutynin (Ditropan)
Hyoscyamine (Levbid)
Hyoscyamine (Levsin)
Hyoscyamine (Urised)
Flavoxate (Urispas)

tion necessitates intermittent catheterization to ensure regular, complete bladder evacuation (Table 16.2).[1]

Surgical Treatment of Benign Prostatic Hypertrophy

The only currently available definitive treatment for BPH is surgery. During a prostatectomy, the urologist removes the obstructing prostatic tissue either through transurethral resection of the prostate (TURP) or by one of the open-operative approaches (suprapubic or perineal). In general, glands that are very large are removed by open prostatectomy, whereas smaller glands are removed by TURP. The open prostatectomy procedure requires a longer hospitalization and recovery period.[7] Indications for surgery in patients with BPH include recurrent epididymitis, obstructive uropathy with renal failure, chronic intolerable symptoms of obstruction, acute urinary retention, and recurrent urinary tract infections.[1,7]

Transurethral Resection of the Prostate

TURP is the most commonly used procedure in the treatment of BPH. The TURP procedure is a surgical resection of prostate tissue under endoscopic control. It requires hospitalization for 4–7 days. General or spinal anesthesia is used. A rigid cystoscope is inserted into the urethra and bladder, and the prostatic urethra is localized. Obstructive prostatic tissue is then removed using a special resection instrument (resectoscope). The area of resection varies with each patient. The trigone and ureteral orifices are carefully avoided to prevent potential complications of vesicoureteral reflux and stress incontinence.[1,6]

Postoperatively, a three-way Foley catheter is used to promote the simultaneous infusion and drainage of an irrigating solution (normal saline) through the bladder. Continuous irrigation mechanically removes clots from the bladder, preventing clogging of the catheter and urinary retention. During continuous irrigation, the drainage bag should be emptied every 1–2 hours. A large drainage bag of 2 liters or greater capacity should be used after prostatectomy. Gentle traction is maintained against the prostatic vascular bed by the inflated catheter to compress vessels of the prostatic urethra, thereby preventing excessive bleeding following TURP.[1]

Complications after TURP include bleeding, infection, bladder spasms, and plasma hypo-osmolality (from absorption of irrigation fluid).[7]

Although some bleeding is to be expected postoperatively, excessive bleeding may also occur after TURP. Significant blood loss is noted as a large volume of blood mixed with urine output, along with a rapid pulse and declining blood pressure. Postoperatively, vital signs should be monitored, and a serum hemoglobin and hematocrit should be obtained and compared with presurgical data.[1]

Flecks of blood and pink-tinged urine are common after catheter removal for approximately 36–72 hours. As hematuria clears, the urine regains its clear, yellow color. The catheter should be reinserted to provide ongoing hemostasis should frank hematuria persist for more than 24 hours after its removal. Dark flecks of blood and minimal hematuria may occur for approximately 10–14 days after definitive catheter removal. This occurs as the scabs from the surgical resection spontaneously fall off.[1]

Unstable bladder contractions may occur after TURP, causing pain and leakage around the catheter. Anticholinergic or antispasmodic medications can be administered to prevent painful bladder spasms.[1]

The transurethral resection (TUR) syndrome is a potentially fatal complication of prostatectomy. Signs of TUR syndrome include bradycardia, tachypnea, vomiting, agitation, and altered alertness during the first postoperative day. TUR syndrome is caused by excessive absorption of bladder irrigating solution. This causes fluid volume excess, with plasma hypo-osmolality and electrolyte imbalance.[1] TUR syndrome cannot be left untreated. Postoperatively, vital signs and electrolytes should be monitored regularly. Irritating solutions and intravenous fluids may require adjustments. Overhydration also requires the judicious use of diuretics.

Long-term complications of TURP include urethral stricture, bladder neck contracture, incontinence, and retrograde ejaculation. Retrograde ejaculation is a frequent consequence of TURP. It is characterized by the ejaculation of semen into the bladder rather than externally through the urethra. This phenomenon occurs because the bladder neck, which is resected as part of the TURP, cannot contract during ejaculation, as is necessary to direct the semen into the urethra. Retrograde ejaculation results in sterility, but does not usually affect orgasms. The consequence of sterility should be discussed with sexually active patients and their partners before TURP. Most patients can resume normal physical and sexual activity approximately 4 weeks after TURP.[7]

Mild stress incontinence may occur after prostatic resection. Often, the leakage is transient and should regress and disappear within the first year after surgery. The stress incontinence that complicates TURP is a treatable condition, managed by physiotherapy, medications, or other means (electrical stimulation, biofeedback) under the care of a qualified specialist. Postoperatively, the patient with dribbling and stress incontinence should be instructed on how to do pelvic exercises that strengthen periurethral muscles. If the incontinence persists, a more formal rehabilitation program should be ordered.[1]

Sphincter damage is a rare complication of TURP. Persistent stress incontinence results from this rare complication.[1]

Last, the patient should be informed about the potential for regrowth of remaining prostatic tissue (usually 10 years or more after surgery). Routine prostate evaluation is necessary even after surgical resection.[1]

Open Prostatectomy
Open prostatectomy is the surgical resection of the prostate gland using a suprapubic, retropubic, or perineal approach. Open prostatectomy

requires a slightly longer hospitalization and recovery period than TURP. This procedure is reserved for those cases of BPH with profound prostatic enlargement that virtually closes the urethral outlet or when BPH is associated with a pathologic bladder condition such as bladder calculi or diverticula. A retropubic prostatectomy is typically reserved for radical surgery when adenocarcinoma is present.[1,6]

Open prostatectomy requires open incision and extensive resection. General anesthesia is required. During the procedure, the bladder is opened and the prostate enucleated with blunt or sharp instruments, leaving the prostatic capsule intact.[1]

Postoperatively, the patient has suprapubic and urethral catheters. The urethral catheter is used primarily for hemostasis of the enucleated prostate capsule, while the suprapubic catheter provides urinary drainage. Continuous or intermittent irrigation of the bladder is required for the first 24 hours after surgery to help evacuate blood clots and prevent urinary retention. Traction on the urethral Foley catheter and balloon provides gentle hemostasis for the vascular bed until active bleeding stops. The catheters typically are removed 36–72 hours after surgery.[1]

Short-term complications of open prostatectomy include bladder spasms, hemorrhage, urinary infection, osteitis pubis, dysuria, and obstruction.

Overdistension of the bladder promotes bladder spasms. These unstable detrusor contractions increase the risk of bleeding and disruption of the surgical site. Anticholinergic medications can be used to inhibit bladder spasms.[1]

Although blood-tinged urine is expected after prostatectomy, passage of excessive, bright red blood may indicate significant, uncontrolled hemorrhage. Uncontrolled bleeding causes hypovolemic shock, which is characterized by a rapid weak pulse and declining blood pressure. The hemoglobin and hematocrit values decline from preoperative data when significant postoperative bleeding occurs. The urologist should be notified immediately if signs of significant bleeding occur. Should hemorrhage occur after catheter removal, the urethral catheter should be reinserted for ongoing hemostasis.[1]

Anti-infective medications are administered immediately after surgery to help prevent urinary tract infection. After catheter removal, the development of signs and symptoms of UTI necessitate reinstitution of antibiotics. Osteitis pubis refers to a postoperative painful infection of the symphysis bone. Anti-infective medications may help prevent and treat this complication.[1]

The patient may have moderate dysuria (discomfort with urination) for several days after catheter removal. Dysuria can be treated with appropriate analgesics and adequate intake of clear liquids. Adequate hydration dilutes the urine minimizing dysuria.[1]

After the catheter has been removed, poor urinary output is an indication of urinary retention, most likely a result of urethral obstruction from clots or debris.[1] This necessitates catheter reinsertion and bladder irrigation to dislodge and remove clots.

Possible long-term postoperative complications of open prostatectomy include urinary stress incontinence, epididymitis, erectile dysfunction, fistula, altered fertility potential, and bladder neck contracture or stricture.

Bladder neck contracture may complicate open prostatectomy. The urologist may need to gently dilate the urethra on one or more occasions to minimize the potential for contracture formation. Strict adherence to postoperative follow-up visits is required.[1]

Open prostatectomy may cause transient or chronic sphincter incompetence with stress incontinence. Stress incontinence is a treatable condition managed by physiotherapy, medications, and if necessary, surgery (artificial urinary sphincter).[1]

Other long-term postoperative complications include erectile dysfunction (due to nerve damage from the surgery itself or scar tissue), altered fertility potential (due to postoperative retrograde ejaculation), and chronic epididymitis.[1]

References

1. Gray M. Obstructive Uropathies. In M Gray (ed), Genitourinary Disorders. St. Louis: Mosby, 1992;160–199.
2. Blaivas JG, Oliver L. Pathophysiology of Urinary Incontinence. In DB Doughty (ed), Urinary and Fecal Incontinence: Nursing Management. St. Louis: Mosby, 1991;23–46.
3. Berry SJ, Coffey DS, Walsh PC, Ewing LL. The development of human benign prostatic hyperplasia with age. J Urol 1984;132:373.
4. Moore KL. The Perineum and Pelvis. In KL Moore (ed), Clinically Oriented Anatomy. Baltimore: Williams & Wilkins, 1980;293–418.
5. Gray ML, Dobkin K. Genitourinary System. In J Thompson (ed), Mosby's Manual of Clinical Nursing. St. Louis: Mosby–Year Book, 1989.
6. Grayhack JT, Kozlwoski JM. Benign Prostatic Hyperplasia. In JY Gillenwater, JT Grayhack, SS Howards, JW Duckett (eds), Adult and Pediatric Urology. Chicago: Mosby–Year Book, 1991.
7. Smolev JK. Bladder Outlet Obstruction. In LR Barker, JR Burton, PD Zieve (eds), Principles of Ambulatory Medicine (2d ed). Baltimore: Williams & Wilkins, 1986;568–573.
8. Webster GD. Urodynamic Studies. In MI Resnick, RA Older (eds), Diagnosis of Genitourinary Disease. New York: Thieme-Stratton, 1982;173–204.
9. Webster GD, Lockhart JL, Older RA. The evaluation of bladder neck dysfunction. J Urol 1980;123:196.
10. Abrams PH. Sphincterometry in the diagnosis of male bladder outflow obstruction. J Urol 1975;116:489.
11. Gray M, Siegel SW, Troy R, et al. Management of Urinary Incontinence. In DB Doughety (ed), Urinary and Fecal Incontinence: Nursing Management. St. Louis: Mosby, 1991;95–150.
12. Jarvis GJ. A controlled trial of bladder drill and drug therapy in the management of detrusor instability. Br J Urol 1981;53:565.
13. Lepor H. What will replace TURP? Contemp Urol 1992;4(2):30.
14. Olin BR. Professional's Guide to Patient Drug Facts. Philadelphia: JB Lippincott, 1990.
15. Skidmore-Roth L. Mosby's 1990 Nursing Drug Reference. St. Louis: Mosby–Year Book, 1990.
16. Physicians' Desk Reference (51st ed). Montvale, NJ: Medical Economics, 1997.

17   Extraurethral Incontinence

Jack L. Rook

Extraurethral incontinence refers to the uncontrolled leakage of urine through some fistulous or ectopic communication that bypasses the normal urethral sphincter mechanism. The urinary leakage is continuous and relatively unaffected by physical exertion. In some cases, extraurethral leakage manifests as a continuous dribble coexisting with a relatively normal voiding pattern, while in other instances, the leakage is severe and replaces normal voiding.

Extraurethral incontinence may be particularly frustrating to treat, as traditional management strategies used with detrusor or sphincter dysfunction are ineffective. The extraurethral leakage is continuous, and even relatively small ectopic fistulae produce a significant volume of urine over the course of a typical day.

As with other forms of incontinence, complications of extraurethral incontinence include urinary tract infection, altered skin integrity, and social isolation.[1]

Pathophysiology

Extraurethral leakage arises from urinary ectopia or urinary fistula. *Urinary ectopia* refers to a congenital defect (epispadia or exstrophy), whereby an ectopic ureter opens into the vagina or urethra (below the urethral sphincter), or part of the bladder is externalized without a urethral sphincter mechanism.

A urinary fistula is an acquired pathological tract that communicates between pelvic organs or between a pelvic organ and the skin. The tract is named by describing its origin and terminal points:

1. A vesicovaginal fistula is a communication between the bladder and vaginal vault.
2. A urethrovaginal fistula is a tract between the urethra and vagina.

3. A urethrocutaneous fistula produces leakage if it bypasses the sphincter mechanism.
4. A vesicocutaneous fistula allows leakage directly from the bladder to the skin.[1]

The most common causes of urinary fistulae are complications of labor and delivery, or as a complication of hysterectomy or other pelvic surgical procedures. Other causes of urinary fistulae are penetrating trauma, perineal wounds, and invasive tumors.[1-3]

History

Patients with extraurethral incontinence report constant urinary leakage ranging in severity from continuous dribbling leakage superimposed on a normal voiding pattern to complete absence of spontaneous voiding with severe continuous leakage requiring diaper containment. The leakage is usually not associated with urgency to void or physical exertion. Some patients may report alterations of skin integrity and social isolation.[1]

Physical Examination

Physical examination may reveal the cutaneous opening of the fistulous tract with leakage through the perineum, penis, or vagina. Examination of the perineal skin may reveal moist, odorous skin with lesions or specific rashes.[1]

Diagnostic Studies and Findings

The cystogram and voiding cystogram demonstrate the bladder or urethral urinary fistula as an extravasation of contrast material through the fistulous tract.

The intravenous pyelogram and intravenous urogram demonstrate ectopic ureter as an extravasation of contrast material through an aberrant tract leading into the vagina or urethra.

An endoscopy may allow direct visualization of an opening to a fistulous tract. A cystourethroscopy may identify a fistula involving the bladder or urethra. An ectopic ureter with an orifice in the urethra can be detected with urethroscopy. An ectopic urethral orifice opening into the vagina may be detected by colposcopy. The methylene blue test (instillation of methylene blue into the bladder) may also be used to detect small vesicovaginal or urethrovaginal fistulae.[1]

Treatment

The treatment of extraurethral incontinence includes conservative measures aimed at containment and skin care until a definitive surgical repair procedure can be performed. Conservative management includes a skin care program, urinary containment, topical application of tetracycline to any fistulous tract, and in some cases, the prophylactic use of anti-infective drugs or an indwelling catheter.[1]

A skin care program includes regular washing, complete drying, application of a moisture barrier or skin sealant, and use of a collection device.[1]

Candidal rashes are managed by routine skin care and local application of an antifungal cream or powder. Ammonia contact dermatitis may result from prolonged exposure of the skin to urine. Regular adherence to a skin care program including complete drying and the use of a moisture barrier and collection device minimizes exposure.[1]

The patient must utilize an appropriate urinary containment device. Individuals with mild extraurethral leakage may require only a small pad, while those with more significant leakage require a diaper. The ideal urinary containment device protects the skin by completely absorbing leakage, thus minimizing the time urine is in contact with the skin.[1]

An indwelling catheter is sometimes required to block or divert urine from a fistula. Depending on its anatomic relation to the fistula, the catheter may ablate, alleviate, or fail to affect incontinence. The indwelling catheter can be left in place until surgical repair is completed or as a permanent management program in nonsurgical candidates.[1]

A potential curative but nonsurgical option is sclerosis of the fistulous tract with a tetracycline-saline solution. Tetracycline is a caustic substance when administered topically. The infusion of this solution into a fistula may produce sufficient scarring to close the fistulous tract and prevent incontinence.[1]

Most patients ultimately require a definitive management program for their extraurethral incontinence. Surgical therapy includes closure or repair of urinary ectopia and closure of urinary fistulae.[1]

The goals of treatment are to ensure adequate containment and to restore and maintain skin integrity while the patient awaits a definitive procedure (surgery or tetracycline administration).

References

1. Gray M. Urinary Incontinence/Voiding Dysfunction. In M Gray (ed), Genitourinary Disorders. St. Louis: Mosby, 1992;90–159.
2. Symmonds RE. Incontinence: vesical and urethral fistulae. Clin Obst Gynecol 1984;27:499.
3. Wheatley JK. Causes and treatment of bladder incontinence. Comp Ther 1983;9:27.

18   Functional Incontinence

Jack L. Rook

Functional incontinence refers to urinary leakage due to a functional deficit (impaired physical mobility, dexterity, or cognition), rather than due to organic dysfunction of the urinary system.[1-4] Functional incontinence is relatively unusual as an isolated finding. More commonly, stress, instability, overflow, and continuous incontinence are complicated or exacerbated by functional deficits. A comprehensive management plan must include measures to alleviate both the primary voiding dysfunction problem and any associated functional aspects of urinary leakage.[2]

The population of patients who may become afflicted with functional incontinence includes those with orthopedic, musculoskeletal, and neurologic deficits.

The management of functional incontinence requires interventions designed to enhance the individual's access to toilet facilities, manipulate clothing to prepare for toileting, and to enhance the individual's perception that maintaining continence is a desirable and attainable goal.

Like all incontinent individuals, the person with functional incontinence faces the potential complications of social isolation, urinary tract infection, altered skin integrity, and upper urinary tract distress.[1]

Pathophysiology

Functional factors that contribute to incontinence include deficits of mobility, dexterity, and cognition. Deficits of mobility include physiologic or environmental factors that limit the patient's access to toilet facilities as needed. Dexterity deficits impair continence by limiting the individual's ability to manipulate clothing before voiding. Deficits in cognition make it difficult for a person to process and synthesize environmental and sensory indicators of the need to void or the steps necessary to complete this task.[2]

Impaired Mobility

Impaired mobility affects the individual's ability to reach the bathroom and maneuver onto the toilet in preparation for voiding. An elderly individual's mobility may be limited by impaired vision, generalized deconditioning, neurologic disorders, and musculoskeletal conditions.[1]

Visual problems may impair the patient's ability to get to and from the bathroom. Poor vision may be a consequence of diabetic retinopathy, macular degeneration, cataracts, glaucoma, and those cerebrovascular accidents with associated cortical blindness or visual perceptual dysfunction. Impaired vision and perceptual problems may impair safe mobility to and from the bathroom.

Generalized deconditioning may have either a cardiovascular or musculoskeletal etiology. The deconditioned patient may be too weak to ambulate to and transfer onto the toilet.

Neurologic conditions that may be associated with mobility deficits include Parkinson's disease, multiple sclerosis, polyneuropathy, peroneal mononeuropathy, cerebral vascular accidents (CVAs), and spinal cord injury.

Patients with Parkinson's disease may have difficulty mobilizing to and from the bathroom. Parkinson's disease, a neurodegenerative brain disorder, can lead to an unsafe, shuffling-type gait. Ten to sixty-five percent of parkinsonian patients may also develop Alzheimer's dementia.[5] Multiple sclerosis patients can have mobility problems (paraparesis, spasticity), as well as neurogenic bladder dysfunction of varying degrees. Some patients with multiple sclerosis also develop cognitive dysfunction. Advanced polyneuropathy can cause impaired motor and sensory function in the lower extremities ultimately leading to gait problems due to weakness and ataxia. More selective nerve injuries such as peroneal mononeuropathy around the fibular head can lead to foot drop with difficulty ambulating and increased potential for falls. Left and right hemispheric CVAs can lead to hemiparetic conditions that may impair mobility.

Musculoskeletal conditions that may impair mobility include lower extremity osteoarthritis or rheumatoid arthritis, intrinsic foot pathology, and amputation. Patients with severe degenerative arthritis of the hips or knees or rheumatoid arthritis (which has a predilection for small joints of the feet) may have mobility problems to and from the bathroom. Some patients have chronic foot pain due to plantar fasciitis or intermittent pain associated with gout, both of which may affect mobility. Last, some patients with severe peripheral vascular disease may have required an amputation (below or above knee) that may impair mobility, particularly in individuals with other medical or orthopedic disorders.

Impaired mobility is also influenced by issues related to access. For example, the paraplegic patient requires a wheelchair-accessible bathroom. Likewise, elderly individuals may be unable to use a toilet that is too low for reasonable access or that has no handrails with which to lower themselves. Other barriers to successful toileting include stairs, poor lighting, and environmental hazards such as slick-soled shoes or loose throw rugs.[1]

Impaired Dexterity

Impaired dexterity also affects an individual's predisposition to incontinence. Once the toilet has been reached, the individual must still be able to manipulate his or her clothing to successfully void. Manipulating zippers, buttons, hooks, undergarments, and other aspects of clothing requires time, dexterity, and visual acuity.[1] Impaired dexterity can occur in patients with a diffuse polyneuropathy who may have developed upper extremity motor and sensory dysfunction. More selective upper extremity nerve entrapments (such as carpal or cubital tunnel syndromes) can result in decreased finger sensation and dexterity. Patients with advanced upper extremity osteoarthritis or rheumatoid arthritis develop chronic joint pain, deformity, and loss of ability to perform fine dexterous activities. Some patients may require splints or casts related to recent trauma or a chronic condition. These may interfere with the ability to manipulate clothing.

Impaired Cognition

Altered cognition also affects urinary continence, as the mentally impaired patient may fail to grasp the significance of urinary urgency or the social significance of continence.[1] Cognitive dysfunction may occur with head injury, a cerebrovascular accident, Alzheimer's disease, or mental retardation. Thirty percent of parkinsonian patients go on to develop Alzheimer's dementia. Patients who have multi-infarct cerebral vascular disease due to atrial fibrillation or hypertension may also have associated significant cognitive impairment. In contrast, patients with brain stem or deep internal capsular strokes typically develop hemiparesis that can impair mobility and lead to functional incontinence without cognitive impairment.

Many patients who have had a cerebral injury also have bladder dysfunction due to cortical loss of inhibition of the pontine micturition center. Patients with frontal lobe CVAs due to occlusion of the anterior cerebral artery are particularly prone to developing this problem.

Spinal Cord Injured Patient

The spinal cord injured (SCI) patient has to deal with issues of mobility, access, and dexterity, which may interfere with successful bladder management. SCI patients have varying toileting abilities depending on the level of injury. Very important functional improvements can occur by addition of a single neurologic spinal cord level. With each additional level added, new muscles are recruited that can aid the patient in assisting a caretaker or actually performing a bladder program (Table 18.1).

History

Patients with functional incontinence related to impaired mobility report difficulty walking or an inability to walk. They either require more time to

TABLE 18.1 Bladder care capabilities as related to spinal cord injury level

Level of injury	Bladder routine	Transfers	Mobility: wheelchair propulsion	Mobility: ambulation	Muscles recruited to assist with bladder care	Muscles missing that can interfere with bladder routine	Potential environmental obstacles
C3–C4	Total dependence: indwelling catheter; intermittent catheterization; sphincterotomy/ condom catheter	Total dependence	Independent with pneumatic or chin-controlled–driven power wheelchair with powered reclining feature	—	—	Upper extremity muscles for transfers; hand intrinsics for catheter manipulation	—
C5	Total dependence: indwelling catheter; intermittent catheterization; sphincterotomy/ condom catheter	Assistance of one person with or without transfer board	Independent in power chair indoors and outdoors; short distances in manual wheelchair with lugs indoors	—	—	Upper extremity muscles for transfers; hand intrinsics for catheter manipulation	—
C6	Total dependence: indwelling catheter; intermittent catheterization; sphincterotomy/ condom catheter	Potentially independent with transfer board	Independent with manual wheelchair with plastic rims or lugs indoors; assistance needed outdoors	—	Starting to recruit triceps (C6–C7) to assist with transfers	Hand intrinsics for catheter manipulation	—
C7	Requires assistance to independence with upper extremity tenodesis splint orthosis; indwelling catheter; intermittent catheterization; sphincterotomy/ condom catheter	Independent with or without transfer board	Independent with manual wheelchair indoors and outdoors except curbs, stairs	—	Triceps (C6–C7) helps transfers be independent; finger flexors with tenodesis splint allows pinching of catheter for intermittent catheterization	Hand intrinsics for fine manipulation of catheter	Patient must manipulate wheelchair to bathroom; narrow hallways; narrow bathroom doors; wheelchair inaccessible bathrooms; absence of hand rails

Level	Bladder management	Transfers	Mobility	Ambulation	Muscle recruitment	Functional status	Architectural barriers
C8–T1	Independent: intermittent catheterization; sphincterotomy/condom catheter; trigger reflex voiding with certain maneuvers	Independent	Independent with manual wheelchair indoors and outdoors including curbs	—	Triceps for transfers; hand intrinsics for fine manipulation of catheter	Trunk muscles/abdominal and back muscles make trunk unstable when sitting without support	Patient must manipulate wheelchair to bathroom; narrow hallways and bathroom doors; wheelchair inaccessible bathrooms; absence of handrails
T2–T10	Independent: intermittent catheterization; sphincterotomy/condom catheter; trigger reflex, voiding with certain maneuvers	Independent7	Independent	Exercise only (not functional with orthosis); requires assist or guarding	Recruiting trunk and back muscles to help stabilize trunk and provide better balance	Lower extremity muscles of ambulation/patient is still wheelchair dependent	Patient must manipulate wheelchair to bathroom; narrow hallways and bathroom doors; wheelchair inaccessible bathrooms; absence of handrails
T11–L2	Independent: intermittent catheterization; sphincterotomy/condom catheter; trigger reflex voiding with certain maneuvers	Independent	Independent	Potential for independent functional ambulation indoors with orthosis; some have potential for stairs using railing	Recruiting pelvic muscles, including hip flexors, which gives patient potential for limited ambulation	Lower extremity muscles for smooth, safe ambulation	Patient must manipulate wheelchair to bathroom; narrow hallways and bathroom doors; wheelchair inaccessible bathrooms; absence of handrails
L3–S3	Independent: intermittent catheterization; Credé's maneuver; deflation of periurethral cuff	Independent	Independent	Community ambulation: independent indoors and outdoors with orthosis	Quadriceps recruited for safer ambulation with knee stabilization utilizing ankle-foot orthosis	Without ankle-foot orthosis, potential for foot drop, which impairs ambulation	Loose rugs; stairs

gain access to the toilet, or they may be unable to gain access at all.[1] Patients may give a history of visual problems, neurological disorders, or a musculoskeletal condition that interferes with gait and mobility.

Functional incontinence can occur due to impaired dexterity. Such patients report difficulty manipulating clothing.[1] The history may include rheumatoid arthritis, osteoarthritis, carpal tunnel or other upper extremity nerve entrapment syndrome, or a diffuse polyneuropathy that may contribute to a dexterity impairment. Polyneuropathy can occur due to diabetes, renal failure, alcoholism, or earlier toxic exposure. Patients with SCI above the C8–T1 level have upper extremity and hand intrinsic muscle weakness, which may impair dexterity to some degree.

The patient with functional incontinence due to impaired cognition is unaware of or unconcerned about their incontinence.[1] The patient's medical history may include conditions that may lead to cognitive impairment such as CVA, organic brain syndrome, Alzheimer's disease, Parkinson's disease, or mental retardation.

Evaluation of the patient's home environment is essential. The evaluation should include information about the size of the house, the presence of stairs, and bathroom location. Flooring (plush carpets, slippery floors, presence of throw rugs), doorway size, adaptive toileting equipment (elevated toilet seat, grab bars), and adequacy of lighting should be assessed during the history.

Physical Examination

The physical examination can begin with a vision screening. Next, patient mobility should be assessed, including transfers from supine to sit and from sit to stand, gait, and the use of any assistive devices. The patient may demonstrate difficulty initiating or stopping ambulation, or they may be completely unable to walk, requiring a wheelchair. The patient's balance should be observed while walking.

During ambulation, any foot dragging should be noted. Foot dragging can occur with polyneuropathy or peroneal mononeuropathy. Lower extremity sensation should be assessed. An ataxia may develop due to impaired sensation from a peripheral neuropathy. An ataxia may also be a central condition due to cerebellar disease. Cerebellar ataxia can be differentiated from a sensory ataxia by the fact those patients with sensory ataxia can compensate using their vision, whereas a cerebellar ataxia persists even with they eyes open.

A complete mental status evaluation should be performed. The patient should be observed for their ability to complete toileting when prompted, even if assisted to sit on the toilet. Patients with cognitive impairment may not be able to process signals of urinary urgency and translate them into appropriate toileting behavior.[1]

An assessment of upper extremity function should include manual muscle testing of arm and hand musculature. Evidence of muscle atrophy may be present in patients with spinal cord injury, nerve entrapment syndromes, or polyneuropathy. Upper extremity sensation should be checked. Impaired sensation (due to polyneuropathy or nerve entrapment) is usually associated with impaired dexterity. Patients with impaired manual dexterity should be observed for the ability to manipulate zippers, buttons, hooks, snaps, Velcro, and laces.

Physical examination of the SCI patient should include evaluation of motor and sensory level and elucidation of the type of neurogenic bladder problem. This ultimately helps in determining the optimal bladder control program. For example, the quadriplegic patient may not be able to manipulate a hand-held catheter to proceed with an intermittent catheterization program. The SCI patient should also be checked for ability to transfer. With sparing of C7 musculature (including triceps), the patient should be able to transfer to and from a commode. However, he or she may still require assistance with toileting activities. The SCI patient should be assessed for the ability to manipulate clothing, and the mobility device should be evaluated as part of the physical examination.

A musculoskeletal examination should follow the neurological assessment. Patients should be checked for scars that suggest prior hip or knee arthroplasty procedures, and amputations should be noted. Patients with below-knee amputation usually mobilize better than do those with higher level amputations. The patient's prosthesis should be evaluated. Some patients require orthotic devices. For example, patients with foot drop or a CVA with increased plantar flexion tone may require an ankle-foot orthoses for safe ambulation. Any deformity due to osteoarthritis or rheumatoid arthritis should be noted, and lower extremity contractures or range of motion deficits that can impair mobility should be assessed.

Evaluation of the upper extremities may display findings consistent with osteoarthritis (Heberden's nodes or Bouchard's deformity involving the fingers) or rheumatoid arthritis (ulnar deviation of the fingers, radial deviation of the wrist, boutonniere or swan-neck deformities of the fingers, and nodules in the upper extremities).

Ideally, a home assessment should be performed to determine the patient's accessibility to his or her own toilet. Environmental barriers may limit or preclude an individual's access to the toilet. Such information is useful in determining the need for a particular assistive device or structural home alterations.

Diagnostic Studies and Findings

Urodynamic and videourodynamic studies typically show normal bladder functioning in patients who have classic functional incontinence. On the other hand, pathologic urinary incontinence may coexist with functional deficits.[1]

Cognitive functioning can be assessed through neuropsychological screening or a full neuropsychological evaluation. Magnetic resonance imaging or computed tomographic scans of the head may demonstrate cerebral atrophy, normal pressure hydrocephalus (a treatable condition), earlier CVA, or multiple earlier CVAs.

X-rays of the lower extremities may demonstrate arthritic disorders or earlier surgical procedure(s), such as knee or hip arthroplasty, which may interfere with mobility. X-rays of the low back may demonstrate severe spinal or pelvic disease that could contribute to back and lower extremity pain, nerve impairment, and impaired mobility.

Electrodiagnostic studies help differentiate between diffuse impairment of the peripheral nervous system (polyneuropathy) and more selective, upper extremity entrapment disorders, such as carpal tunnel syndrome. Both may impair dexterity. Lower extremity testing may help differentiate between polyneuropathy, spinal stenosis, and lumbosacral radiculopathy, all of which can impair mobility.

Treatment

The treatment of functional incontinence involves measures to improve mobility, dexterity, and mentation and motivation. Goals of treatment for patients with functional incontinence should include[1,2]

1. Overcoming impaired mobility so that the patient develops the ability to maneuver into the bathroom and onto the toilet seat in a reasonable period of time
2. Removal of any barriers to toilet access
3. Providing adequate equipment for the patient's toilet (handrails, elevated seat), and if necessary, an alternative to a conventional toilet (e.g., bedside commode or hand-held urinal)
4. Ensuring that hallway and bathroom lighting is adequate
5. Ensuring that clothing can be manipulated and removed without assistance in a reasonable amount of time for toileting
6. Providing the patient with a regular unassisted toileting schedule or a program with prompting and assistance as needed

Mobility Deficits

Impaired mobility is a common finding in patients with functional urinary incontinence. Some patients may be confined to a wheelchair. Others may ambulate only with assistive devices such as braces or a walker. The elderly person's mobility may be limited by arthritis or impaired vision. Environmental barriers to the toilet, such as loose throw rugs, stairs, and poor lighting, may compromise the mobility of a borderline impaired individual.[1,2] Therapeutic intervention for these individuals focuses on improving their mobility and access to toilet facilities. Referral to physical therapy may help maximize the patient's strength, mobility, and balance. The therapist should also help the patient manipulate their home environment to improve access to bathroom facilities. Adequate lighting in corridors and bathroom facilities must be provided. Loose throw rugs should be eliminated.[1,2]

Those individuals who require assistive devices such as a wheelchair or walker may require physical alterations of his or her home to provide for increased mobility. Such alterations may include widening doorways or installing handrails to facilitate transfers. Handrails enhance access to toileting by helping individuals raise and lower themselves onto the commode.[2] A raised toilet seat minimizes the distance the trunk must be raised or lowered during transfers.[1]

The patient's mobility and access to bathroom facilities are particularly likely to be impaired at night because of disorientation on awakening and poor lighting. For women, a bedside commode, and for men, a hand-held urinal may help facilitate nocturnal voiding, bypassing the need to reach a distant toilet. The bedside commode should have four sturdy legs with rubber pads that prevent it from sliding, arm rails that the patient can use to help seat herself, and legs that can be adjusted to a proper height to facilitate transfers from bed to commode and back. The hand-held urinal gives the male patient immediate access to a receptacle for voiding. The patient may require assistance emptying and cleaning the commode or hand-held urinal.[1,2]

A nurse or therapist should help the patient with limited mobility obtain appropriate assistive devices, such as a cane, orthotic(s), a walker, or a wheelchair. These devices allow the otherwise immobile patient to maneuver and control the environment, including access to the toilet. The patient should be encouraged to use nonskid walking or running shoes, as slick-soled shoes or house slippers limit mobility by impairing balance and increase the risk of a serious fall.[1,2]

The patient may need to obtain eyeglasses or hearing aids, both of which increase sensory input.[1]

Dexterity Deficits

Because deficits in dexterity may also contribute to incontinence, the patient with impaired dexterity should consult an occupational therapist for appropriate therapy, including exercise and the use of assistive devices.

The patient should also wear clothing that maximizes their dexterity. Easily managed clothing reduces the time required to prepare for urination. Excessive clothing layers and even underwear may need to be eliminated. Clothing can also be modified so that fewer fine motor movements are required to prepare for voiding: zippers are easier to manipulate than buttons; Velcro fasteners and elastic waistbands are even easier to manipulate than zippers.[1,2]

Impaired Cognition

Altered cognition may profoundly affect urinary continence, as a patient may lack the motivation or orientation to control voiding. To manage the patient with altered mentation, a scheduled prompted voiding program or an individualized pattern of prompted toileting should be designed. The nursing staff or caregiver should help the patient to the bathroom or bedside commode and encourage him or her to void every 2 hours or as indicated by the individualized program. Prompting the patient provides both a visual and audible stimulus for toileting, and assistance to the toilet can be provided as needed.[1,2]

A behavior modification program may help to encourage toileting behaviors in mentally impaired individuals with no obvious underlying voiding dysfunction and adequate mental facilities to integrate social and sensory input into effective toileting behaviors. Providing rewards helps to reinforce appropriate toileting behaviors that promote continence.[1]

References

1. Gray M. Urinary Incontinence/Voiding Dysfunction. In M Gray (ed), Genitourinary Disorders. St. Louis: Mosby, 1992;90–155.
2. Gray M, Siegel SW, Troy R, et al. Management of Urinary Incontinence. In DB Doughty (ed), Urinary and Fecal Incontinence: Nursing Management. St. Louis: Mosby, 1991;95–150.
3. Gray ML. Functional Incontinence. In JM Thompson (ed), Mosby's Manual of Clinical Nursing, (2d ed), St. Louis: Mosby–Year Book, 1989.
4. Kim MJ, McFarland GH, McLane AM. Pocket Guide to Nursing Diagnoses (3d ed), St. Louis: Mosby–Year Book, 1989.
5. Mayeux R, Chen J, Mirabello E, et al. An estimate of the incidence of dementia in idiopathic Parkinson's disease. Neurology 1990;40:1513.

19   Prostate Cancer

Jack L. Rook

Adenocarcinoma of the prostate is the most common malignancy affecting men in the United States, accounting for approximately 20% of all malignant tumors diagnosed in men and 10% of all cancer-related deaths. It is the second most common cause of cancer-related deaths for this group. Unsuspected or undiagnosed prostate adenocarcinomas were found microscopically at autopsy in approximately 30% of all men over 50 years of age who died of unrelated causes, and in about 60% of men over 80 years of age.[1-3]

The cause of prostate adenocarcinoma remains unclear. A genetic predisposition has been suspected, and racial differences in its occurrence have been noted. Black men tend to have prostate adenocarcinoma at an earlier age, with higher tumor stages and higher mortality than white men. In contrast, Native Americans, Oriental Americans, and Hispanics have a lower incidence of prostate cancer than either white or black males.[1,2]

The pathophysiologic significance of prostate cancer lies in the tumor's propensity for local growth, invasion of adjacent structures, and metastases to distant organ systems.[1]

Prostate adenocarcinomas originate as a firm, single or multifocal nodule, usually within the posterior lobe of the gland near the outer margin of the stroma. As the tumor grows, it causes symptoms of bladder outlet obstruction and obstructive uropathy. As the tumor spreads locally and disrupts the prostatic capsule, it may involve the facial envelope surrounding the seminal vesicles and the bladder base, contributing to bladder outlet and ureteral obstruction. Extension to the membranous urethra occurs in very advanced cases.[1]

Cancer of the prostate metastasizes via both hematogenous and lymphatic routes. Metastases to the vertebral column and pelvis occur via the valveless venous communications between the prostatic plexus of veins and the vertebral venous plexus. Straining during urination, necessary because of the obstructive prostatic cancer tissue, causes the blood draining the prostatic venous plexus to reverse its flow and pass via the lumbar veins into the vertebral venous plexus.[3]

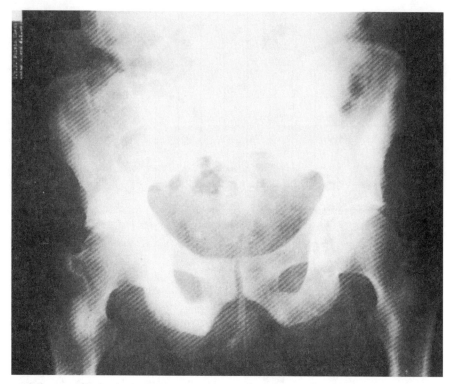

FIGURE 19.1   *Plain x-ray of the pelvis showing sclerotic (osteoblastic) metastases from carcinoma of the prostate in the right pubic bone. (Reprinted with permission from A Cuschieri, GR Giles, AR Moossa [eds]. Essential Surgical Practice [3d ed]. Oxford: Butterworth–Heinemann, 1995;1517.)*

Prostate cancer cells also spread via the pelvic lymphatics (lymphogenous metastases), to lymph nodes around the internal iliac and common iliac arteries and the aorta.[3] Lymphatic metastases can involve the pelvic region (obturator, hypogastric, external iliac, common iliac, presacral, and presciatic nodes), inguinal, and distant (periaortic, mediastinal, and supraclavicular) nodes.[1]

Tumor cells from the prostate may also pass via the pelvic veins to the inferior vena cava, the right heart, the lungs, the left heart, and then throughout the body. Distant organ prostate metastases most commonly involve the skeleton, lungs, adrenal glands, and kidneys. Prostatic cancer cells are more apt to produce bone metastases than organ metastases. The bony metastases are more likely to demonstrate an increase in bone density (osteoblastic) than bone destruction (osteolytic) (Figure 19.1).[1,3] Staging systems for prostate adenocarcinoma are useful in determining treatment options and as a guideline for prognosis. The modified Jewett-Strong-Marshall system and the tumor, node, metastases system defined by the American Joint Committee for Cancer are the common classification systems used for prostate cancer.[1]

The modified Jewett-Strong-Marshall system defines four stages of tumor, A through D.

TABLE 19.1 Staging of prostatic carcinoma

Stage	Clinical findings
A	Clinically undetectable; found on pathologic examination after prostatectomy performed for obstructive symptoms
A1	Focal, well differentiated
A2	Diffuse, poorly differentiated
B	Limited to prostate on rectal examination
B1	Solitary nodule <1.5 cm, one lobe
B2	One whole lobe or both lobes
C	Locally extending outside of prostatic capsule
D	Distant organ metastases
D1	Limited to pelvic lymph nodes
D2	Distant organ and bone metastases

1. *Stage A prostate carcinoma* refers to disease that is unsuspected on rectal examination, but which is discovered at the time of prostatectomy done for obstructive symptoms. If less than 5% of the available tissue is cancerous, and if it is well differentiated, then the disease is considered stage A1 and no further therapy is required. If a larger percentage of the tissue is cancerous, or if it is less well differentiated, the classification becomes stage A2.[4]
2. *Stage B carcinoma* is defined as disease limited to the prostate gland, detected clinically either as a nodule or diffuse hardness on digital rectal examination. Stage B1 tumors have a nodule of 1.5 cm or less, while stage B2 tumors are multifocal nodules larger than 1.5 cm, involving most of a single lobe of the prostate, or parts of both lobes.[1,4]
3. Stage C tumors have spread beyond the prostatic capsule. This stage has the most extensive localized prostatic cancer spread.[1,4]
4. Men with stage D tumors have organ metastases. Stage D1 tumors are limited to pelvic lymph nodes, and stage D2 tumors have advanced to the bones, liver, or lungs (Table 19.1).[1,2,4]

The tumor, node, metastases staging system for prostate carcinoma uses "T" for tumor, "N" for node, and "M" for metastases. T1 tumors are comparable to stage A and T2 tumors are comparable to stage B malignancies of the Jewett-Strong-Marshall system. T3 and T4 tumors have spread beyond the prostatic capsule. The addition of the letter N to the descriptor indicates nodal involvement, and the letter M indicates distant organ metastases.

In addition to staging systems, prostate carcinomas are further classified by the Gleason grading system, which is used to describe the malignant potential of the tumor. The Gleason system utilizes grading scores up to 10, with scores of 2 through 4 indicating a well-differentiated tumor, and scores of 8 through 10 defining poorly differentiated, aggressive tumors.[1,5]

Complications of prostate adenocarcinoma include bladder outlet obstruction, ureteral obstruction, painful bony metastases, lung and liver dysfunction related to metastases, and death. The local invasion produces bladder outlet obstruction and obstructive uropathies, and distant metastases may cause pain, organ dysfunction, and ultimately death.[1]

TABLE 19.2   Survival with appropriately managed prostatic cancer

Stage	Percentage survival, 5 years	Percentage survival, 15 years
A1	Normal life expectancy	Normal life expectancy
A2	50	—
B1	85–90[a]	50
B2	20[b]	1
C	50	—
D	50 (3 yr)	—

[a]Survival is better with stage B1 tumors than stage A2 probably because the cancer can be detected on examination and may therefore be detected earlier; also A2 is a larger, more poorly differentiated cancer, than B.
[b]Untreated.

It is difficult to accurately assess the influence of prostate cancer on longevity, as this disease typically occurs in older men who often also have coexisting diseases that may influence longevity. The best estimates for survival with various stages of prostatic cancer, and with appropriate treatment are listed in Table 19.2.

History

Carcinoma of the prostate may present with obstructive symptoms that often progress rather quickly, in contrast to those seen in patients with benign prostatic hypertrophy, whose symptoms of outlet obstruction may progress over several years.[4] Early on, altered patterns of urinary elimination including diminished force of stream, postvoid urinary dribble, diurnal frequency, nocturia, and feelings of incomplete bladder emptying, are suggestive of bladder outlet obstruction. With advanced cases of urinary retention, flank pain may indicate hydronephrosis.[1]

The onset of back or bone pain, anorexia, and weight loss suggests metastatic disease. Patients with the chronic bone pain of skeletal metastases complain of dull, aching discomfort aggravated by movement or exertion.[4]

Physical Examination

The physical examination of the patient with urinary retention and suspected prostate carcinoma should include an observation of the urinary stream, assessment of postvoid residuals, an abdominal examination, pelvic lymph node palpation, skeletal palpation for pain, and a prostate examination. A neurologic examination in advanced disease may suggest spinal cord injury due to vertebral metastasis.

Tumor enlargement causes the urinary stream to be poor with prolonged voiding time and significant postvoid residual volume (greater than 100 ml or 25% of total bladder capacity).[1]

The abdominal examination may demonstrate an enlarged bladder or renal enlargement due to chronic obstruction. On percussion of the patient's back, costovertebral angle tenderness and flank pain may be associated with obstruction. Vertebral bone pain upon percussion of lumbar vertebrae suggest advanced (metastatic) disease.[1]

The posterior surface of the prostate is palpable through the rectum. Palpating the prostate rectally provides information about its size and consistency. Digital examination of a malignant prostate reveals asymmetric posterior lobe enlargement and specific hard nodules. The patient with evidence of asymmetric, nodular prostate enlargement on digital examination should be advised to seek prompt evaluation and care from a urologist.[1,3]

Laboratory Data

Once asymmetric, nodular prostate enlargement is discovered on prostate examination, further evaluation and biopsy are indicated. The following laboratory workup should be considered in suspected cases of prostate carcinoma:

1. Transrectal prostatic ultrasound may demonstrate an increased volume of prostate gland noted with cancerous tissue.
2. Serum prostate specific antigen (PSA) is elevated (greater than 2.5 ng/ml) in prostate cancer. However, a mild elevation of PSA (less than or equal to 10 ng/ml) may also be noted with benign prostatic hypertrophy.
3. Serum alkaline phosphatase is elevated with advanced disease.
4. Intravenous pyelogram and intravenous urogram may demonstrate evidence of obstructive uropathy at the level of the bladder outlet or ureterovesical junction.
5. Radionuclide bone scan shows bony metastases (Figure 19.2).
6. Plain x-rays of bones show bony metastases (see Figure 19.1).
7. Chest x-ray may demonstrate lung metastases.
8. Computed tomography can be used to detect metastases to the pelvis, sternum, or vertebral column not evident on radionuclide bone scan. This procedure may also reveal enlarged lymph nodes.
9. Magnetic resonance imaging may be used to detect bone metastases, enlarged lymph nodes, and the extent of local tumor spread (Figures 19.3 and 19.4).
10. Lymphangiography helps demonstrate lymphatic node metastases.[1]

Treatment

The treatment for prostate carcinoma should begin with prophylactic screening measures to aid in early detection of the disease. Once identified, available treatment for prostate cancer and its complications includes conservative measures for urinary retention caused by the tumor, medications for urinary retention and bone pain, surgery, radiation therapy (external beam vs. radioactive seeds), chemotherapy, hormonal therapy, and orchiectomy.

The therapy for prostatic carcinoma may be approached on the basis of the disease stage (see Table 19.1).

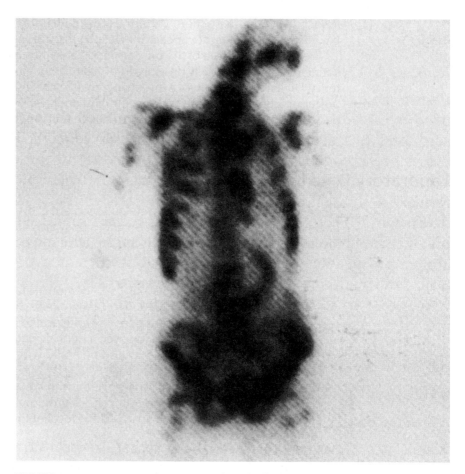

FIGURE 19.2   *Bone scan of a patient with multiple "hot spots" due to metastases from carcinoma of the prostate. (Reprinted with permission from A Cuschieri, GR Giles, AR Moossa [eds]. Essential Surgical Practice [3d ed]. Oxford: Butterworth–Heinemann, 1995;1516.)*

Stage A prostate carcinoma refers to disease unsuspected on rectal examination, but which is discovered by the pathologist at the time of prostatectomy performed for obstructive symptoms. Once identified, the urologist or oncologist initiates a metastatic evaluation by obtaining a serum acid phosphatase, bone scan, intravenous pyelogram, and abdominal-pelvic computed tomography scanning to check for lymph node involvement. If there is no evidence of metastatic disease or lymph node involvement, the prostatic tissue that has been resected should be reexamined to determine the percentage of cancerous tissue. If less than 5% of the available tissue is cancer, and if it is well differentiated, then stage A1 disease is present. With stage A1 disease, no further therapy is required, but careful urological follow-up every three to six months for three years and then yearly is recommended to evaluate for recurrence. If greater than 5% of the tissue is cancerous or if it is less well differentiated, the classification is stage A2. With this stage, definitive radiotherapy is the

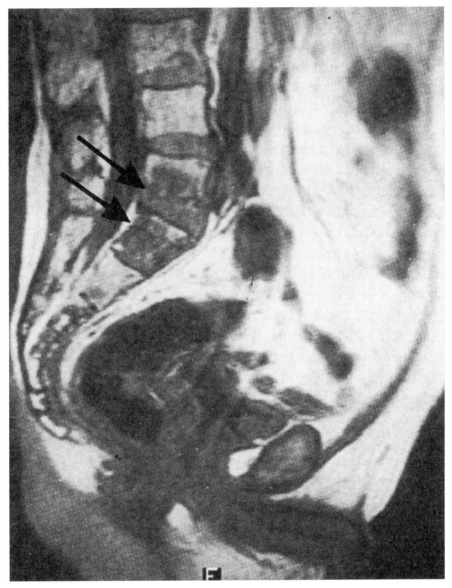

FIGURE 19.3 *Magnetic resonance imaging scan of the pelvis shows metastases* (arrows) *from carcinoma of the prostate. (Reprinted with permission from A Cuschieri, GR Giles, AR Moossa [eds]. Essential Surgical Practice [3d ed]. Oxford: Butterworth–Heinemann, 1995;1516.)*

recommended treatment. Radiation cystitis and proctitis occur with this form of treatment in approximately 25% of cases. Some urologists and oncologists recommend radical prostatectomy for those under age 60 with well-differentiated stage A2 carcinoma of the prostate.[4,6,7]

Stage B tumor is defined as disease limited to the prostate gland, which is detected clinically either as a nodule or as diffuse hardness of a lobe on digital examination. If less than one lobe is involved, and if a patient

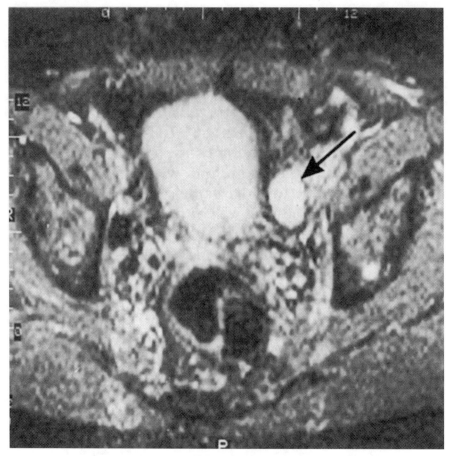

FIGURE 19.4 *Pelvic magnetic resonance imaging scan showing enlarged lymph nodes* (arrow) *in the left side of the pelvis due to carcinoma of the prostate. (Reprinted with permission from A Cuschieri, GR Giles, AR Moossa [eds]. Essential Surgical Practice [3d ed]. Oxford: Butterworth–Heinemann, 1995;1517.)*

under 70 years of age has no contraindicating medical diseases, he is a candidate for curative radical prostatectomy.[4]

Extensive localized prostate cancer, stage C, is best treated by definitive radiotherapy. Transurethral resection of the prostate may also be needed if bladder outlet obstruction is present.[4,8]

Metastatic, stage D prostate cancer is best managed by hormonal therapy or orchiectomy. Estrogen therapy with diethylstilbestrol (1–3 mg per day), and orchiectomy give similar results, producing an 85–90% partial response rate in previously untreated symptomatic patients. The average duration of response is 18 months, although prolonged remissions have been documented. There is no advantage to combining orchiectomy and estrogen therapy. Generally, estrogen therapy (which causes salt and water retention) should be avoided in patients who have a poorly controlled, edema-forming illness such as severe congestive heart failure or nephrotic syndrome.[4]

A Prostate Screening Program

A prostate screening program should be an important part of a man's health care program. Men of any age may develop prostate cancer, although the risks increase after age 40. Several screening modalities can be used. A digital examination performed by a urologist or a trained nurse specialist should be the initial screening tool. Suspicious digital examination is further evaluated by transrectal prostatic ultrasound and transrectal or transperineal biopsy as indicated. Measuring PSA serves as a sensitive screening method. The PSA may be elevated even before the onset of clinically apparent symptoms.[1]

Educational seminars for prostate cancer should emphasize the following:

1. The American Cancer Society recommends all men over age 40 should have a digital rectal examination annually.
2. The early stages of prostate cancer are asymptomatic.
3. Early disease can be detected by digital rectal examination, increasing the probability of cure.
4. Obstructive voiding symptoms do not necessarily indicate cancer (also caused by benign prostatic hypertrophy), but, nonetheless, require prompt medical evaluation.
5. A screening program, including community seminars, may be targeted to occur during prostate awareness week, the last week in September.[1]

Conservative Measures to Treat Altered Patterns of Urinary Elimination Related to Prostate Gland Enlargement

The patient with urinary retention due to prostate carcinoma should void on a regular basis, approximately every two hours. Double voiding helps to maximize bladder evacuation and reduce residual urinary volumes. A fluid management program to ensure adequate fluid intake while avoiding bolus fluid consumption (which predisposes the patient to acute urinary retention) should be instituted.[1] Such measures are helpful until definitive surgical intervention can occur.

Pharmacologic Treatment of Retention

Alpha-blocking agents (prazosin, terazosin, or doxazosin) should be administered as directed. Alpha blockers inhibit alpha-adrenergic tone in the prostatic urethra, possibly reducing urinary retention related to prostate carcinoma.[1]

Treatment of Bone Pain

The pain related to skeletal metastases from prostate cancer is chronic, dull, boring, and located in affected bones. Exertion and movement typically aggravate the pain. The patient with bony metastases should restrict excessive movement if bone pain is severe or if the risk of pathologic fracture is significant.[1]

Narcotic analgesic agents should be used to manage severe bony pain. In some instances, nonsteroidal anti-inflammatory agents may offer relief from skeletal discomfort. Analgesics should be administered as needed to relieve pain.

External beam radiation therapy directed at skeletal metastases may be used to reduce the size and discomfort associated with them.[1] A thoracolumbosacral orthosis may provide spinal stability so as to help prevent pathologic fractures.

Surgery for Prostate Cancer

Definitive surgery is ultimately required to remove cancer tissue, stage the tumor, and relieve obstruction. Surgical procedures include radical prostatectomy (for resection of localized tumor); implantation of interstitial radioactive seeds; pelvic lymphadenectomy (primarily a staging procedure); and orchiectomy as an alternative to hormone therapy.[1] The various surgical procedures are usually followed by hormone therapy, radiation therapy, or chemotherapy.

Radical prostatectomy is the surgical removal of the prostate, seminal vesicals, and prostatic capsule followed by reanastomosis of the urethra to the bladder. Radical prostatectomy eliminates bladder outlet obstruction through resection of the prostate and its capsule. Different surgical approaches can be used, depending on the extent of the patient's tumor and the surgeon's familiarity with and preference for a given technique. The most commonly used approaches are suprapubic, retropubic, perineal, and transcoccygeal. Lymphadenectomy may also be performed during the procedure.[1]

Indications for radical prostatectomy include prostate cancers contained within the capsule (stages A1, A2, B1, and B2). Contraindications include advanced stage lesions that have penetrated the capsule (stage C, D1, and D2).[1]

Postoperatively, a catheter is left in the urethra for 10–14 days to ensure bladder drainage as the urethrovesical junction heals. The patient should consume a low-residue diet and take stool softeners for the first several weeks after surgery. This helps soften the stool, preventing the need to strain while defecating, which diminishes the risk of disrupting the urethrovesical anastomosis before adequate wound healing. Bladder spasms after radical prostatectomy may also potentially compromise urethrovesical integrity. Anticholinergic and antispasmodic medications inhibit unstable contractions while the catheter is in place.[1]

Complications that can occur after radical prostatectomy include impotence (erectile dysfunction), incontinence, infection, and separation of urethra and bladder.[1]

Sexual dysfunction and infertility may occur as a consequence of radical prostatectomy, orchiectomy, or hormonal therapy for prostate carcinoma. The patient who undergoes radical prostatectomy or surgical orchiectomy should be informed preoperatively that infertility is to be expected. Postoperative erectile dysfunction can be minimized by the use of nerve-sparing radical prostatectomy procedures or by subsequent treatment using surgical or pharmacologic measures. Sexual dysfunctions (erectile dysfunction, infertility, ejaculatory dysfunction, and altered libido) should be treated by a qualified specialist.[1]

Some dribbling incontinence or stress incontinence may occur after radical prostatectomy, related to reconstruction of the sphincter during the procedure. Pelvic floor muscle exercises and alpha sympathomimetic agents may help to reduce or ablate stress incontinence in affected patients.[1]

Hormonal Therapy for Prostate Cancer

Hormonal therapy using estrogens and antiandrogens after prostatectomy works by suppressing the growth of any residual tumor.

Estrogens (diethylstilbestrol, others) are used as a palliative therapy of advanced prostate cancer. Prostate tumor cell growth is stimulated by the male hormone testosterone. With androgenic hormone–dependent conditions, such as metastatic carcinoma of the prostate, estrogens counter the androgenic influence by competing for receptor binding sites. As a result of this treatment, metastatic lesions may show improvement. Side effects of estrogen therapy include an increased risk of cardiovascular disease, peripheral edema, change in body habitus, gynecomastia, and increased risk of thromboembolism.

Antiandrogens (ketoconazole, aminoglutethimide, spironolactone, flutamide, megestrol acetate, cyproterone acetate, others) work either by inhibiting androgen synthesis, or by competition for androgen-binding sites. Side effects of antiandrogens include nausea and vomiting, gynecomastia, hepatotoxicity, and hypocalcemia.

Orchiectomy is an alternative to hormone therapy.[1]

Radiation Therapy

External beam radiation therapy is used to impede or eradicate prostate cancer and its metastatic lesions. External beam radiotherapy affects rapidly proliferating cells, including tumor cells and normal components of gastrointestinal and bladder mucosa. Symptoms of diarrhea, altered appetite, nausea, and cystitis may occur due to bowel or bladder mucosal compromise.[1]

Interstitial radiation therapy uses radioactive seeds, which are surgically implanted to deliver radiation to the prostate. Interstitial radiation therapy attacks rapidly proliferating malignant and normal cells near and inside the prostate gland, and this form of radiotherapy may also cause diarrhea, proctitis, and irritative voiding symptoms.[1]

Chemotherapy

Chemotherapy is used to inhibit or eradicate advanced prostate malignancies. Chemotherapy, like radiotherapy, attacks both neoplastic and

TABLE 19.3   Treatment for prostate cancer

A prostate screening program
    Educational seminars
    Digital examination
    Serum markers (prostate-specific antigen)
Conservative measures for altered patterns of urinary elimination related to prostate
        gland enlargement (until definitive surgical intervention)
    Double voiding
    Fluid management program
Pharmacologic treatment of retention
    Alpha-blocking agents
Treatment of bone pain
    Nonsteroidal anti-inflammatory drugs
    Opioids
    Radiation therapy
    Thoracolumbosacral orthosis
Surgery for prostate cancer
    Radial prostatectomy
    Implantation of interstitial radioactive seeds
    Pelvic lymphadenectomy (staging)
    Orchiectomy
Hormonal therapy for prostate cancer
    Estrogens
    Antiandrogens
    Orchiectomy as an alternative to hormone therapy
Radiation therapy
    External beam
    Interstitial (seeds)
Chemotherapy

normal cells that reproduce rapidly. Side effects of chemotherapy include nausea, vomiting, suppressed appetite, and alopecia.[1]

Table 19.3 summarizes the treatment modalities used in the management of prostate carcinoma.

References

1. Gray M. Genitourinary Cancer. In M Gray (ed), Genitourinary Disorders. St. Louis: Mosby, 1992;200–257.
2. Kozlowski JM, Grayhack JT. Carcinoma of the Prostate. In JY Gillenwater, JT Grayhack, SS Howards, JW Duckett (eds), Adult and Pediatric Urology. Chicago: Mosby–Year Book, 1991.
3. Moore KL. The Perineum and Pelvis. In KL Moore (ed), Clinically Oriented Anatomy. Baltimore: Williams & Wilkins, 1980;293–418.
4. Smolev JK. Bladder Outlet Obstruction. In LR Barker, JR Burton, PD Zieve (eds), Principles of Ambulatory Medicine (2d ed). Baltimore: Williams & Wilkins, 1986;568–576.
5. Narayan P. Neoplasms of the Prostate Gland. In EA Tanagho, JW McAninch (eds), Smith's General Urology. Norwalk, CT: Lange Medical Publishers, 1992.

6. Whitmore WF Jr, Batata M, Hilaris B. Prostate Irradiation: Iodine-125 Implantation. In DE Johnson, ML Samuels (eds), Cancer of the Genitourinary Tract. New York: Raven, 1979.
7. Walsh PC, Lepor H, Eggleston JC. Radical prostatectomy with preservation of sexual function: Anatomical and pathological considerations. Prostate 1983;4:473.
8. Catalona WJ, Scott WW. Carcinoma of the prostate: A review. J Urol 1978;119:1.

II   Wound Care

Section Editor: Lyn D. Weiss

20 Anatomy and Physiology of Human Skin

Daniel Mendez

The skin is the largest organ system of the body. It is continuous with the mucosae of the alimentary, respiratory, and urogenital tracts. The skin forms about 8% of the total body mass and its thickness ranges from about 1.5 to 4.0 mm, variations being due to maturation, aging, and regional specialization.[1] It consists of an epithelium (the epidermis), a connective tissue matrix (the dermis), and adipose tissue (hypodermis) (Figure 20.1). The skin forms a protective barrier between the individual and the external environment. Within limits, it impedes the penetration of microorganisms, and protects against mechanical, chemical, thermal, and radiation damage. It is also an important primary site of immuno-surveillance. Skin is involved in sociosexual communication from close and distant contact. It provides personal identification and individual identity or self-image.

Anatomy

Epidermis

The epidermis is a dynamic structure capable of acting as a semi-impermeable barrier and that reacts to exogenous stimuli. It consists of stratified, squamous epithelium that keratinizes and gives rise to other structures (nails, hair, sebaceous apparatus, and sweat glands) (Figure 20.2). It is approximately 0.4–1.5 mm in thickness.[2] The majority of cells in the epidermis are keratinocytes. These cells are organized into four layers that are named for either their position or a structural property. The purpose and ultimate goal of the epidermis is to produce a semi-impermeable membrane called the *stratum corneum* (horny layer). The process of migration of keratinocytes from the basal layer to the environment takes approximately 28 days.[3]

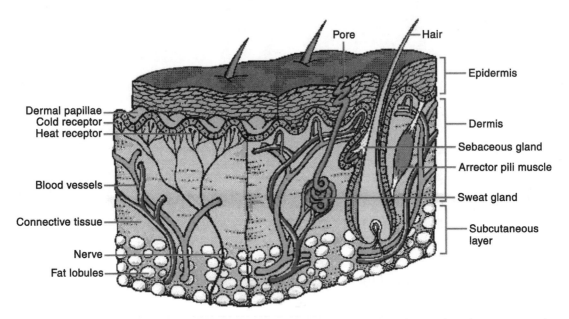

FIGURE 20.1   *Cross-section of skin. (Reprinted with permission from Microsoft Encyclopedia Encarta. Redmond, WA: Microsoft, 1998.)*

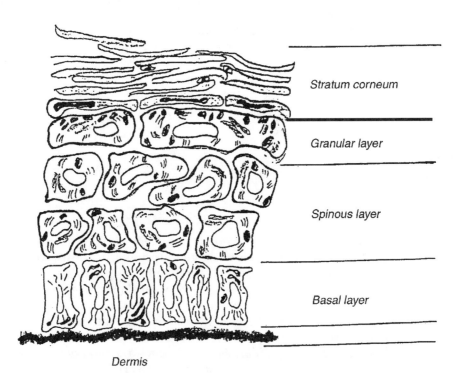

Stratum corneum

Granular layer

Spinous layer

Basal layer

Dermis

FIGURE 20.2   *The four stages of differentiation in the adult epidermis. In the skin of the palms and soles we can find the stratum lucidum, not present in this diagram.*

Layers of the Epidermis

Basal Cell Layer (Stratum Germinativum)   The basal cell layer is composed of two distinct cells, the keratinocytes and the melanocytes. The keratinocytes attach to the basement membrane zone and also to each other by intercellular bridges, or desmosomes. Basal cells contain a large nucleus and a prominent nucleolus. Golgi, rough endoplasmic reticulum, mitochondria, lysosomes, and ribosomes are present in the cytoplasm. In addition there are membrane-bound vacuoles that contain pigmented melanosomes transferred from melanocytes by phagocytosis. The keratin filaments are collected into fine bundles that organize around the nucleus and insert into desmosomes and hemidesmosomes.

Microfilaments (actin, myosin, and alpha-actinin) and microtubules are present in basal cells. They assist in the upward movement of cells as they differentiate.[2] The basal cell layer is the primary location of mitotically active cells of the epidermis.

Squamous Cell Layer (Stratum Spinosum)   The cells on this layer are polygonal in shape and gradually flatten as they approach the surface. The cells of the upper spinous layers contain new organelles known as lamellar granules. As in the basal cells, the keratin filaments are around the nucleus and insert into desmosomes peripherally. The "spines" of spinous cells are the abundant desmosomes, calcium-dependent cell surface modifications that promote adhesion of epidermal cells and resistance to mechanical stresses.[2] Four integral membrane glycoproteins provide adhesive properties on the external surface of the desmosome.

Granular Cell Layer (Stratum Granulosum)   Granular cell layer cells are flattened and filled with irregularly shaped and dark-staining keratohyaline granules. Keratohyaline granules are composed primarily of an electron-dense (13) protein, profilaggrin, and keratin intermediate filaments. By this layer, the squamous cells have lost all their intracellular machinery, including nuclei, Golgi apparatus, ribosomes, and mitochondria.[3]

Horny Cell Layer (Stratum Corneum)   Complete transition from a granular to a cornified cell is accompanied by a 45–86% loss in dry weight.[2] The horny cell layer is characterized by strength, flexibility, elasticity, toughness, and a dry surface that discourages growth of microorganisms. The flattened, polyhedral-shaped, horny cell is the largest of the epidermis. High molecular mass keratins (>60 kDa), stabilized by intermolecular disulfide bonds, account for up to 80% of the cornified cell. Cells survive for approximately 14 days on this layer and eventually fall away. The desmosomes undergo proteolytic degradation in the outermost stratum corneum cells.

Nonkeratinocytes Cells of the Epidermis

Melanocytes   Melanocytes are dendritic pigment-synthesizing cells derived from the neural crest and are confined mainly to the basal layer. Other sites for melanocytes are the hair follicles, dermal-epidermal junction, mucous membranes, the central nervous system (leptomeninges), eye, inner ear, oral cavity, and cochlea. Each melanocyte is associated with about 36 keratinocytes. Melanocytes contact keratinocytes in the basal and more superficial layers but do not form junctions with them at any level. Differentiation of the melanocyte correlates with the acquisition of its primary functions: melanogenesis, arborization, and transfer of pigment to keratinocytes.

Melanosome is a distinctive, melanin-producing organelle of the melanocyte. The size of melanosomes is determined genetically; black skin typically contains larger melanosomes than more lightly pigmented skin. Melanocytes also contain vimentin-positive and keratin-negative intermediate filaments. They divide within the epidermis at a rate that keeps pace with the turnover of keratinocytes and increase their rate of proliferation when stimulated by ultraviolet B.

Merkel Cells Merkel cells are slow adapting, type I mechanoreceptors located in sites of high tactile sensitivity.[2] Their specific localization in epidermal appendages has caused some speculation that they may stimulate the development of these structures.

Langerhans' Cells Langerhans' cells are bone marrow-derived, antigen-presenting cells that are involved in a variety of T-cell responses. They account for 2–8% of the total epidermal cell population. Langerhans' cells are mostly localized in the basal and spinous layers of the epidermis.[1] They do not form junctions with keratinocytes or melanocytes. The Langerhans' cell is present not only on the epidermis, but also populates areas like the oral cavity, esophagus, vagina, spleen, thymus, lymph nodes, and the normal dermis.[2]

Dermal-Epidermal Junction (Basement Membrane Zone) The dermal-epidermal junction or basement membrane zone (BMZ) forms an interface between the epidermis and dermis. The BMZ includes several ultrastructural components: the inner portion of the basal cell plasma membrane, the lamina lucida, the lamina densa and the sublamina densa or reticular lamina (Figure 20.3). The structures of the BMZ are almost entirely a product of the basal keratinocytes, with minor contributions from the dermal fibroblasts.

Basal Cell Membrane The outermost portion of the BMZ contains the basal keratinocytes. Hemidesmosomes are found along the dermal side of this membrane. Carter et al.[4] have identified a glycoprotein ligand named *epiligrin*, which is associated with the X6 4 integrin and the X3 1 integrin. This molecule may be the adhesive that helps to bind epidermal cells to adjacent structures on the basement membrane.

Lamina Lucida The lamina lucida begins at the inner portion of the basal cell membrane and is 20–40 mm wide.[3] It is the primary location of several noncollagenous glycoproteins: laminin, entactin-nidogen, and fibronectin. This is the weakest area of the BMZ. It separates easily with heat and suction, with treatment using salt solutions and proteolytic enzymes, and in disease.[2]

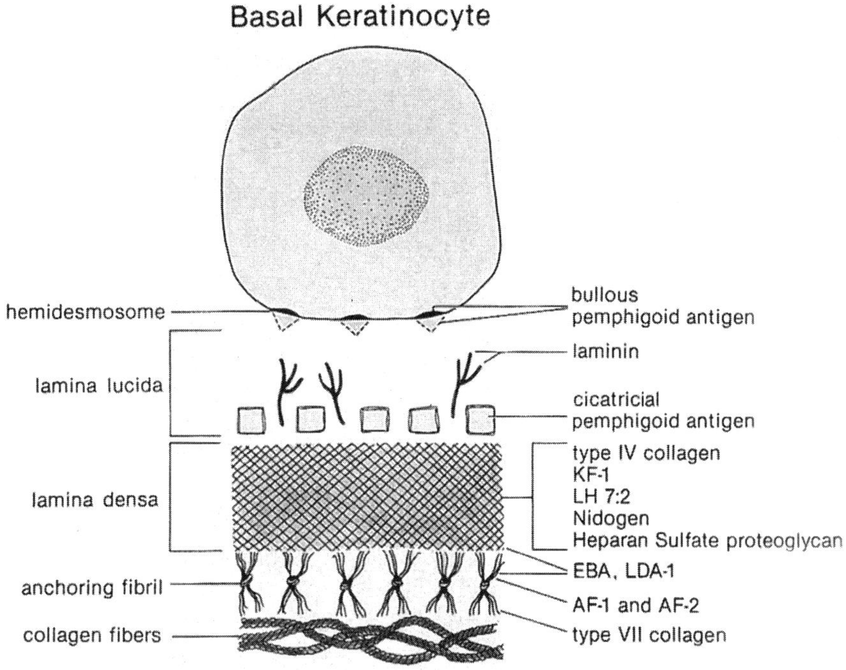

Basal Keratinocyte

FIGURE 20.3 *Basement membrane zone. A number of antigens are now recognized, many of which are associated with specific diseases. (Reprinted with permission from WM Sams, PJ Lynch [eds]. Principles and Practice of Dermatology [2d ed]. New York: Churchill Livingstone, 1996;9.)*

Lamina Densa   The lamina densa is 30–60 mm wide.[3] Also sometimes referred to as the basal lamina. The primary component of this lamina is type IV collagen.

Sublamina Densa   The sublamina densa consists of interstitial collagens (types I, III, V, and VI) and procollagens (types I and III) that in addition to the first fibers of the elastic system bind the epidermis to the dermis through the BMZ.

Dermis   The dermis is an irregular, moderately dense, integrated system of fibrous and filamentous connective tissue. It contains an amorphous ground substance consisting of glycosaminoglycans, glycoproteins, and bound water. This ground substance accommodates nerve and vascular networks, epidermally derived appendages, fibroblasts, macrophages, mast cells, and other blood-borne cells (including lymphocytes, plasma cells, and other leukocytes) that enter the dermis in response to diverse stimuli. The dermis is vital for the survival of the epidermis. The dermis can be divided into two zones: a narrow superficial papillary layer and a deeper reticular layer (Figure 20.4).

Dermal Collagen   Collagen is the most common protein in the body. It is the major dermal component, making up approximately 70% of the dry

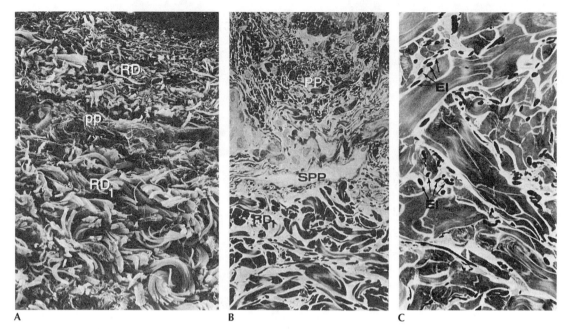

FIGURE 20.4　Papillary and reticular dermis shown in scanning electron **(A)** and light **(B,C)** micrographs. In **(A)** the fine papillary network is seen beneath the epidermis extending to a vascular boundary created by vessels of the subpapillary plexus as shown in **(B)**. The upper portion of the reticular dermis has smaller collagen bundles than the deep reticular dermis. Elastic fibers border the collagen bundles. **(A)** ×525, **(B)** ×300, **(C)** ×700 in the original magnifications. (PD = papillary, RD = reticular dermis, E = epidermis, SPP = subpapillary plexus, RD_1 = upper portion of the reticular dermis, El = elastic fibers.) (Reprinted with permission from TB Fitzpatrick, AZ Eisen, K Wolff, et al. Dermatology in General Medicine [4th ed, vol 1]. New York: McGraw-Hill, 1993;120.)

weight of the skin. It has incredible tensile strength.[3] A single fiber 1 mm in diameter is capable of withstanding a static load of up to 20 kg. The interstitial collagens (types I, III, and V) account for the greatest portion of collagen in the adult dermis. Type I collagen makes up about 80–85%, type III 15–20%, and type V less than 5% of interstitial collagen. Type VI collagen is abundant in the dermis, forming a microfibrillar network, enmeshing nerves and vessels. Type IV collagen is confined to the basal lamina of the BMZ, vessels, and epidermal appendages, and type VII collagen form anchoring fibrils at the BMZ. The collagen molecule is produced by fibroblasts, which synthesize the three-polypeptide chains that wrap around one another in a triple helix. All chains are composed of glycine and other amino acids, typically proline and hydroxyproline.

Elastic Tissue　The elastic connective tissue is assembled in a continuous network that extends from the lamina densa of the BMZ throughout the dermis and into the connective tissue of the hypodermis. Elastic fibers are also present in the walls of cutaneous vessels and lymphatics and in the sheaths of hair follicles. By dry weight, elastic connective tissue accounts for 4% of the dermal matrix protein.[2] Elastic fibers are also produced by fibroblasts and their major component is elastin, a substance with a well-characterized molecular structure and an amorphous appearance.

Microfibrils are embedded within and collected on the surface of the elastin matrix. Elastic fibers turn over very slowly in the skin, are damaged by solar radiation, and become dysmorphic with aging.

Ground Substance   Ground substance is the amorphous substance that bathes the structural components of the dermis. Proteoglycans and glycosaminoglycans are the molecules of the ground substance. They account for only 2% of the dry weight of skin. A more recently recognized macromolecule of the dermis is fibronectin, which apparently functions as an adhesive protein to attach cells, especially fibroblasts, to collagen.

Major Regions of the Dermis

The dermis is organized into papillary and reticular regions.

Papillary Layer
The papillary layer is immediately below the epidermis. It is characterized by small bundles of small-diameter collagen fibrils and oxytalan elastic fibers. The papillary dermis is specialized to provide mechanical anchorage, metabolic support, and trophic maintenance to the overlying tissue, as well as housing rich networks of sensory nerve endings and blood vessels. Capillaries extending from the subpapillary plexus project toward the epidermis within the dermal papillae, fingerlike projections of papillary dermis that interdigitate with the rete pegs. Rete pegs project from the epidermis into the dermis.

Reticular Layer
This layer is composed primarily of large-diameter collagen fibrils organized into large fiber bundles. Other branching elastic fibers form a structure around the collagen fiber bundles. The two systems are integrated and can provide the dermis with strong and resilient mechanical properties.

Cells of the Dermis

Fibroblasts   Fibroblasts are responsible for the synthesis and degradation of fibrous and nonfibrous connective tissue matrix proteins.

Monocytes, Macrophages, and Dermal Dendrocytes   Monocytes, macrophages, and dermal dendrocytes constitute the mononuclear phagocytic system of cells in the skin.

Blood Vessels   Arteries supplying the dermis rise from the subcutaneous fat to the subpapillary area, where they branch to form a reticular plexus. From the reticular plexus individual capillaries supply each dermal papilla (forming the papillary plexus). Capillaries from this plexus loop into the dermal papillae and later form the superficial venous plexus. This venous plexus is closely associated with the arteriolar plexus. These vessels provide nutrition for the tissues. The skin as a whole, however, does not require the abundance of vessels to meet its metabolic needs. The vasculature is also involved in the regulation of temperature, blood pressure, wound repair, and numerous immunologic events.

Nerves

The innervation of the skin contains somatic sensory and sympathetic autonomic fibers. The sensory fibers alone or in conjunction with specialized structures can provide a wealth of information about touch, pain, temperature, itch, and mechanical stimuli. Large, myelinated cutaneous branches of musculocutaneous nerves that arise segmentally from spinal nerves innervate the skin. The free nerve endings are the most widespread and more important sensory receptors of the body. They are common in the papillary dermis just beneath the epidermis.

The corpuscular receptors have a capsules and inner core. The main receptors are the Meissner's corpuscles that function as mechanoreceptors and the Pacinian corpuscles that are mainly located on weight bearing surfaces of the body.

Lymphatics

Water, proteins, macromolecules, cell fragments, mobile inflammatory and tumor cells leave the interstitial space partially or exclusively through the most peripheral part of the lymph vessel system. The lymphatic vessels are divided into two networks[5]:

1. A superficially spread, subpapillary fine-meshed area
2. A part lying at greater depth, which wholly fills the reticular dermis

These drain into somewhat larger vessels that disappear into the subcutis, taking a curving course. There they discharge into larger collecting lymphatics.

Epidermal and Dermal Appendages

A number of glands, follicles, and muscles can be found in the skin, described in the following sections.

Eccrine Glands
Eccrine glands are found in abundance throughout the skin surface, with the exception of the vermilion of the lips, labia minora, and glans penis. They are found in highest concentration on the palms and soles and in the axillae. Their secretory coil is located deep in the dermis and transmits sweat directly to the skin surface via a duct composed of two layers of cells (clear-serous cells and dark-mucoid cells).

Apocrine Glands
Apocrine glands are found primarily in the axillae and anogenital region. They are classified as a type of sweat gland and serve mainly as scent glands. Their activity is controlled mainly by adrenergic nerves and response to emotional stimuli. Apocrine glands do not become active until puberty.

Hair Follicles
The hair follicle is an invagination of the epidermis containing a hair, which may extend deeply into the hypodermis, or may be more superfi-

cial within the dermis. The hair follicle usually buds downward at an angle from the epidermis. Hair growth proceeds through distinct phases: anagen phase, catagen phase, and telogen phase. In anagen the hair is actively growing, followed by the involuting or catagen phase when hair growth ceases and the follicle shrinks. During the final phase, the telogen phase, the inferior segment of the follicle is absent. Mature hair is called *terminal*, and the fine hair over much of the body surface (forearm and abdomen) is called *vellus*.

Arrector Pili Muscles

Each hair follicle has a smooth muscle attached to its base on a diagonal link. These muscles are virtually vestigial in humans. They contract in exposure to cold or in response to fright and give the appearance of "goose bumps."

Sebaceous Glands

Sebaceous glands are small saccular structures lying in the dermis. They are found on all parts of the body except the palms and soles. These glands empty into the outer portion of the hair follicle, except on the labia minora, inner aspect of prepuce, nipple, and areola, where they open directly to the surface. Their secretory product is called *sebum*. This secretion may become impacted within the duct and may lead to a comedo, which when inflamed and infected, is the primary lesion of acne.

Nail Unit

The nail unit has five components.

- The nail plate, a horny, rectangular-shaped plate on the extensor surface of each digit's end
- The matrix, a proximal nail fold
- The nail bed, on which the nail plate rests
- The hyponychium, which underlies the free distal edge of the nail plate
- The cornified cells of the nail plate, formed from the nail matrix, which lies 2–4 mm proximal to the cuticle[3]

The nails in humans serve for protection and as tools for scratching and as a window into an array of systemic diseases.

Hypodermis

The hypodermis is mainly an adipose tissue–rich subcutaneous region. It is structurally and functionally well connected with the reticular dermis through nerve and vascular networks and the continuity of epidermal appendages.

The tissue of the hypodermis insulates the body, serves as a reserve energy supply, cushions and protects the skin, and allows for its mobility over underlying structures. It has a cosmetic effect in molding body contours.

Physiology

Epidermis

The cells of the stratum corneum are organized into geometric stacks, which are embedded in a lipid-enriched intercellular matrix. This layer protects the body's aqueous interior from excessive water loss in a dry environment. It also protects against the entrance of microorganisms, as well as the penetration of natural and man-made toxins.[6] The melanocytes of the epidermis synthesize ultraviolet-absorbing pigments (melanin), and the Langerhans' cells play a role in cutaneous immuno-surveillance, protecting the organism against antigens that breach the stratum corneum.

Epidermal Differentiation (Keratinization)

In the process of keratinization, the epidermal basal cells multiply and eventually cornify to form the stratum corneum. This process involves synthesizing proteins designed for this purpose and also the dissolution of normal cellular components. Four events are involved in this differentiation. The first event is keratinization, the synthesis of the principal fibrous protein of the keratinocyte. Keratin filaments not only impart structural and chemical integrity, but also filter incidental ultraviolet radiation and act as an absorptive element for water and other small molecules.

Keratohyalin disposition is the second major event, and is associated with the synthesis of the stratum corneum basic protein filaggrin. These molecules enhance the water holding capacity of the stratum corneum. The absence of this water is associated with inflexibility, cracking, sealing, and flaking of the skin.

The third event is the formation of an insoluble cornified envelope that provides a rigid structural ectoskeleton. This ectoskeleton provides a highly resistant barrier to external assault (organic solvents, acid and alkaline solutions, and proteolytic enzymes).

The last event is the generation of the lipid-enriched intercellular domains of the stratum corneum. The lamellar bodies produce this lipid content. Three of the most abundant lipid species in the stratum corneum are cholesterol, ceramides, and free fatty acids.[7] The stratum corneum is viewed currently as a layer of protein-enriched corneocytes embedded in a lipid-enriched, intercellular matrix.[8] This two-compartment model is responsible for epidermal waterproofing. The structural integrity protects against invasion by microorganisms and blocks the penetration of macromolecules. The continuous shedding of the outer layer of corneocytes (desquamation) helps to remove adherent microorganisms.

The stratum corneum is not a perfect shield. For this reason, the epidermis has developed a range of second-line biochemical and cellular defenses, which include cytokines, prostaglandins, antioxidants, xenobiotic-metabolizing enzyme system, Langerhans' cells, and the T lymphocytes.

Cytokines

Cytokines are polypeptides produced by keratinocytes, melanocytes, and Langerhans' cells. These cytokines play a role in normal regulation of the epidermis, inflammatory processes, and wound repair in the skin.

Antioxidants

Free radicals can cause various degrees of cellular damage. The epidermis processes an antioxidant mechanism designed to protect the skin from both external and internal environments.

Immune System

Lymphocytes are the principal effector cells of the immune system. Langerhans' cells of the epidermis are accessory cells, which function to present antigens to T lymphocytes. This process leads to a localized immune response within the skin.[6]

Protection from Ultraviolet Irradiation

The skin has two barriers to protect against ultraviolet radiation, a protein barrier in the stratum corneum and a melanin barrier. Melanin is synthesized by melanocytes and transferred to surrounding keratinocytes in secretory granules known as melanosomes. Both of these barriers function by absorbing incident radiation, thereby dissipating the excess energy before absorption by DNA, critical cellular proteins, and membrane lipids.

Protection from Low-Voltage Electric Current

Protection from low-voltage electric current is provided by the highly resistant stratum corneum due to its low water content. The low water content helps to resist the conduction of electrical current through the skin.

Protection from Extremes in Ambient Temperature

The skin, the subcutaneous tissues, and especially the fat of the subcutaneous tissue are heat insulators for the body. Having insulation beneath the skin allows an effective means of maintaining normal internal core temperature, while allowing the temperature of the skin to approach that of the surroundings.[9]

The skin also provides thermoregulation by either dissipating heat from the body or retaining heat within the body. The skin controls body temperature by[9]

1. Conduction (heat lost from the body by direct conduction from the surface of the body to other objects)
2. Convection (removal of heat from the body by convection air currents as the air adjacent to the skin rises as it becomes heated)
3. Evaporation (0.58 calories of heat is lost for each gram of water that evaporates, mainly through sweat, a product of the sweat glands), and
4. Radiation (loss of heat in form of infrared heat rays)

Basement Membrane Zone

In normal skin the BMZ provides cohesion between the dermis and epidermis. It serves as a support for the epidermis, determines the polarity and growth and directs the organization of the cytoskeleton in basal cells, provides developmental signals of morphogenetic events during development and wound healing, and serves as a semipenetrable barrier.

The lamina densa functions as a barrier and filter that restricts the passage of molecules with a molecular mass of >40 kDa, but is penetrated by melanocytes and Langerhans' cells during development.[2]

Dermis

The dermis makes up the bulk of the skin and provides its pliability, elasticity, and tensile strength. It protects the body from mechanical injury, binds water, aids in thermal regulation, and includes receptors of sensory stimuli.

Elastic fibers in the dermis return the skin to its normal configuration after being stretched or deformed. The proteoglycans and glycosaminoglycans[2] of the dermal matrix can bind up to 1,000 times their own volume and thus regulate the water binding capacity of the dermis and influence dermal volume and compressibility. They also influence proliferation, differentiation, tissue repair, and morphogenesis.

References

1. Williams PL (ed). Gray's Anatomy (38th ed). New York: Churchill Livingstone, 1995.
2. Karen AH, Klaus W. The Structure and Development of Skin. In TB Fitzpatrick (ed), Dermatology in General Medicine (4th ed). New York: McGraw-Hill, 1993.
3. Sams WM Jr. Structure and Function of the Skin. In WM Sams Jr, P Lynch (eds), Principles and Practice of Dermatology (2d ed). New York: Churchill Livingstone, 1996;1–23.
4. Carter WG, Ryan MC, Gahr PS, et al. Epiligrin, a new cell adhesion ligand for integrin alpha-3 beta-1 in epithelial basement membranes. Cell 1991;65:599.
5. Lubach D, Ludemann W. Recent findings on the angioarchitecture of the lymph vessel system of human skin. Br J Dermatol 1996;135:733.
6. Elias PM, Jackson SM. What Does Normal Skin Do? In KA Arndt (ed), Cutaneous Medicine and Surgery (vol 1). Philadelphia: WB Saunders, 1996.
7. Elias PM. The stratum corneum revisited. J Dermatol 1996;23:756.
8. Elias PM. Stratum corneum architecture, metabolic activity. Exp Dermatol 1996;5:191.
9. Guyton A, Hall J. Textbook of Medical Physiology (9th ed). Philadelphia: WB Saunders, 1996.

21 Classification of Wounds

Mery Elashvili

Wounds can generally be classified into two categories: acute and chronic. Acute wounds benefit from the normal reparative process that results in the timely restoration of anatomic and functional integrity, but this process does not achieve anatomic and functional integrity with chronic wounds. Acute wounds usually occur in healthy people and close by primary or secondary intention. Chronic wounds usually occur in patients with chronic debilitating diseases. The wounds usually fail to heal until the underlying cause is corrected. Correction of the underlying cause and stimulation of wound healing is essential to the treatment of chronic wounds. With proper management, most chronic wounds heal, but wound recurrence is common. Skin ulcers are the most common chronic wounds and are discussed here. Acute wounds are beyond the scope of this text.[1,2]

Causative Factors

Chronic wounds are generally caused by one of 7 factors. It should be noted that chronic wounds may result from a combination of factors.[3]

1. Vascular: arterial occlusion, venous insufficiency, antiphospholipid syndrome, cryofibrinogenemia or cryoglobulinemia, sickle cell disease or embolic disease
2. Inflammatory processes: pyoderma gangrenosum, necrobiosis lipoidica diabeticorum, panniculitis, dysproteinemias, idiopathic leukocytoclastic vasculitis, periarteritis nodosa, Wegener's granulomatosis, lymphomatoid granulomatosis, erythema elevatum diutinum
3. Pressure necrosis: decubitus ulcers, neuropathic ulcers
4. Physical agents: radiation, heat, frostbite
5. Infectious: bacterial, fungal, mycobacterial, tertiary syphilis, viral
6. Tumors: lymphomas, metastases, primary skin tumors

Pressure ulcers are the most common types of chronic wounds. They occur in patients who are paralyzed, debilitated with chronic diseases, or unconscious.

Staging

Staging of pressure ulcers was developed as a tool for communication and assessment to classify the degree of tissue damage. The recommendations regarding staging put forth here are consistent with those of the National Pressure Ulcer Advisory Panel Consensus Development Conference,[4] as derived from previous staging systems proposed by Shea[5] and the Wound Ostomy and Continence Nurses Society.[6]

Staging of Pressure Ulcers

Stage I

Stage I is nonblanchable erythema of intact skin, the heralding lesion of skin ulceration. In individuals with darker skin, discoloration of the skin, warmth, edema, induration, or hardness may also be indicators.[7]

Stage II

Stage II is partial-thickness skin loss involving epidermis, dermis, or both. The ulcer is superficial and presents clinically as an abrasion, blister, or shallow crater.[7]

Stage III

Stage III is full-thickness skin loss involving damage to or necrosis of subcutaneous tissue that may extend down to, but not through, underlying fascia. The ulcer presents clinically as a deep crater with or without undermining of adjacent tissue.[7]

Stage IV

Stage IV is full-thickness skin loss with extensive destruction, tissue necrosis, or damage to muscle, bone, or supporting structures (tendon and joint capsule). Sinus tracts also may be associated with stage IV ulcers.[7]

Shea Classification

The Shea classification, a classification from which others have been derived, may also be used.[5]

Stage I

Stage I is limited to the superficial epidermis and dermal layers; shows an irregular, ill-defined area of soft-tissue swelling, erythema, and increased warmth; and is reversible.

Stage II

Stage II involves the epidermal and dermal layers and extends into the adipose tissue.

Stage III

Stage III extends through superficial structures down to and including muscle. It is a full-thickness skin defect.

Stage IV

Stage IV involves destruction of all soft tissues down to bone and communication with bone or joint structures.

While the staging of wounds is important, the limitations of any type of classification should be noted. Because skin remains intact in stage I, there is no ulceration of the skin. This type of lesion is hard to assess in dark-pigmented patients. Nevertheless, identification of a stage I ulcer is critical in preventing and assessing wounded skin. If eschar is present, it must be removed before accurate staging can be determined. A deep wound may be covered by a superficial eschar.[7] In the presence of a cast, the skin has to be assessed under the edges of the cast. The health care provider must be alert to patients complaining of pressure-induced pain, and determine if the cast has to be changed to relieve the pressure.[7] The clinician must be especially careful in patients with insensate skin. When evaluating a patient, any support stockings or orthotic devices must be removed in order to adequately assess the skin.[7]

Closed pressure sores are a separate entity, which characterize the innocent clinical presentation that conceals a deep, potentially rapidly fatal lesion. Prolonged pressure and shear stress causes an ischemic necrosis of the subcutaneous fat without skin ulceration, leading to the development of a bursa-like cavity filled with necrotic debris. This can create a small defect on the skin, which drains to the larger base. Eventually, the wound becomes contaminated with bacteria. Because of the extent and depth of tissue damage, these wounds are usually graded as stage III or stage IV pressure sores.[5]

References

1. Greenfield LJ, Mulholland M, Oldham KT, Zelenock GB (eds). Surgery: Scientific Principles and Practice (2d ed). Philadelphia: Lippincott–Raven, 1997.

2. Yarkony GM, Kirk PM, Carlson C, et al. Classification of pressure ulcers. Arch Dermatol 1990;126:1218.
3. Eaglestein WH, Falanga V. Chronic wounds. Surg Clin North Am 1997;77:689.
4. National Pressure Ulcer Advisory Panel. Pressure ulcers, prevalence, cost and risk assessment: consensus development conference statement. Decubus 1989;2:24.
5. Shea JD. Pressure sores: classification and management. Clin Orthop Rel Res 1975;112:89.
6. International Association of Enterostomal Therapy. Dermal wounds: pressure sores: philosophy of the IAET. J Enterostom Ther 1988;15:4.
7. U.S. Department of Health and Human Services. Public Health Service. Treatment of Pressure Ulcers. Clinical Practice Guideline. Washington, DC: Agency for Health Care Policy and Research, 1994.

22   Wound Healing

Nashin Manohar

It is important to grasp the fundamental physiology of wound healing for a clearer understanding of the pathophysiologic processes that impair healing. Wound healing response can be divided into the following distinct but overlapping phases[1]:

- Inflammatory-exudative phase
- Proliferative-granulation phase
- Maturation-remodeling phase
- Wound contraction–remodeling phase

Phases of Wound Healing

Inflammatory-Exudative Phase

The inflammatory-exudative phase begins immediately on injury and lasts several days. It is characterized by increased vascular permeability, chemotaxis of cells from circulation into wound milieu, and local release of cytokines and growth factors.

Inflammation
Injury to tissues results in disruption of blood vessels and extravasation of blood constituents.[2] The rupture of blood vessels exposes the subendothelial collagen to platelets and results in aggregation of platelets and activation of the intrinsic part of the coagulation cascade.[2] Hemostasis is re-established via the formation of blood clot and provides a provisional extracellular matrix for cell migration.[2] The contact between collagen and platelets and the presence of thrombin, fibronectin, and their fragments result in the release of cytokines and growth factors from platelet alpha granules. These growth factors include platelet-derived growth factor,

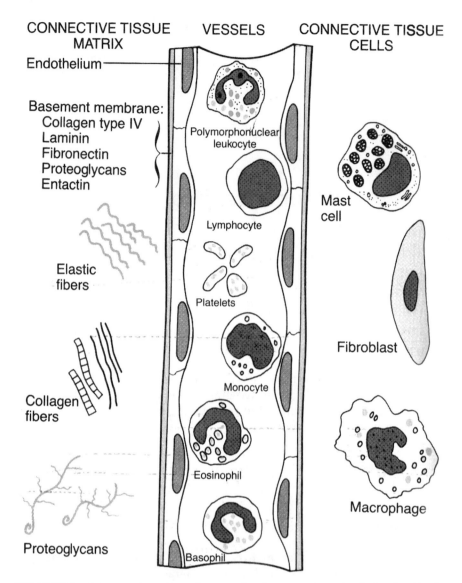

CONNECTIVE TISSUE MATRIX   VESSELS   CONNECTIVE TISSUE CELLS

Endothelium

Basement membrane:
Collagen type IV
Laminin
Fibronectin
Proteoglycans
Entactin

Polymorphonuclear leukocyte

Elastic fibers

Lymphocyte

Platelets

Collagen fibers

Monocyte

Eosinophil

Proteoglycans

Basophil

Mast cell

Fibroblast

Macrophage

FIGURE 22.1 *Intravascular cells and connective tissue matrix and cells involved in the inflammatory response. (Reprinted with permission from RS Cotran, V Kumar, SL Robbins. Robbins Pathological Basis of Disease [4th ed]. Philadelphia: WB Saunders, 1989;52.)*

transforming growth factor, platelet-activating factor, fibronectin, and serotonin. The locally formed fibrin clot serves as a scaffold for invading cells such as neutrophils, monocytes, fibroblasts, and endothelial cells.[1] The early cocktail of growth factors "kick starts" the wound closure process: It provides chemotactic cues to recruit circulating inflammatory cells to the wound site, initiates the tissue movements of re-epithelialization and connective tissue contraction, and stimulates the characteristic wound angiogenic response (Figure 22.1).[1,3]

Chemotaxis

Chemotaxis is defined as the unidirectional migration of cells towards an attractant or, more simply, as locomotion oriented along a chemical gradient.[2,4] Neutrophils, monocytes, and lymphocytes are attracted to wound sites by a huge variety of chemotactic signals. These include not only growth factors released by degranulating platelets, but also cues as diverse as peptides cleared from bacterial proteins and the by-products of the proteolysis of fibrin and other matrix components. Both neutrophils and monocytes are recruited from the circulating blood in response to molecular changes in the surface of endothelial cells lining capillaries at the wound site. Initially, selectin adhesion molecules are expressed on endothelial cell surfaces to allow adhesion of leukocytes to endothelium. Integrin receptors expressed on neutrophil cell surfaces help facilitate the activated leukocytes to adhere to the extracellular matrix. Neutrophils normally begin arriving at the wound within minutes of injury. Unless a wound is grossly infected, the neutrophil infiltration ceases after a few days, and expended neutrophils are themselves phagocytosed by tissue macrophages. Macrophages continue to accumulate at the wound site by recruitment of blood-borne monocytes and are essential for effective wound healing; if macrophage infiltration is prevented, then wound healing is severely impaired.[3]

Chemotaxis of cells into the wound milieu is followed by functional activation. Local mediators induce the phenotypic altering of cellular, biochemical, and functional properties. Activation may induce new cell surface antigen expression, increased cytotoxicity, increased production and release of cytokines, and other phenotypic alterations.[1]

The initial and brief release of factors from platelets is a first and strong stimulus of macrophage activation. The phagocytosis of cellular debris such as fibronectin or collagen also contributes to their activation.[1]

Activation of macrophages leads to release of cytokines, which mediate phagocytosis, angiogenesis, and fibroplasia. Activated macrophages can activate other cells such as lymphocytes via cytokines. The lymphocytes in turn release lymphokines such as interferons and interleukins. Released interferon-gamma acts back on macrophages and monocytes to induce the release of other cytokines such as tumor necrosis factor–alpha and interleukin-1. This ensures a prolonged presence of cytokines in the wound[1] (Table 22.1 and Figure 22.2).

Proliferative-Granulation Phase

The proliferative-granulation phase occurs 3–4 days after injury. This phase is characterized by a rapid increase in the number of fibroblasts, epithelial cell mitosis, and synthesis of extracellular collagen and proteoglycans. Re-epithelization of the wound begins within hours of injury and intensifies during this phase as cells migrate along the new fibrin bridge. Epithelial migration continues until cells touch one another, causing contact inhibition and signaling the end of epithelial expansion and the beginning of keratinization.[1]

There is also a proliferation and ingrowth of capillaries. Angiogenesis

TABLE 22.1   Hemostatic and platelet-derived factors associated with wound healing

Factor	Function
Hemostatic factors	
Fibrin, plasma fibronectin	Coagulation, chemoattraction, adhesion, scaffolding for cell migration
Factor XIII (fibrin-stabilizing factor)	Induces chemoattraction and adhesion
Circulatory growth factors	Regulation of chemoattraction, mitogenesis, fibroplasias
Complement	Antimicrobial activity, chemoattraction
Platelet-derived factors	
Cytokines, growth factors	Regulation of chemoattraction, mitogenesis, fibroplasias
Fibronectin	Early matrix, ligand for platelet aggregation
Platelet-activating factor	Platelet aggregation
Thromboxane A_2	Vasoconstriction, platelet aggregation, chemotaxis
Platelet factor IV	Chemotactic for fibroblasts and monocytes, neutralizes activity of heparin, inhibits collagenase
Serotonin	Induces vascular permeability, chemoattractant for neutrophils
Adenosine dinucleotide	Stimulates cell proliferation and migration, induces platelet aggregation

SOURCE: Adapted with permission from RS Cotran, V Kumar, SL Robbins. Robbins Pathological Basis of Disease (4th ed). Philadelphia, WB Saunders, 1989.

involves chemotactically stimulated migration, which causes the wound to become filled with granulation tissue (such as fibroblasts, macrophages, and new capillaries). Angiogenesis begins approximately 48 hours after injury and ingrowing fibroblasts produce collagen, elastin, and proteoglycans within 3–4 days. The interdigitation of collagen in the midportion of wound with collagen along the wound edges forms a source of intrinsic strength.[1]

Fibroblasts and endothelial cells are the primary cells proliferating during this phase. Fibroblasts migrate into the wound site from the surrounding tissue. Endothelial cells proliferate from intact venules close to the wound and form new capillaries by the process of angiogenesis. The growth factors and cytokines responsible for the proliferation of these two cell types derive

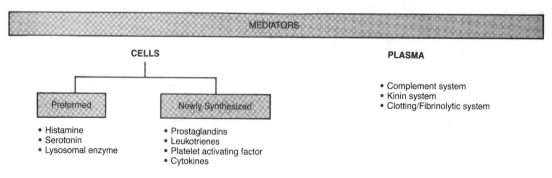

FIGURE 22.2   *Chemical mediators of inflammation. (Reprinted with permission from RS Cotran, V Kumar, SL Robbins. Robbins Pathological Basis of Disease [4th ed]. Philadelphia: WB Saunders, 1989;52.)*

mainly from platelets and activated macrophages. Some of them are stored in the fibrin clot, which is invaded by the cells. Mesenchymal cells can also be induced to release growth factors and cytokines.[1]

Fibroblasts in the surrounding tissue need to become activated from the quiescent state. Many of the growth factors (such as platelet-derived growth factor and epidermal growth factor) induce chemotaxis, proliferation of fibroblasts, and are strong stimulators of replication.[1]

In excisional wound healing, epithelial cells start proliferating a few days after wounding from the wound edges or uninjured epithelial islands within the wound. The stimuli for epithelial cell proliferation are not yet fully understood.[1]

Maturation-Remodeling Phase

The maturation-remodeling phase is characterized by the deposition of collagen in the wound. From a clinical viewpoint, this is the most important phase of healing. The rate, quality, and total amount of matrix deposition determine the strength of the scar. Three main events occur in this phase: deposition of matrix, collagen synthesis, and the change in the structure of the matrix.[1] The details of these phases are beyond the scope of this chapter.

Initially, the wound matrix is composed mainly of fibrin and fibronectin originating from hemostasis and macrophages. Glycosaminoglycans, proteoglycans, and other proteins, such as SPARC (secreted protein acidic, rich in cysteine), are synthesized next, and they support future matrix deposition and remodeling. Subsequently, collagens become the predominant scar protein.[1]

Net collagen synthesis is increased for at least 4–5 weeks after wounding. The increased rate of collagen synthesis during healing is due not only to an increased number of fibroblasts but also to a net increase of collagen production per fibroblast.[1]

The structure of the matrix changes with time as well. The collagen derived from granulation tissue is different from collagen derived from nonwounded skin, with greater hydroxylation and glycosylation of lysine. Despite a long, ongoing remodeling phase (up to 1 year), the collagen fibers in the healed scar tissue never become as organized as in the intact dermis.[1] In the first 3 weeks, a wound gains about 20% of its final strength. Fibrillar collagen accumulates rapidly and remodels by contraction of the wound. Thereafter, the rate at which a wound gains tensile strength is slow, with a much slower rate of collagen accumulation and remodeling, the formation of larger collagen bundles, and an increase in the number of intermolecular cross-links.[1] According to Singer and Clark, "wounds never attain the same breaking strength (the tension at which skin breaks) as uninjured skin. At maximal strength, a scar is only 70% as strong as normal skin."[2]

Wound Contraction–Remodeling Phase

The wound contraction–remodeling phase is characterized by a reduction in the number of fibroblasts, macrophages, and wound vascularity. During remodeling, the size of the scar is determined by wound tension, pressure, patient age, and oxygen supply to the area. Mechanical stress promotes collagen synthesis and deposition, often yielding a hypertrophic scar. Hypoxia also stimulates collagen formation and deposition. As the scar matures, it usually becomes denser as a result of loss of fluid and volume.[1]

Wound contraction is the approximation of the wound edges, and wound contracture is the shortening of the scar itself. During the second week of healing, the appearance of the myofibroblasts indicates the beginning of connective tissue compaction and contraction of the wound. The contraction requires stimulation by transforming growth factor–beta-1 or –beta-2 and platelet-derived growth factor, attachment of fibroblasts to the collagen matrix through integrin receptors, and cross-links between individual bundles of collagen. The myofibroblasts contain large bundles of actin-containing microfilaments disposed along the cytoplasmic face of the plasma membrane of the cells and by cell-cell and cell-matrix linkages.[2]

Summary

Even with improvements in diagnostics and therapy, wound failure remains a clinical problem. The approach to a nonhealed wound is an interdisciplinary challenge. A better understanding of the complex wound-healing cascade and factors that can impede wound healing helps our approach to wound healing and its possible failure. Manipulations of the growth factors, mediators, and parenchymal cells offer future therapeutic strategies.[1]

References

1. Witte MB, Barbul A. General principles of wound healing. Surg Clin North Am 1997;77(3):509.
2. Singer AJ, Clark RAF. Cutaneous wound healing. N Engl J Med 1999;2:738.
3. Cotran RS, Kumar V, Robbins SL. Inflammation and Repair. In Robbins Pathologic Basis of Disease (4th ed). Philadelphia: WB Saunders, 1989;39–86.
4. Koopman CF Jr. Cutaneous wound healing (an overview). Otolaryngol Clin North Am 1995;28(5):835.

23   Etiology of Chronic Skin Wounds

Mery Elashvili

Intrinsic versus Extrinsic Factors

Chronic skin ulcerations usually develop in patients with spinal cord injury, coma, or in those who are debilitated. Etiologic factors can be divided into extrinsic and intrinsic factors. Extrinsic factors include pressure, shear, friction, immobility, and incontinence. Intrinsic factors include age, infection, malnutrition, anemia, vascular status, mental status, comorbid medical disorders, immune status, and medications.[1-4]

Body Loading

The primary factor in the development of a pressure sore is excessive body loading, which is sustained for a protracted time period. "Where there is no pressure, there is no sore."[5] There are three types of body loading:

1. Pressure (load applied perpendicularly)
2. Friction (the force of two surfaces moving across each other)
3. Shear (load applied parallel to the plane)

These forms of body loading go hand to hand in the development of pressure sores. Sustained for prolonged periods of time, body loading induces trauma and ischemia to the tissue. The greater the pressure, friction, and shear forces, the less time is required to produce ischemia. Ischemia alone or associated with a large but evenly distributed pressure source requires considerable time to produce degeneration. However, when localized pressure is applied, trauma is evident at a lower value of time and pressure.[6]

Whether the pressure is localized or uniform is significant in terms of friction and shear formation. Localized pressure generates a larger shear value, whereas a uniform pressure distribution does not. As the pressure gradient becomes steep, friction and shear stressors become greater.[5,7]

Kosiac noted that whereas 70 mm Hg pressure over a 2-hour period produced moderate skin changes, 115 mm Hg over a 3-hour period produced marked changes.[8,9] Dinsdale found that 450 mm Hg pressure causes full-thickness ulceration.[10] Daniel documented that 500 mm Hg pressure for 4 hours or 100 mm Hg pressure for 10 hours produced muscle damage.[11] The pressure required for skin damage is much higher.[12] Davis found that externally applied pressure was approximately twice as effective as shear in reducing pulsatile blood flow.[13] The combination of pressure plus shear was found to very effectively cause occlusion and subsequent pressure sore development.

Kosiac concluded that tissue degeneration takes place simultaneously at all levels, including the skin.[8] Clinically, impending necrosis only becomes apparent when the skin becomes inflamed. Frank ulceration, when it occurs, tends to dissect almost completely to the bony prominence, lending further evidence that necrosis had been taking place at all levels. Rudd[14] and Daniel[11] note that subcutaneous tissue and muscles are more easily damaged by pressure than is the overlying skin.

Local Factors and Infection

Local factors including moisture from perspiration, urine, or feces can lead to maceration of the skin, cellulitis, rash, or skin infections. Moisture or local factors may precipitate development of pressure ulcers or complicate an already ischemic and necrotic wound. Patients with decubitus ulcers are prone to local and systemic infections. Because these ulcers are commonly located in proximity to the anus, anaerobic conditions are frequently present, due to tissue necrosis and incontinence. Robson found that pressure sores had one hundred times more bacterial growth than did wounds not subjected to increased pressure.[15] In these patients, the tissue was compromised because of chronic fibrosis, inflammation, and atrophy, which resulted in decreased phagocytosis. Because the local cutaneous layer was destroyed, there was an impaired local defense mechanism, with formation of granulation tissue.

Infection is the single most important local cause for delayed wound healing. The most commonly isolated types of bacteria are *Pseudomonas*, *Escherichia coli*, *Proteus*, enteric gram-negative facultative organisms, gram-negative anaerobes, and especially *Bacteroides*. Local wound care and systemic antibiotics are helpful for the prevention and treatment of bacteria and for the prevention of seeding from another focus. Osteomyelitis is a common complication and impairs the chances of a local cure. Foreign bodies and often sutures constitute impediments to healing by serving as sources for bacterial contamination. Removal of all extraneous foreign bodies and judicious use of sutures are desirable to facilitate wound healing.[16]

Age

As we age, it takes longer for wounds to heal secondary to an overall decrease in the supply of blood to the skin and an increase in systemic disease. The wound contraction time is lengthened, healing rate is slower, final epithelization occurs later, and the breaking strength and bursting force of wounds are less.[17]

Temperature

Infection is the single most important local cause for delayed wound healing. An increase in body temperature leads to an increased blood flow by four- to fivefold, increases cellular metabolism, and in conjunction with other causes of tissue ischemia, may further compromise the metabolism and survival of tissue. Locally increased temperature during sitting or lying down, in combination with pressure, shear, and friction, promote skin ulceration in debilitated patients. Composition and conformity of seat cushions and mattress surfaces are very important, as they may retain heat and moisture.[18]

Malnutrition

Malnutrition is one of the most reversible factors in the etiology of pressure sores. Recognition of existing malnutrition is a necessary first step in the prevention and management of patients with pressure sores. Malnutrition decreases wound healing and diminishes resistance to infection. Nutritional deficiencies increase the length of hospitalization and increase mortality. Mulholland found that the depth and multiplicity of ulcers were related to hypoproteinemia.[19] The required time-pressure interval for development of decubiti decreases when protein malnutrition is present. Daniel documented that normal skin is highly resistant to pressure, as compared with the tissue wasting that was seen in paraplegic pigs and was associated with a significant decrease in pressure-duration threshold.[11]

Perkash demonstrated that patients having both anemia and decubitus ulcers had decreased serum iron binding capacity, thus demonstrating a decreased visceral protein status.[20] The presence of decubitus results in further worsening of a patient's metabolic status due to a large protein loss from the wound. Mulholland observed that discharge from decubitus ulcers had a high protein content.[19] Approximately 30 g of protein is lost daily from large wounds. When plasma protein decreases, there is a subsequent decrease in oncotic pressure. This promotes edema, increases the amount of interstitial fluid, increases the distance from the capillary to the cells, decreases diffusion of oxygen and nutrients to the cell, and impairs cell metabolism. All of these factors contribute to the production of ischemic ulcers.

Several studies have documented that secretory immunoglobulins, serum complement, and opsonic activity are depressed in ischemic ulcers.[21] Daly documented that balanced nutrition is effective in restoration of immunocompetence.[22] Zinc, vitamin A, and pyridoxin deficiencies result in a depression of the cell-mediated immune system. Zinc therapy is associated with restoration of immunocompetence, weight gain, and rapid healing of pressure ulcer.[23] Malnutrition results in wasting of respiratory muscles. In debilitated patients, a decreased respiratory effort increases susceptibility to respiratory infections and atelectasis, which further leads to decreased tissue oxygenation.[23] Poor nutritional status affects myocardium by decreasing cardiac output and stroke volume, increasing vascular resistance, and decreasing oxygen content in cells. These factors increase tissue necrosis and interfere with wound healing.[23]

Inadequate and improper diets can lead to severe malnutrition; decreases in collagen synthesis, fibroblast proliferation, humoral and cell-mediated antibody responses; and lowered resistance to bacterial infections. Inadequate protein intake decreases collagen formation, whereas a high protein diet increases the tensile strength of wounds. In protein-starved animals, supplementation with the amino acids methionine and cystine has been found to promote wound healing.[16] Vitamin A and iron play a role in collagen formation. Vitamin A also promotes collagenase production. Vitamin B plays a role in the function of white cells and formation of antibodies. Vitamin C plays a role in conversion of proline to hydroxyproline and lysine to hydroxylysine that can promote collagen formation. Vitamin D enhances new bone formation. Vitamin K plays a role in the formation of clotting factors VII, IX, and X. Patients who are zinc deficient were found to have delayed wound healing. Zinc deficiency delays epithelialization and retards fibroblasts.[17]

Anemia

Anemia is a significant factor in determining the potential occurrence of cellular hypoxia and necrosis. The possibility of tissue survival increases if the hemoglobin content and oxygen supply is normal. If oxygen content is decreased, tissue metabolism is compromised.[12] Matheson and Lipschitz recommend transfusion in patients with chronic ulcers to keep the hemoglobin level at least 15 g per 100 ml.[24] To promote wound healing, blood transfusion may be needed in severely anemic patients. Patients with chronic ulcers often present with anemia due to chronic infections, decreased appetite, and loss of serum from the wound. In different studies it was shown that anemia with a hematocrit below 50% of normal reduces the tensile strength in healing wounds.[25] Hemoglobin should be maintained at 10–12 g/dl for adequate tissue oxygenation.[26] Anemia can also lead to tissue hypoxia, higher infection rates, and wound fragility. Blood delivers immune factors to the local area. Cardiac output and blood volume must be maintained at near-normal levels to promote wound healing.[17]

Vascular Status

Adequacy of blood supply to a wound is an important influence. Arterial disease that limits blood flow and venous abnormalities that retard drainage impair wound healing. Chronic pathologic changes in the skin due to vascular insufficiency make the skin extremely vulnerable to injury. Trauma, whether mechanical, thermal, chemical, or surgical, increases the likelihood of decubiti. It has been established that venous stasis is produced because of ambulatory venous hypertension. In the studies of Browse et al., it was documented that with high venous pressure, vessels become dilated and intercellular capillary pores increase in size.[27,28] This allows the escape of fibrinogen. Fibrinogen then changes to fibrin, which surrounds capillaries and acts as a barrier to the diffusion of oxygen from the capillaries to the cells. This compromises cell metabolism, which makes the tissue more susceptible to the injury. In addition, high resistance opens arteriovenous shunts proximally to the diseased skin. This diversion of arterial flow further deprives the skin of needed oxygen and nutrients.

Ulceration of the skin occurring in arterial diseases is due to peripheral ischemia. Ischemia is commonly caused by a reduction of blood flow to the skin due to acute or subacute arterial occlusion or arteritis. In arterial disease, blood flow is significantly altered if occlusion exceeds 20% of arterial diameter. However, even 50% occlusion will not affect tissue oxygenation if a good collateral system is present.[23] In normal capillaries effective filtration pressure is 35 mm Hg. The critical closing pressure for arterioles is 20 mm Hg and for capillaries it is 5 mm Hg.[23] As per Kosiak, pressures greater than 35 mm Hg applied to the body surface result in closure of the capillary circulation with necrosis of the skin and development of ischemic ulcers.[9] When capillary pressure drops below this, normal tissue perfusion stops and necrosis develops. In this situation, any trauma to the area may precipitate the formation of ulcers.

Concurrent Diseases

Chronic wound formation is very often related to specific diseases such as diabetes mellitus, syringomyelia, syphilis, and severe peripheral neuropathy. The mechanism of skin ulcer formation is associated with trauma or local pressure, which initiates tissue breakdown and is maintained by repeated mechanical injury. Impairment of healing occurs in approximately 10% of diabetic patients. The activation of inflammatory cells and chemotaxis is decreased. This results in less efficient killing of bacteria with subsequently more infections and reduced collagen deposition. Leukocyte function is altered with reduced fibroblast proliferation and collagen deposition. The increase in occlusive vascular disease results in reduced skin blood flow, poor tissue perfusion, and peripheral neuropathy.[17]

Neuropathic patients frequently have a reduction or loss of skin sensitivity. These patients do not feel pressure, and repeated injuries make them prone to skin ulcerations. Most often, this type of ulcer develops on the plantar aspect of the foot. This area is more subject to trauma, and most neuropathies affect the distal aspect of the extremity more than the proximal aspect.

There are several biomechanical factors that contribute to the formation of plantar ulcers.[23] A necrotic blister can become an ulcer by friction of the skin between bone, shoe, and ground. The impact of the body weight at heel-contact produces repeated tissue damage and ulceration. In addition, thrust during walking or running causes intermittent and concentrated pressures, especially under the metatarsal heads before toe-off. Because skin is more resistant to trauma than the subcutaneous tissue, the subcutaneous tissue may develop a deep focus of necrotic tissue formation. Finally, horizontal movement of the skin during walking can tear previously scarred tissue because of a loss of elasticity. In patients with sensory loss, one long walk is more likely to produce an ulceration than a number of short walks.[23] Plantar ulceration may develop in any foot with neurological deficit, but occurs most often in the diabetic patient. The high incidence of chronic cutaneous wounds in diabetic patients often relates to the combination of neuropathy, vasculopathy, impaired host defense against infection, and metabolic problems. Good control of blood sugars plays a major role in preventing and treating skin ulcerations in diabetic patients.

Chronic skin sores are very common in patients with organic mental syndrome, depression and other psychiatric problems, chronic pain syndrome, spinal cord injury, strokes, head injury, and coma. These patients spend long periods of time in bed and frequently stay in one position for hours. They almost always have cognitive deficits and perceptual impairment, may develop heterotopic ossification, are at high risk of developing contractures, have limited mobility, and have less potential to relieve ischemia that may develop as a result of remaining in one position too long. Patients with mental status changes may have increased motor activity or agitation that requires the use of restraints. The most common cause of decubiti in these patients is friction created by the use of such restraints. In the late phases of rehabilitation, pressure problems are associated with wheelchair use, and proper positioning is very important to maintain proper posture. A patient's ability to change and control body position and the degree of physical activity is very important in relieving localized pressure, friction, and shear, and thereby reduces the potential for pressure sore development.

Immune Status

The immune system mediates an inflammatory response. Leukopenia itself at the time of insult has little effect on the wound, because the macrophages are sufficient. However, the absence of neutrophils or defects in leukocyte chemotaxis and phagocytosis predisposes a wound to infection. The circulating blood volume delivers the necessary components to the local area. Anemia leads to tissue hypoxia, higher infection rates, and wound fragility. Thus, cardiac output and blood volume must be maintained at near-normal levels to promote wound healing.

Smoking

Smoking and nicotine patches inhibit oxygen delivery to the tissue via sympathomimetic vasoconstriction. Smoking also elevates carboxyhemoglobin levels in the blood, shifting the oxygen delivery curve to the left due to the high affinity carboxyhemoglobin has for oxygen. This results in less available oxygen to the wound. Smoking has been shown to substantially increase wound infections and severely impair wound healing.[2]

Medications

Corticosteroids impair wound healing by reducing inflammation which further decreases cell migration, proliferation, and angiogenesis. It can be partially reversed by vitamin A administration. Low doses (less than 10 mg of prednisone per day) have minimal effects on wounds, but doses of 40 mg or more per day adversely affect healing by reducing

1. Granulation tissue and fibroblast proliferation
2. Motility and phagocytosis of polymorphonuclear leukocytes
3. Lymphocytes
4. Blood and nutrient supplies
5. Synthesis of collagen
6. Glycosaminoglycan
7. Macrophage functioning

Anticoagulants increase the risk of bleeding, infection, and wound dehiscence. Nonsteroidal anti-inflammatory drugs lower the tensile strength of wounds and raise the risk of bleeding with hematoma formation and infection.[17]

Antimetabolite drugs may reduce tensile strength through their action during the proliferative phase of healing. It is therefore advisable to withhold chemotherapeutic agents during the first 7–10 postoperative days. Immunosuppressive agents such as azathioprine and cyclosporin A may diminish the inflammatory response. Colchicine has been used with penicillamine or beta-aminopropionitrile in the treatment of keloids and hypertrophic scars.

Radiation

The effect of radiation upon wound healing is dose dependent. Above 4,000 rads, desquamation, bullae, and ulceration occur. Therapeutic radiation in the total dose of 6,000 rads leads to erythema, swelling, and tenderness. Chronic changes include loss of hair, dryness, telangiectasias, ischemia, dermal fibrosis, and epidermal fragility. The long-term effects of radiation include easily damaged skin with little angiogenesis or inflammatory response and severely impaired healing.[16]

In concluding this discussion of factors affecting wound healing, it should be stressed that wound healing involves multiple issues of considerable clinical importance. Scrupulous attention to all of the factors that may hamper wound healing is the responsibility of the clinician.

References

1. Schwartz S (ed). Principles of Surgery (7th ed). New York: McGraw-Hill, 1999.
2. Greenfield LJ, Mulholland M, Oldham KT, Zelenock GB (eds). Surgery: Scientific Principles and Practice (2d ed). Philadelphia: Lippincott–Raven, 1997.

3. Kloth LC, McCulloch JM, Feeder JA. Wound Healing: Alternatives in Management. Philadelphia: FA Davis; 1990.
4. Eaglestain WH, Falanga V. Chronic wounds. Surg Clin North Am 1997;77:689.
5. Bennett L, Kavner D, Lee BY, Trainer FA. Shear versus pressure as causative factor in skin blood flow occlusion. Arch Phys Med Rehabil 1979;60:347.
6. Husain T. Experimental study of some pressure effects on tissues, with reference to the bed sore problem. J Pathol Bacteriol 1953;66:347.
7. Bennett L, Kavner D, Lee BY, et al. Skin blood flow in seated geriatric patients. Arch Phys Med Rehabil 1981;62:392.
8. Kosiak M. Etiology and pathology of ischemic ulcers. Arch Phys Med Rehabil 1959;40:62.
9. Kosiak M. Etiology and pathology of ischemic ulcers. Arch Phys Med Rehabil 1961;42:19.
10. Dinsdale SM. Decubitus ulcers: role of pressure and friction in causation. Arch Phys Med Rehabil 1974;55:147.
11. Daniel RK, Priest DL, Wheatley DC. Etiologic factors in pressure sores: an experimental model. Arch Phys Med Rehabil 1981;62:492.
12. Morris PJ, Malt RA (eds). Oxford Textbook of Surgery. New York: Oxford University Press, 1994.
13. Davis DL. Digital artery blood flow and digital pad opacity during vasoconstriction. J Blood Vessels 1976;13:58.
14. Rudd TN. The pathogenesis of decubitus ulcers. J Am Geriatr Soc 1962;10:48.
15. Robson MC, Krizek TJ. The Role of Infection in Chronic Pressure Ulceration. In S Fredricks, GS Brody (eds), Symposium on the Neurologic Aspects of Plastic Surgery. St. Louis: CV Mosby, 1978;242–249.
16. Cotran RS, Kumar V, Robbins SL. Inflammation and Repair. In Robbins Pathologic Basis of Disease (5th ed). Philadelphia: WB Saunders, 1999.
17. Koopman CF Jr. Cutaneous wound healing (an overview). Otolaryngol Clin North Am 1995;28:835.
18. Fisher SV, Szymke TE, Apte SY, Kosiak M. Wheelchair cushion effect on skin temperature. Arch Phys Med Rehabil 1978;59:68.
19. Mulholland JH, Tui C, Wright AM, et al. Protein metabolism and bed sores. Ann Surg 1943;118:1015.
20. Perkash A, Brown M. Anemia in patients with traumatic spinal cord injury. Paraplegia 1982;20:235.
21. Neumann CG, Laulor GJ Jr, Stiehm ER, et al. Immunologic responses in malnourished children. Am J Clin Nutr 1975;28:135.
22. Daly JM, Dudrick SJ, Copeland EM. Effects of protein depletion and repletion on cell mediated immunity in experimental animals. Ann Surg 1978;188:791.
23. Lee BY. Chronic Ulcers of the Skin. New York: McGraw-Hill, 1985.
24. Matheson AT, Lipschitz R. Nature and treatment of tropic pressure sores. S Afr Med J 1956;30:1129.
25. Narsete TA, Orgel MG, Smith D. Pressure sores. Am J Fam Pract 1983;28:135.
26. Elliot TM. Pressure ulceration. Am J Fam Pract 1982;25:171.
27. Browse NL. Venous Insufficiency: Nonoperative Management. In NU

Ban, JL Glover, RW Holder, DA Triplett (eds), Thrombosis and Athero-sclerosis: Prevention, Diagnosis and Management. Chicago: Year-Book, 1982;275–281.

28. Browse NL, Burnand KG. The Postphlebitic Syndrome. In JJ Bergan, JST Yao (eds), Venous Problems. Chicago: Year-Book. 1978;395–404.

24   Pressure Ulcers

Anna Dacanay

Pressure ulcers are localized areas of tissue necrosis, which usually occur over bony prominences. The skin may be intact or may be open. Damage to the underlying tissue develops secondary to an externally applied pressure for a prolonged period of time. The term *pressure ulcer* may be interchangeably used with pressure sore, bedsore, decubitus ulcer, ischemic ulcer, or dermal ulcer. Because pressure is a critical factor in the development of these wounds, the term pressure ulcers is recommended to describe these lesions.[1]

Pressure Ulcer Statistics in the United States

Pressure ulcers are a significant health care problem in the United States. Approximately two million Americans suffer from pressure ulcers.[2] The pressure ulcers occurrence rate varies greatly by practice settings and is estimated as follows:

1. In hospitals or acute care settings, the incidence rate is 3.0–29.5% and the prevalence rate is 3–14%.[3,4]
2. In long-term care facilities, the incidence rate is 10.8% and the prevalence rate is 15–25%.
3. In critical care units, the incidence rate is 33% and the prevalence is 44%.[5]
4. In orthopedic and fracture cases, the incidence is 0.9–1.0 per 100 patients and the prevalence is 23% (nonacute rehabilitation setting).
5. In the spinal cord injury (SCI) population, the incidence ranges from 25% to 85% and the prevalence is 20–66%.
6. In the rehabilitation setting the incidence rate is 4% with a prevalence rate of 27%,[6] and home care has a 17–29% incidence rate and an 8.7–20.0% prevalence rate.[7]

The estimated cost of treatment ranges from $2,000 to $30,000 per ulcer in an acute care setting,[8] with an estimated $6.4 billion being spent annually in hospitals alone. One study showed the average cost of medical treatment of a single pressure sore is estimated at $58,000.[9] Miller and Delozier estimated the 1992 Medicare treatment cost of pressure ulcers.[10] They found that the mean hospital charge for patients with primary diagnosis of pressure ulcers was $21,675 and estimated that physician charges were $2,900 per case. The charges for 34,000 inpatients with a primary diagnosis of pressure ulcer totaled $836 million. To illustrate the cost of pressure ulcers as a secondary diagnosis, hip-fracture patients with and without pressure ulcers were compared. An average of $10,986 in additional hospital charges was attributed to the pressure ulcers. When estimated physician fees of $1,200 per case were included, the total cost of pressure ulcers as complications of hip fracture was $84 million. A recent study estimates the cost of managing pressure ulcers from their initial occurrence in a long-term care setting through their natural history, including hospital treatment of complications.[11] Thirty patients in the 1-year study developed 45 ulcers. The mean length of treatment for an ulcer was 116 days. The mean cost of treatment was $489 per ulcer. With addition of hospital expenditures, this increases to $2,731 per ulcer. The mean cost of treatment per patient was $4,647. Excluding hospital cost, the mean treatment cost was $1,284 per patient. Eight percent of the total cost of pressure ulcer treatment was generated by the 4% of patients who needed hospitalization for the pressure ulcers. This study suggests that, in the absence of complications, pressure ulcers can be treated successfully and cost effectively in long-term care.

Risk Factors

Most of the risk factors for the development of pressure ulcers have been discussed extensively in Chapter 21 of this book. Ulcer development depends on the pressure exerted and the tissue response to it. Intrinsic and extrinsic factors influence tissue response to pressure. The intrinsic factors most commonly associated with pressure ulcer development include impaired mobility and activity levels, incontinence, nutritional status, altered sensory perception, and altered levels of consciousness. Extrinsic factors include pressure, shear, friction, and moisture (external insults to the skin).[12,13]

These factors may also be grouped into biomechanical, biochemical, and medical factors. Biomechanical factors include pressure, shear, friction, moisture, and temperature. Mechanical injury to the skin from friction and shearing forces occurs during repositioning and transfer activity. Prolonged positioning, deteriorated or inappropriate seating device, or improper sitting or lying postures cause moderate to large compression forces and sustained load leading to mechanical deformation of the flesh. This leads to pressure induced vascular ischemia, tissue hypoxia, and necrosis. Incontinence and excessive perspiration cause an increase in skin moisture and may promote adherence to bed linen and clothing. This leads to maceration through direct trauma or exposure to pressure. Increased skin temperature and humidity contribute to an increase in metabolic demands, dry the tissue, and lead to skin breakdown. Incontinence can also cause chemical irritation of the epidermis, which can predispose to infection.[14]

Biochemical factors include decreased fat distribution, poor circulation, decreased collagen metabolism, heterotopic ossification, anemia, and poor nutritional status. Nutrition is important in maintaining tissue integrity. Decreased protein intake delays wound granulation, contributes to negative nitrogen balance, and promotes tissue edema. This in turn decreases skin elasticity, increases skin fragility, and makes skin susceptible to inflammation. Deficiencies relating to anemia, such as iron, folate, and vitamin B_{12}, and decreased oxygenation of tissues prevent ulcer healing and promote further skin breakdown. Inadequate intake of vitamin C and zinc impairs wound healing.

Age and existing medical conditions may increase susceptibility to pressure ulceration. Those with increased susceptibility include elderly, disabled, bed- or chair-bound persons, especially those who have sustained SCI or stroke. Patients who are immobile or deconditioned secondary to trauma (hip fracture, post surgery, traumatic brain injury) or illness (multiple sclerosis, patients on steroids or chemotherapy) are at increased risk for pressure ulcers. In addition, comorbidities such as infection, malnutrition, anemia, diabetic neuropathy, depression, or altered mental status increase the risk for development of pressure ulcers. Patients with spasticity due to inflammation or infection can develop muscle contractures and joint deformities that can compromise patient care and lead to skin breakdown.[5,14,15]

Certain medical conditions predispose patients to other types of wounds or ulcers, and they need to be differentiated from pressure ulcers (especially when predominant in the leg area). Patients with a history of venous insufficiency (either with obvious varicosities or a past history of thrombophlebitis), immobility of calf muscles, leg fracture, increased intra-abdominal pressure, congestive heart failure, obesity, pregnancy, tumors, or arteriovenous shunting are at risk for venous ulcers. Characteristic pruritic patches of stasis dermatitis at the medial aspect of the lower leg above the malleolus often precede ulceration. Arterial ulcers are common in patients with a history of atherosclerosis, previous vascular surgery, cardiac disease, hypercholesterolemia, or smoking. Depending on the level of occlusion, intermittent claudication, atrophic changes, or absent pulses accompany these ulcers. Diabetic ulcers, on the other hand, are common in patients with longstanding diabetes, poorly controlled blood glucose levels, loss of protective sensation, and joint deformity. These ulcers are usually located at the heel or metatarsal heads and are due to increased plantar pressure.

Risk Assessment

Pressure ulcer risk assessment requires a comprehensive and systematic approach including skin assessment, staging, and evaluation of factors most commonly associated with pressure ulcer development. (For information in staging of pressure ulcers, see Chapter 21.)

Wound Assessment and Documentation

A thorough assessment of alterations in skin integrity includes information about type, stage, size, location of wound, wound bed characteristics, and periwound status. Wounds are staged according to assessment parameters as defined by the Agency for Health Care Policy Research (AHCPR).[12] Documentation of the above information facilitates effective management of pressure ulcers.[16]

Skin inspection is the basis of prevention. Special attention should be given to skin over bony prominences. Areas at particularly high risk in the chair-bound person include ischial tuberosities, thoracic spine, feet, and heels. On the other hand, sacrum and greater trochanter ulcers are common in the bed-bound and tetraplegic patients. Other common sites include malleoli, tibial crests, patella, anterior superior iliac spine, elbows, shoulders, scapulae, costal margins, ear, and occiput.[5,17] Infants are especially at risk for occipital skin breakdown because of the relative size of the head to the body. Potential signs of tissue breakdown should be noted. These include color variation (redness, skin discoloration), blisters, rashes, swelling, temperature variation, pimples, ingrown hair, bruises, surface breaks, or dry, flaky skin. Periwound skin condition must be checked for evidence of atrophy and maceration.

Initial assessment of pressure ulcers includes determination of location, stage, size, presence or absence of granulation tissue, and epithelialization, accurate measurement of length, width, and depth of ulcer, and a full description of the appearance of any sinus tract, tunneling, necrotic tissue, or exudate. Signs of infection such as redness, warmth, swelling, pain, and induration must be noted.[18] Eschar must be removed before staging of ulcer can be determined. Valuable aids for the evaluation and reassessment of ulcer appearance are the use of a ruler, plastic or transparent measuring scale, and photographs.

Individual risk factors should be reviewed. This entails obtaining a thorough history and physical examination. Medical conditions including nutritional, immunological, vascular, and endocrine abnormalities, and psychosocial conditions must be assessed. Pressure ulcer–related pain or other complications such as infection should be taken into consideration. Laboratory and bacteriology workup may be required in the presence of infection. Imaging studies such as x-ray, magnetic resonance imaging, and bone scan may be used to rule out osteomyelitis, heterotopic ossification, and formation of abscesses.

Pressure ulcer risk assessment must be done systematically. A validated risk assessment tool is used to identify at-risk individuals. Several risk assessment instruments have been developed and published. The currently used scales are the Braden and Norton scales.

The Braden scale (Figure 24.1) is a helpful screening instrument for pressure ulcer risk. It assesses six factors: sensory perception, moisture, activity, mobility, nutrition, and friction or shear. Each area is scored on a scale of 1 to 3 or 4, with a total possible score of 23 points. The higher the Braden score the lower the risk. A score of 23 indicates the lowest risk for pressure ulcer development. Its validity has been examined in various patient care settings, and its reliability among raters is generally good.[19]

6. SKIN INTEGRITY RISK ASSESSMENT (DAILY) (7a-3p)
CIRCLE DATA WHICH BEST DESCRIBES THE PATIENT'S SKIN CONDITION. (BRADEN SCALE)

SENSORY PERCEPTION
1. completely limited
2. very limited
3. slightly limited
4. no impairment

MOISTURE
1. constantly moist
2. very moist
3. occasionally moist
4. rarely moist

ACTIVITY
1. bedfast
2. chairfast
3. walks occasionally
4. walks frequently

MOBILITY
1. completely immobile
2. very limited
3. lightly limited
4. no limitation

NUTRITION
1. very poor
2. probably inadequate
3. adequate

FRICTION & SHEAR
1. problem
2. potential problem
3. no apparent problem

PRESSURE ULCER RISK
 6-15 HIGH RISK
16-17 MODERATE RISK
18-19 LOW RISK
20-23 NO RISK (PREVENTATIVE)

Skin score_____

FIGURE 24.1   *Braden Scale. (Reprinted with permission from South Nassau Communities Hospital, Oceanside, NY.)*

The Norton scale (Figure 24.2) was the first pressure ulcer risk assessment scale developed. It assesses five factors: general physical condition, mental condition, activity, mobility, and incontinence. Each area has 4 components with a descending value from 4 to 1. The maximum patient score is 20 and the minimum score is 5. A descending scale or value corresponds with a decline in the patient's condition and therefore is more highly associated with a risk of developing ulcers. It is basic, simple, and easy to use. Its predictive validity is confined to the elderly population. Inter-rater reliability has not yet been fully established.[20]

Current assessment tools still require further research testing and outcome studies to provide data on their effectiveness. Prospective studies suggest that additional risk factors such as diastolic blood pressure, age, or dry skin may need to be included in these scales. Some factors may be more important in different health care settings. For example, fecal incontinence may be a greater risk factor in the acute care hospital. Elevated body tempera-

		Norton Risk Assessment Scale									
		Physical condition		**Mental condition**		**Activity**		**Mobility**		**Incontinent**		**Total score**
		Good	4	Alert	4	Ambulant	4	Full	4	Not	4	Total score
		Fair	3	Apathetic	3	Walk/help	3	Slightly limited	3	Occasional	3	
		Poor	2	Confused	2	Chairbound	2	Very limited	2	Usually/Urine	2	
		Very bad	1	Stupor	1	Bedbound	1	Immobile	1	Doubly	1	
Name	Date										

FIGURE 24.2   *Norton Scale. (Reprinted with permission from D Norton, R McLaren, AN Exton-Smith. An Investigation of Geriatric Nursing Problems in Hospital. London: National Corporation for the Care of Old People [now Centre for Policy on Ageing], 1962.)*

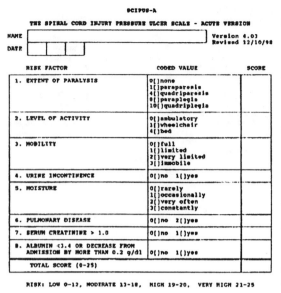

SCIPUS-A

THE SPINAL CORD INJURY PRESSURE ULCER SCALE - ACUTE VERSION

NAME _____ Version 4.03
                            Revised 12/10/98
DATE ___ ___ ___

RISK FACTOR	CODED VALUE	SCORE
1. EXTENT OF PARALYSIS	0[ ]none 1[ ]paraparesis 4[ ]quadriparesis 8[ ]paraplegia 10[ ]quadriplegia	
2. LEVEL OF ACTIVITY	0[ ]ambulatory 1[ ]wheelchair 4[ ]bed	
3. MOBILITY	0[ ]full 1[ ]limited 2[ ]very limited 3[ ]immobile	
4. URINE INCONTINENCE	0[ ]no 1[ ]yes	
5. MOISTURE	0[ ]rarely 1[ ]occasionally 2[ ]very often 3[ ]constantly	
6. PULMONARY DISEASE	0[ ]no 2[ ]yes	
7. SERUM CREATININE > 1.0	0[ ]no 1[ ]yes	
8. ALBUMIN <3.4 OR DECREASE FROM ADMISSION BY MORE THAN 0.2 g/dl	0[ ]no 1[ ]yes	
TOTAL SCORE (0-25)		

RISK: LOW 0-12, MODERATE 13-18, HIGH 19-20, VERY HIGH 21-25

NURSE ASSESSOR'S SIGNATURE: _____

Operational Definitions

1. EXTENT OF PARALYSIS
   0-none
   1-paraparesis
   4-quadriparesis
   8-paraplegia
   10-quadriplegia

2. LEVEL OF ACTIVITY
   0-ambulatory-can walk with/without assistance
   1-wheelchair mobile- sits out of bed only, cannot bear own weight and/or must be assisted into chair or wheelchair
   4-bed mobile-confined to bed during entire 24 hours of the day

3. MOBILITY
   0-full-independent in moving, no limitations, able to control and move all extremities at will
   1-slightly limited- requires assistance when moving
   2- very limited
   3-immobile-complete immobility, unable to change position does not make even slight changes in body or extremity position without assistance, completely dependent on others for movement

4. URINE INCONTINENCE-incontinent of urine at least once a day, absence of control

5. MOISTURE
   0-rarely
   1-occasionally
   2-very often
   3-constantly

6. PULMONARY DISEASE (ICD CODES 450,460-519,796.0)

7. SERUM CREATININE > 1.0

8. SERUM ALBUMIN <3.4 gm/dl OR DECREASE FROM ADMISSION BY MORE THAN 0.2 g/dl

Most recent values should be used for all risk factors.

PRESSURE ULCER (ICD-9 CODE=707.0)
"a lesion on any skin surface that results from pressure and which may include reactivity hyperemia and blistered, broken, or necrotic skin".

FIGURE 24.3 *Spinal Cord Injury Pressure Ulcer Scale–Acute Version. (Reprinted with permission from CA Salzberg. The spinal cord injury pressure ulcer scale active version and operational definitions. Wounds 1999;11[2]:54–55.)*

ture, decreased blood pressure, and decreased dietary intake may be more important in a long-term care setting. Identifying setting-specific risk factors and incorporating them into risk assessment and risk reduction programs may decrease the incidence of pressure ulcers.[21] Furthermore, there is a need for validation of assessment tools for specific types of patient population. The Spinal Cord Injury Pressure Ulcer Scale (SCIPUS) and SCIPUS-Acute (SCIPUS-A) were developed for SCI patients.[22] SCIPUS-A (Figure 24.3) is intended for use in the newly diagnosed SCI patient. Patients at high risk for pressure ulcer within 30 days after an acute SCI can be identified using this new scale. SCIPUS (Figure 24.4) is used for subsequent hospitalizations. Preliminary studies suggest that SCIPUS-A is an accurate predictor of pressure ulcer development in this population compared with Braden or other widely used scales. However, it remains to be validated with prospectively collected data.

Patients must be assessed for pressure ulcer risk on admission to any health care setting, because pressure ulcers often occur within the first few weeks of admission. Patients should be reassessed periodically as their condition changes. Skin inspection must be a part of the patient's daily routine. Patients must learn techniques for self-inspection as well as assessment by the clinical staff. It may be incorporated during morning care and at least every shift or when the patient is turned or receives a specific treatment.

PRESSURE ULCER RISK ASSESSMENT SCALE
FOR THE SPINAL CORD INJURED

Version 1.16
Revised 10/25/94

NAME

DATE

RISK FACTOR	CODED VALUE	SCORE
1. LEVEL OF ACTIVITY	0[]ambulatory 1[]wheelchair 4[]bed	
2. MOBILITY	0[]full 1[]limited 3[]immobile	
3. COMPLETE SCI	0[]no 1[]yes	
4. URINE INCONTINENCE OR CONSTANTLY MOIST	0[]no 1[]yes	
5. AUTONOMIC DYSREFLEXIA OR SEVERE SPASTICITY	0[]no 1[]yes	
6. AGE (years)	0[]≤34 1[]35-64 2[]≥65	
7. TOBACCO USE/SMOKING	0[]never 1[]former 3[]current	
8. PULMONARY DISEASE	0[]no 2[]yes	
9. CARDIAC DISEASE OR ABN. EKG	0[]no 1[]yes	
10. DIABETES OR GLUCOSE ≥110 mg/dl	0[]no 1[]yes	
11. RENAL DISEASE	0[]no 1[]yes	
12. IMPAIRED COGNITIVE FUNCTION	0[]no 1[]yes	
13. IN A NURSING HOME OR HOSPITAL	0[]no 2[]yes	
14. ALBUMIN <3.4 OR T.PROTEIN <6.4	0[]no 1[]yes	*
15. HEMATOCRIT <36.0% (HGB <12.0)	0[]no 1[]yes	
TOTAL SCORE (0-25)		

RISK: LOW 0-2, MODERATE 3-5, HIGH 6-8, VERY HIGH 9-25

NURSE ASSESSOR'S SIGNATURE: _____

Operational Definitions

1. **LEVEL OF ACTIVITY**
   0-ambulatory-can walk with/without assistance
   1-wheelchair mobile- sits out of bed only, cannot bear own weight and/or must be assisted into chair or wheelchair
   4-bed mobile-confined to bed during entire 24 hours of the day
2. **MOBILITY**
   0-full-independent in moving, no limitations, able to control and move all extremities at will
   1-limited-(slightly to very) requires assistance when moving
   3-immobile-complete immobility, unable to change position does not make even slight changes in body or extremity position without assistance, completely dependent on others for movement
3. **COMPLETE SCI**-Complete transection of spinal cord
4. **MINIMALLY CONTROLLED URINARY BLADDER**-incontinent of urine at least once a day, absence of control
   CONSTANTLY MOIST-skin is kept moist almost constantly by perspiration, urine, etc. Dampness is detected every time patient is moved or turned
5. **AUTONOMIC DYSREFLEXIA (ICD 358.9)**
   SEVERE SPASTICITY (ICD 780.3)
6. **AGE** in years at time of the assessment
7. **TOBACCO USE/SMOKING STATUS**
   0-never-smoked <10 packs in lifetime
   1-former-smoked >10 packs in lifetime & stopped >2 months
   3-current-smokes on a regular basis
8. **PULMONARY DISEASE (ICD CODES 450,460-519,796.0)**
9. **CARDIAC DISEASE OR ABNORMAL EKG**-documented cardiac disease, congestive heart failure, or an abnormal EKG) (ICD CODES 390-459)
10. **DIABETES OR GLUCOSE ≥ 110 (ICD CODES 250.0-250.9)**
11. **RENAL DISEASE (ICD CODES 580.0-589.9)**
12. **IMPAIRED COGNITIVE FUNCTION (ICD CODES 290.0-319.9)** (dementia, decreased level of consciousness, cerebral hemorrhage, cerebrovascular accident, narcotic poisoning, using sedatives or tranquilizers, disoriented, non-responsive)
13. **CURRENTLY RESIDES IN A NURSING HOME OR HOSPITAL**
14. **SERUM ALBUMIN <3.4 gm/dl OR TOTAL PROTEIN <6.4 g/dl**
15. **HEMATOCRIT < 36.0% (HGB < 12.0 gm/dl)**

Most recent values should be used for all risk factors.

PRESSURE ULCER (ICD-9 CODE=707.0)
"a lesion on any skin surface that results from pressure and which may include reactivity hyperemia and blistered, broken, or necrotic skin." (13)

FIGURE 24.4 *Spinal Cord Injury Pressure Ulcer Scale. (Reprinted with permission from CA Salzberg. Pressure ulcer risk assessment scale for the spinal cord injured and operational definitions. Am J Phys Med Rehabil 1996;75[2]:98.)*

Ulcer healing should be assessed at least weekly. Indicators of a deteriorating pressure ulcer include increases in exudate and wound edema, loss of granulation tissue, or a purulent discharge. The frequency of monitoring should be determined by the clinician based on the patient's condition, condition of the ulcer, the rate of healing, and the type of health care setting. Treatment plans and implementation strategies must be modified as necessary. Documentation must be done at regular intervals and should include risk assessment, skin evaluation, therapies designed to maintain intact skin, patient's response to alterations in therapy, the rationale for the alteration(s), and the outcome of the skin care program.[1]

Treatment Options

Local wound care consists of daily cleansing, dressing, and débridement.

Wound Cleansing

Pressure ulcers heal best when they are clean. All dead tissue, wound debris, and old dressing materials should be removed at each dressing change. Cleaning usually involves selecting a wound cleansing solution and a mechanical means of delivering it to the wound. Routine cleansing should be performed with as little chemical and mechanical trauma as possible.

The cleansing solution of choice is usually normal saline because it is physiologic and safe. Commercial wound cleansers often contain chemicals to enhance their cleaning ability, which may harm sensitive healing tissues. Antiseptic solutions such as hydrogen peroxide and povidone-iodine solution are not appropriate for irrigating open wounds and are cytotoxic to normal tissue.[12]

Enough irrigation force should be used to clean the ulcer adequately without traumatizing the wound bed. Moreover, excessive pressure can increase risk of infection by driving surface bacteria into the wound tissue. Irrigation pressure of 4–15 psi is recommended.[12] Whirlpool treatment may be considered for a noninfected large ulcer filled with debris.

Dressings

Pressure ulcers require special dressings to maintain their physiologic integrity and to heal faster. An ideal dressing should protect the wound, be biocompatible, and provide ideal hydration. The condition of the ulcer bed and the function of the desired dressing dictate the type of dressing needed.

The most common types of dressings that support moist wound healing are transparent films, hydrocolloids, hydrogels, alginates, polyurethane foams, combinations of these, or continuously moist saline gauze.

A draining ulcer requires an absorptive dressing. A moist dressing should be applied to a dry wound. A dressing that retains moisture should cover a moist wound that is not draining. Wound cavities need to be filled with dressings to prevent abscess formation and to inhibit the ulcers from closing at the surface (called *wall off*) before new tissue fills the cavity. Overpacking a wound may increase internal pressure on the tissue bed and cause further tissue injury.[12,18,23]

Débridement

Moist, necrotic tissue slows wound healing by providing a medium for bacterial growth. Removal of such tissue facilitates ulcer healing. Four methods of débriding necrotic tissue are available.

Sharp Débridement
A wound care specialist uses a sterile scalpel or other cutting instrument to surgically remove necrotic tissue. This is the fastest way to remove dead tissue and is the treatment of choice if there are signs of advancing cellulitis or sepsis. It is nonselective, painful, and requires specialized skills and possibly an operating room.

Mechanical Débridement
The most common débridement is the application of a wet-to-dry dressing. The gauze is moistened with 0.9% sodium chloride and placed on the wound bed. After the dressing has adhered to the tissue and dried com-

pletely, it can be removed, and necrotic tissue may be pulled away with it. This method of débridement is economical and easy to administer. However, it is nonselective, removes both viable and nonviable tissues, and is potentially traumatic to granulation tissue (especially to new epithelial tissue.) It is painful and takes longer than sharp débridement. Wet-to-dry dressings are ineffective as a débridement method if the dressing never dries out or is "soaked" off.

Other mechanical methods include forceful scrubbing with coarse materials or application of dextranomer beads into a wound bed to absorb exudate, bacteria, and other debris. The beads may be difficult to apply and remove and are expensive. Hydrotherapy and wound irrigation can be used to débride wounds and soften eschar. Pressurized hydrotherapy may be done with a whirlpool. Wound irrigation with a 19-gauge Angiocath attached to a 35-ml syringe provides enough force to remove eschar, bacteria, and debris.[23]

Chemical Débridement

In a chemical débridement, topical biologic enzymes are applied on the wound surface. These enzymes break down necrotic tissue and promote débridement and the growth of granulation tissue. The enzymes selectively débride necrotic tissue and can be combined with other forms of débridement. Chemical débridement should be considered when patients cannot tolerate surgery, are in long-term care facilities, or are receiving care at home. It should only be used when the ulcer does not appear to be infected. It requires a longer treatment period than sharp débridement. This treatment should be used only on necrotic tissue and must be discontinued when the wound is free from dead tissue.

Autolytic Débridement

The ulcer is covered with dressing materials that retain wound moisture, thus allowing the body's own enzymes contained in the wound fluid to digest dead tissue. This method may be used in combination with sharp débridement and selectively débrides necrotic tissue. It may be appropriate for patients who are unable to tolerate other forms of débridement. Autolytic débridement takes longer than other débridement methods. Progress should be visible within two to three days. An increase in cloudy drainage is usually a normal finding. Occlusive dressings should not be used for autolytic débridement of an infected wound.

Periwound Skin Protection

Measures to prevent injury to the periwound area from maceration, mechanical stripping, and shearing must be employed. These involve application of an appropriate dressing to the wound bed in combination with nonadherent wraps to the atrophied periwound skin. Polyurethane foam dressings and absorption dressings may be used for draining ulcers to prevent periwound skin maceration. Skin sealants, solid form skin barriers, or petrolatum ointments protect skin from exudate or solutions used in wound care.

Topical Agents

Growth factors (epidermal and fibroblast) and extracts of autologous human platelets (platelet-derived growth factor) are undergoing clinical trials for their use in pressure ulcer healing.[12] Other topical agents whose therapeutic efficacy are being studied are sugar, vitamins, honey, insulin, yeast extract, and elements like zinc, magnesium, gold, and aluminum. Phenytoin, as a topical agent, has been used in the healing of pressure sores, venous stasis, and diabetic ulcers, traumatic wounds, and burns.[24] It may promote wound healing by stimulation of fibroblast proliferation, facilitation of collagen deposition, glucocorticoid antagonism, and antibacterial activity. Most studies suggest it is effective in wound healing and deserves further investigation.

Adjuvant Therapy

Physical modalities may be used in conjunction with conventional local wound care treatments to augment the healing process. Most of these modalities have been and continue to be tested but are still not established for routine use.

Electrotherapy

Research studies suggest that certain physiologic changes occur at the tissue and cellular level in a wound when exposed to exogenous electrotherapy. Electrical currents have influenced migration of neutrophilic granulocytes and macrophages when applied to wound tissue. In addition, electric currents inhibit mast cells from migrating into the wound area.[25] In vitro studies show increased DNA and protein synthesis of fibroblasts in response to electrical stimulation.[26] Improved peripheral blood flow and preliminary evidence of bactericidal and bacteriostatic effects on microorganisms known to infect chronic wounds have been also reported.[27]

High-voltage pulsed current has been used for wound healing. Treatment is generally delivered at 75–200 volts and 80–100 pulses per second. The maximum total current reaching the tissue is approximately 2.5 mA when standard-size electrodes are used. The active electrode is placed over saline-soaked gauze on the wound bed for 45–60 minutes, five to seven times per week. Other types of current utilized are alternating current (the most commonly used is the transcutaneous electrical nerve stimulator) and pulsed electromagnetic energy.[27]

Ultrasound

Ultrasound (US) has been used, mostly with positive results, in the treatment of animals with experimental wounds.[28] Research on cultured fibroblasts indicates that US can enhance collagen production. US can assist tissue healing and produce a healed wound with greater strength and elasticity than tissue not exposed to the treatment. However, there have also been negative results reported. A placebo-controlled trial was utilized to study the effects of

US on 40 patients with pressure ulcers not extending beyond the dermis.[29] US was administered three times a week for a minimum of 5 minutes per treatment. No effort was made to control the type of dressings or other topical agents used on the ulcers. Eighteen ulcers were followed until the wound healed. Survival analysis revealed no significant difference in the healing times for ulcers treated with US as compared with those in the placebo-treated group. These findings of mixed results call for further studies to clarify the role of US in pressure ulcer treatment.[27,28]

Hydrotherapy

Hydrotherapy has traditionally been used as a component of wound care in many different wound and burn conditions for its apparent cleansing properties. Its use in pressure ulcer treatment is well known, and it is part of the AHCPR Clinical Practice Guideline.[12] Literature supporting its efficacy is limited and mainly anecdotal. However, a randomized, controlled, prospective study published in 1998 provided evidence that the daily use of whirlpool treatment, when added to a conservative treatment regimen, does indeed enhance the healing rate of wounds.[30] Whirlpool therapy is not without risks, including potential damage to the granulation tissue due to the turbulence of the water and cross-contamination from patient to patient because of difficulty in disinfecting the whirlpool agitators between treatments. Therefore, ongoing assessment of the wound is essential.[27]

Hyperbaric Oxygen Therapy

The rationale for hyperbaric oxygen therapy in chronic wounds is to intermittently increase the tissue oxygen tension to optimize fibroblast proliferation and white blood cell killing capacity during periods of hyperoxia and to stimulate angiogenesis.[31] Hyperbaric oxygen is provided through either a full-body pressurized chamber or topical oxygen therapy. Reports in the literature have been limited to case series and case control studies with small sample sizes involving patients with diabetic foot ulcer, venous ulcers, burns, and osteomyelitis.[27] The studies demonstrated improved wound healing with hyperbaric oxygen. Preliminary studies are encouraging, but more controlled investigations of its effects on pressure ulcer healing need to be conducted.

Negative Pressure with External Application of a Vacuum

The use of negative pressure with vacuum sealing techniques on soft-tissue defects has been described since the early 1990s. When applied to soft-tissue defects, negative pressure results in a significant increase in granulation tissue production in the animal model and increase in skin perfusion in healthy forearm tissue.[32,33] A prospective clinical trial studied the effect of vacuum sealing techniques on sacral pressure ulcers, acute traumatic soft-tissue defects, and infected soft-tissue defects.[34] The use of vacuum sealing techniques following débridement and irrigation decreased the dimensions of the initial wound, facilitated granulation tissue production, and improved maintenance of a relatively clean wound bed.

Other Modalities

Other physical and chemical modalities that have been described in the literature with positive results on pressure ulcer healing are ice therapy, ultraviolet light, and maggot débridement.

Ice Therapy
Ice is useful in decreasing swelling and increasing blood flow in the capillaries, hence aiding in tissue repair. Theoretically, this could lead to a possible acceleration in the rate of repair of pressure ulcers.[35]

Ultraviolet Light
Ultraviolet light increases the amount of fibronectin present in the wound environment, improving the microenvironment for cell migration and stimulating contraction, thus decreasing the size of the wound. In one study there was an increase in the healing of chronic wounds as well as a decrease in the time to healing of superficial pressure ulcers following exposure to ultraviolet light.[36]

Maggot Débridement
Maggot débridement therapy involves the topical application of blow fly larvae to treat human wounds. It has been found to be effective in the treatment of wounds that are recalcitrant to antibiotic and surgical intervention. Surface areas of necrotic wounds are débrided at a faster rate compared with conventional dressings.[37] It has the potential to halt or reverse the progression of pressure ulcers. Clinical effects of maggot débridement therapy are mediated through débridement, disinfection, and promotion of wound healing. Maggots produce these effects by liquefaction and removal of necrotic tissue; killing of bacteria by ingestion, digestion, and antibacterial secretions; and stimulation of healthy granulation tissue.[38]

Therapeutic Positioning

Interventions to reduce pressure over bony prominences are of primary importance in the prevention and treatment of pressure ulcers. A turning schedule must be established for patients who are confined to bed. Two hours in a single position is the maximum duration of time recommended for patients with normal circulatory capacity.[1]

Immobilized patients need to be maintained in proper alignment. For positioning, the rule of 30 is used. The head of the bed is elevated to 30 degrees or less, and the body is placed in a 30-degree laterally inclined position, when repositioned to either side. If the head of the bed is elevated beyond 30 degrees (e.g., for eating, watching television), the duration of this position needs to be limited to minimize both pressure and shear forces. In the 30-degree laterally inclined position, the hips and shoulders are tilted 30 degrees from supine and pillows or foam wedges are used to keep the patient properly positioned without pressure over the greater trochanter or sacrum. If tolerated, the prone position may also be used. Pillows under the calf may be used to elevate the heels off the bed surface. Cushioning devices should be placed between the legs or ankles to maintain alignment and prevent apposition of bony prominences. During transfers, it is important not to drag the patient across the bed. A draw sheet under the patient and two people to lift the patient should be employed. An over-the-bed trapeze may help some patients lift their buttocks off the bed independently and avoid abrasive friction burns and shear forces. Side rails help increase bed mobility.[5,18,23]

Patients who are chair-bound for long periods of time must be repositioned every hour. They need appropriate seating surfaces, capable of safely reducing pressure while still providing adequate stability and support. Patients who are temporarily chair-bound must use good body posture and alignment. The top of the thighs must be kept horizontal to distribute weight equally along the posterior surface of the thighs. If the knees are higher than the hips, the body weight is shifted to the ischial tuberosities, placing them at greater risk for pressure ulcers. Those who are able must be instructed to reposition themselves at 15–20 minute intervals. If patients have enough upper body strength, they may do push-ups, supporting their weight on the arms of the chair. Standing and scheduled walks are encouraged for ambulatory patients. Cushions that furnish maximum pressure reduction over the ischial tuberosities and provide adequate support and comfort should be considered.

Research has focused on comparison of tissue interface pressures of various support surfaces.[13] These studies employed the latest technology, from sensors to laser Doppler blood flow, as well as computerized pressure mapping measurement systems. However, continued research should address the accuracy of tissue interface pressures in determining prevention of pressure ulcers and in advancing new technologies to decrease capillary closing pressure.

Commercially available pressure-reducing mattresses include foam, static air, alternating air, gel, and water. No one support surface works consistently better than others. When using a mattress overlay, a hand check should be done to determine whether the pressure reduction is adequate. If the overlay compresses enough for the patient to rest on the underlying mattress, the patient is said to be *bottoming out*.[18] Patients with large stage III or stage IV ulcers may benefit from a low air loss bed or an air fluidized bed.[12] Preliminary results of research by the author suggest that an alternating pressure relief wheelchair cushion can substantially reduce pressure under the ischial tuberosities to near capillary closing pressure for a limited time.[39] Appropriate seating surfaces should be capable of safely reducing pressure while still providing adequate stability, support, and durability for everyday use. Donut cushions are to be avoided because they can cause tissue ischemia in the area supporting the donut.

Continence Management

Patients who have bladder or bowel incontinence must have an adequate evaluation to identify whether any reversible causes exist.

Reversible causes include urinary tract infection, medications, confusion, fecal impaction, polyuria due to glycosuria or hypercalcemia, or restricted mobility due to restraints. Incontinent patients should be checked frequently. Prevention of wound infection and skin maceration by management of excessive moisture can be achieved through cleansing at appropriate intervals and the use of skin barriers and absorbent materials. Briefs, diapers, and absorbent pads may be used if they are the types that trap moisture away from the patient. Male patients may use a Texas catheter, while an indwelling catheter may be indicated for patients with stage III or IV ulcers. Diversion procedures such as colostomy or urostomy may be considered for severe cases. A bowel-training program must be instituted for SCI patients.[1,5]

Patient and Caregiver Education

Responsibility for pressure ulcer prevention is shared by physicians, nurses, physical and occupational therapists, nutritionists, pharmacists, enterostomal nurses, administrators, patients, and their families. Education of health care professionals and patients is essential for the prevention and early treatment of pressure ulcers.

Staff education must focus on these topics:

- Normal and healthy skin (including anatomy and physiology)
- Pathophysiology and etiology of pressure ulcers
- Principles of wound healing
- Components of skin assessment
- Pressure ulcer risk factors
- Role of nutrition in ulcer management
- Staging and appearance of pressure ulcers
- Prevention strategies and options
- Management of tissue loads including positioning and turning techniques
- Characteristics of different pressure reducing devices and support surfaces
- Update on treatment options for ulcer care
- Principles of bacterial and infection control
- Documentation of skin assessment and skin care program (including intervention and outcome)

Educational programs should be implemented regularly and updated frequently to integrate new technologies and new products developed for wound care and pressure relief. Updating facilitates clarification of information regarding the latest research and techniques available for pressure ulcer care. The effectiveness of these programs needs evaluation. All possible measures to ensure the staff's retention of the knowledge and skills gained should be part of an educational program.

Patient and family education centers must teach the etiology of pressure ulcers, skin inspection, local wound care (including safe and proper cleansing and dressing procedures), importance of healthy diet and nutrition, reduction of risk factors, therapeutic positioning, use of pressure relieving devices, as well as pain, skin, and health status changes that must be reported to health care professionals. The patient and his or her caregiver must be encouraged to actively participate in decision making regarding pressure ulcer prevention and treatment. All measures to ensure patient and family understanding and compliance of the management must be taken.

References

1. National Pressure Ulcer Advisory Panel. Statement of Pressure Ulcer Prevention 1992 at www.iglou.com/npuap/positn1.htm.
2. Staas WE Jr, Cioschi HM. Pressure ulcers—a multifaceted approach to prevention and treatment. West J Med 1991;154:539.
3. Barczak CA, Barnett RI, Childs EJ, Bosley LM. Fourth national pressure ulcer prevalence survey. Adv Wound Care 1997;10:18.
4. National Pressure Ulcer Advisory Panel. Pressure Ulcers: Incidence, Economic Risk Assessment, Consensus Development Conference Statement. Rockville, MD: National Pressure Ulcer Advisory Panel, 1989;5–6.
5. Tan JC. Pressure Ulcers: Practical Manual of Physical Medicine and Rehabilitation. St. Louis: Mosby, 1998;431–444.
6. Baggerly J, DiBlasi M. Pressure sores and pressure sore prevention in a rehabilitation setting: building information for improving outcomes and allocating resources. Rehabil Nurs 1996;21:321.
7. Warren L. Protocols for Prevention of Pressure Ulcers in Home Care at www.ehob.com/clinicals/home_care_protocol.pdf.
8. National Pressure Ulcer Advisory Panel. Pressure ulcer prevalence, cost and risk assessment: consensus development conference statement. Decubitus 1989;2:24.
9. Relethford JH, Standfast SJ. Spinal Cord Injury in New York State. Injury Control and Disability Prevention Program, NY State Dept. of Health, December 24, 1990.
10. Miller H, Delozier J. Cost Implications of the Pressure Ulcer Treatment Guideline. Columbia, MD: Center for Health Policy Studies, 1994.
11. Xakellis GC, Frantz R. The cost of healing pressure ulcers across multiple health care settings. Adv Wound Care 1996;9(6):18.
12. Bergstrom N, Bennet MA, Carlson CE, et al. Treatment of Pressure Ulcers: Clinical Practice Guideline No. 15. Rockville, MD: Agency for Health Care Policy and Research, US Department of Health and Human Services. AHCPR Publication No. 95-0652, 1994.
13. Salcido R, Hart D, Smith AM. The Prevention and Management of Pressure Ulcers. In RL Braddom (ed), Physical Medicine and Rehabilitation. Philadelphia: WB Saunders, 1996;630–644.
14. Garber SL, Blair SL, Krouskop T. Pressure Ulcers. In SJ Garrison (ed), Handbook of Physical Medicine and Rehabilitation Basics. Philadelphia: JB Lippincott, 1995;297–318.

15. Allman RM. Pressure ulcer prevalence, incidence, risk factors, and impact. Clin Geriatr Med 1997;13(3):421.
16. Strayer LS, Martucci NM. Promoting skin integrity: an interdisciplinary challenge. Rehabil Nurs 1997;22(5):259.
17. Kosiak M. Etiology and pathology of ischemic ulcers. Arch Phys Med Rehabil 1959;40:62.
18. Maklebust J, Sieggreen MY. Attacking On All Fronts: How to Conquer Pressure Ulcers. Nursing 96 SpringNet Continuing Education 1996 at www.nursingmanagement.com/ce/p612a.htm.
19. Capobianco ML, McDonald DD. Factors affecting predictive validity of Braden scale. Adv Wound Care 1996;9(6):32.
20. Norton D. Calculating the risk: reflections on the Norton scale. Adv Wound Care 1996;9(6):38.
21. National Pressure Ulcer Advisory Panel. Prevention Monograph on Pressure Ulcer Research: Etiology, Assessment, and Early Intervention at www.iglou.com/npuap/prevmon.htm.
22. Salzberg CA, Byrne DW, Kabir R, et al. Predicting pressure ulcers during initial hospitalization for acute spinal cord injury. Wounds 1999;11(2):45.
23. Mylan Laboratories Inc. Wound Care Guide at www.dowhickam.com/woundcare.
24. Anstead GM, Hart LH, Sunahara JF, Liter ME. Phenytoin in wound healing. Ann Pharmacother 1996;30:768.
25. Weiss DS, Eaglstein WH, Falanga V. Exogenous electric current can reduce formation of hypertrophic scars. J Dermatol Surg Oncol 1989;15:1272.
26. Bourguignon GJ, Bourguignon LYW. Electrical stimulation of protein and DNA synthesis in human fibroblasts. FASEB J 1987;1:398.
27. Frantz RA. Adjuvant therapy for ulcer care. Clin Geriatr Med 1997;13(3):553.
28. ter Riet G, Kessels AGH, Knipschild P. A randomized clinical trial of ultrasound in the treatment of pressure ulcers. Phys Ther 1996;76(12):1301.
29. McDiarmid T, Burns PN, Lowith GT, et al. Ultrasound and the treatment of pressure sores. Physiother 1985;71:66.
30. Burke DT, Ho CHK, Saucier MA, Stewart G. Effects of hydrotherapy on pressure ulcer healing. Am J Phys Med Rehabil 1998;77(5):394.
31. Knighton DR, Silver IA, Hunt TK. Regulation of wound healing angiogenesis effect of oxygen gradients and inspired oxygen concentration. Surgery 1981;90:262.
32. Dersch T, Morykwas M, Clark M, Argenta L. Effects of negative and positive pressure on skin oxygen tension and perfusion. Fourth Annual Meeting of Wound Healing Society, San Francisco, 1994.
33. Morykwas MJ, Argenta LC. Use of negative pressure to decrease bacterial colonization in contaminated open wounds. Annual Meeting, Federation of American Societies for Experimental Biology, New Orleans, 1993.
34. Mullner T, Mrkonjic L, Kwasny O, Vecsei V. The use of negative pressure to promote the healing of tissue defects: a clinical trial using the vacuum sealing technique. Br J Plas Surg 1997;50:194.
35. Karadakovan A, Basbakkal Z. Ice therapy for pressure sores. Rehabil Nurs 1997;22(5):257.
36. Morykwas MJ, Mark MW. Effects of ultraviolet light on fibroblast

fibronectin production and lattice contraction. Wounds 1998;10(4):111.

37. Sherman R, Wyle F, Vulpe M. Maggot débridement therapy for treating pressure ulcers in spinal cord injury patients. J Spinal Cord Med 1995;18:71.

38. Sherman RA. Maggot débridement in modern medicine. Infect Med 1998;15(9):651.

39. Weiss LW, Ezra A, Shah M, Jacknow L. Trial of an alternating pressure relief wheelchair cushion for the reduction of seating pressure. Paper presented at the American Academy of Physical Medicine and Rehabilitation Annual Conference, Washington, DC, November, 1999.

25   Venous Ulcers

Rajshree Puri

Venous Ulcers

Venous ulcers are one of the most common vascular disorders. They account for 60–90% of chronic leg ulcers and affect 1% of the general population.[1] They are nearly seven and one-half times more likely to affect people over the age of 65. The male to female ratio in the affected population is 1 to 3.[1]

Pathophysiology of Venous Ulcers

The venous system in the lower extremity consists of three sets of veins, deep, superficial, and perforating. The deep veins are under high pressure, are embedded in the muscle, and carry most of the venous return to the heart. The deep veins include the anterior tibial, posterior tibial, and peroneal.

The superficial veins are under much lower pressure and lie outside the fascia. The superficial system includes the greater and lesser saphenous veins. The perforating veins penetrate the fascia and connect the high-pressure deep veins to the low-pressure superficial veins at varying intervals from the ankle to the knee.[1]

When the leg muscles contract, the calf muscle pump helps to propel the blood towards the heart. Both the superficial and deep veins have one-way valves that prevent retrograde flow back towards the feet during muscle relaxation.

Approximately 50% of the patients with acute deep vein thrombosis develop post-thrombotic syndrome as a result of chronic venous insufficiency. The underlying pathology consists of recanalization of the deep veins with persistent deformity and incompetence of the valves. This results in a long column of blood, unrestrained by valvular support that transmits pressures of over 100 mm Hg to the venules. This increased pressure promotes both fluid and protein loss into the tissues. In contrast to normal patients, who reduce their distal venous pressure with exercise, patients with post-thrombotic syndrome gain no benefit from their muscle pump.[2]

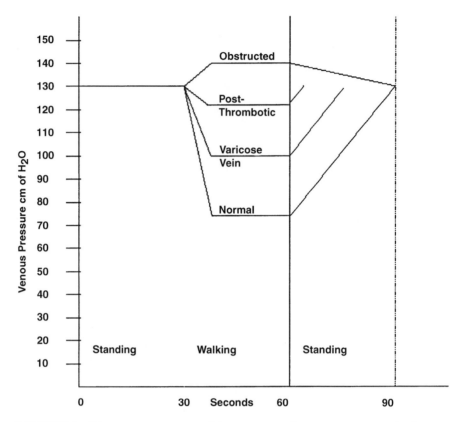

Ambulatory Venous Pressure Changes

FIGURE 25.1 *Direct measurement of the responses in venous pressure in the superficial veins at the ankle. (Reprinted with permission from SI Schwartz, GT Shires, FC Spencer, AC Galloway. Venous and lymphatic disease. In Principles of Surgery. New York: McGraw-Hill, 1994;1005.)*

In the standing position, the venous pressure in the superficial veins at the ankle is slightly higher than hydrostatic pressure in a column extending from the ankle to the heart. This pressure is approximately the same for normal persons and for those with venous insufficiency or chronically obstructed veins in which collaterals have formed. With walking, however, normal persons demonstrate a rapid decrease in venous pressure and a slower return to normal when exercise stops. Patients with varicose veins show a lesser decrease in pressure with walking but a more prompt return to normal following cessation of exercise. Patients with post-thrombotic veins demonstrate little if any decrease in venous pressure with walking and a rapid return to normal. Patients with obstructed veins show an increase in pressure with walking and a slow return to normal (Figure 25.1).[2]

The perforating veins allow blood to move from superficial veins to the deep veins. If the valves are incompetent, there is back-flow of blood from deep veins (high pressure) to superficial veins (low pressure) resulting in high ambulatory venous pressure in the superficial veins. As pressure increases over time, the superficial veins become dilated and tortuous, causing development of varicosities. This increased pressure is then transmitted to the local capillary system, which becomes abnormally dilated and permeable. Consequently fluid and proteins leak out into the interstitium.

Broadly Accepted Theories for Pathophysiologic Basis

Two theories are broadly accepted as the pathophysiologic basis of venous ulceration.[1,3]

Fibrin Cuff Theory
Fibrinogen, one of the larger proteins, polymerizes into fibrin, which adheres to the capillaries and creates a fibrin cuff. This fibrin cuff remains in place because of inadequate fibrinolysis and acts as a barrier to the absorption of oxygen and nutrients from the capillary.[4] This creates tissue anoxia, cellular death, and ulceration. The etiologic significance of the human fibrin cuff theory remains ill defined. Layer and colleagues performed a double-blind prospective, placebo-controlled study in 75 patients with venous ulceration and found no benefit of a fibrinolytic agent—stanozolol—in reducing the ulcer size over a 2-year follow-up period.[5]

Trap Theory
The entrapment of white blood cells creates impedence in the microcirculation, which creates tissue anoxia and free radical injury. The leukocyte activation results in the release of proteolytic enzymes, superoxide radicals, tumor necrosis factor, and other chemotactic substances that mediate tissue injury, liposclerosis, and finally, ulceration. A study of 19 patients with liposclerosis and venous ulceration reported an eightfold increase in the number of leukocytes in the skin of patients with liposclerosis and a 40-fold increase in patients with healed venous ulcers.[6] Immunohistologic analysis has demonstrated that most of these cells are macrophages, with no excess of neutrophils when compared with normal limbs.

Although the exact mechanism of venous ulceration is not known, valvular incompetence is almost always present. Risk factors for venous ulcers include

- History of deep vein thrombosis and postphlebitis syndrome
- Pregnancy
- Chronic heart failure
- Obesity
- Muscle weakness
- Professions involving long periods of standing

Clinical Manifestations

The clinical history and physical examination are important in distinguishing between primary (familial) and secondary (postphlebitic) venous insufficiency.

Primary venous insufficiency usually involves more than one family member and presents in the second or the third decade of life. The incidence of venous ulceration in these patients approaches 15% in most series.[7] The secondary or postphlebitic venous insufficiency usually presents in patients who have already had at least one or two episodes of deep vein thrombosis. The incidence of ulceration in these patients approaches 50%. Bauer and associates reported that about three-fourths of these patients have advanced stasis changes and one-half have ulceration within 10 years after an episode of acute thrombophlebitis.[8] Usually, some traumatic insult to the postphlebitic extremity creates a nidus for stasis ulceration.

Characteristics of Venous Ulcers

Location
The venous ulcers are usually located above the medial malleoli and on the medial side of the leg. Rutherford and colleagues have described this area as a *gaiter zone*.[9]

Pain
Most venous ulcerations are painless, although patients complain of a subjective feeling of heaviness, dullness, and cramping in the affected leg. These symptoms are exacerbated by prolonged standing or sitting and are relieved by rest and elevation. In peripheral arterial disease, pain is present on exercise and is exacerbated by elevation of legs.

Hyperpigmentation
Hyperpigmentation is a characteristic of venous ulcers. Deposits of hemosiderin in macrophages cause this brownish discoloration. A pruritic eczematous reaction (stasis dermatitis) is common. The term *lipodermatosclerosis* is used to describe the hyperpigmentation, accompanying erythema, and induration surrounding the venous ulceration.

Varicose Veins
Varicose veins may also be present in patients with venous ulceration. The varicosities of the greater saphenous veins are present on the medial aspect of the leg and the varicosities of the lesser saphenous veins appear around the popliteal region and ankle.

Edema
Edema is another common finding in patients with venous ulceration. This symptom is exacerbated by prolonged standing and is relieved by elevation of the leg. In the early stages of the disease, the edema is pitting. Later, as fibrosis develops in the subcutaneous tissue and the elasticity of the skin is reduced, the edema becomes brawny.

Differential Diagnosis

The three types of commonly occurring leg ulcers include ischemic ulcers, neurotrophic ulcers, and venous stasis ulcers.[3]

1. Ischemic ulcers are usually found in the distal lower extremity, over the dorsum of the foot or the toes. They are generally painful, especially at night. This pain is typically relieved by dependency, which is characteristic of the ischemic rest pain syndrome. Grossly, these ulcers have irregular edges with poor granulation tissue and other trophic changes of chronic ischemia. These ulcers exhibit little or no bleeding.
2. Neurotrophic ulcers are associated with calluses at pressure points such as the plantar aspects of the first to the fifth metatarsophalangeal joints. They are commonly associated with diabetes and are less painful but bleed briskly when débrided. Neurotrophic ulcers classically are punched-out lesions that can be accompanied by deep sinuses.
3. Venous stasis ulcers occur in the previously described gaiter zone, and are characterized by a moderate amount of pain, which is relieved by limb elevation. These ulcers are solitary and shallow, with irregular borders. They are frequently associated with a reasonably healthy granulating base and a surrounding zone of stasis dermatitis.

Diagnostic Testing

Several bedside tests have been proposed to assist in the diagnosis and mapping of chronic venous insufficiency. The retrograde filling or Brodie-Trendelenburg tourniquet test helps differentiate between valvular and perforator incompetence.[2,3,10] First, the patient is placed in a supine position and the leg veins are emptied by elevating the legs and stroking them firmly to the groin. A high thigh tourniquet is applied to occlude the superficial venous system below the saphenofemoral junction. The patient then stands quickly, and the pattern of saphenous vein filling is noted. If the superficial veins below the tourniquet fill quickly, perforating veins or the lesser saphenous vein are incompetent. If the veins remain empty and fill only when the tourniquet is released, the saphenofemoral junction is incompetent.

Perthes' Test

In Perthes' test, while the patient stands, a tourniquet is applied around the thigh, tightly enough to occlude the long saphenous vein but not the deep veins. The patient walks for 5 minutes. If the fullness of the varicose veins disappears, then the valves of the perforating veins are competent and the deep veins are patent. If the fullness of the varicose veins remains unchanged or increases, then the valves of the perforating veins are incompetent. Aggravation of the varicosities with significant calf pain suggests occluded deep veins.

Variant of Perthes' Test

In another variant of Perthes' test, a tourniquet is applied over the proximal superficial veins immediately below the knee and the patient is then asked to walk for several minutes while the ankle veins are observed. If the varices disappear, the saphenous vein is presumed to be the cause because the blood was cleared by competent perforating veins through the deep venous system. If the varices becomes more prominent with exercise and the patient complains of leg pain, deep venous insufficiency with incompetent perforating veins is suggested.

Mahorne-Ochsner Test

The Mahorne-Ochsner test, also called the *comparative tourniquet test*, uses a tourniquet placed sequentially on the upper thigh, middle thigh, and just below the knee. This enables the examiner to locate the incompetent perforator veins more exactly.[3]

Unfortunately, these bedside tourniquet tests have proven to be of limited value.

Doppler Ultrasound

Doppler ultrasonography is a technique performed at the bedside to determine venous patency and valvular competence. Reflux retrograde flow can be observed at the femoral level during a Valsalva maneuver or at the popliteal level with the patient standing and the calf alternatively compressed and released. It is used to assess coexisting arterial ischemia and to verify the local pulses in the presence of gross edema.[1,3]

Color Flow Duplex Imaging

Color flow duplex imaging provides images of regional flow and is used to identify areas of valvular incompetence.

Photoplethysmography

Photoplethysmography uses a transducer and infrared light to measure subcutaneous vascular volume and can provide a reliable index of valvular incompetence. The venous refilling time, after the calf muscle exercise empties the vein, is considerably shortened in the presence of valvular incompetence.

Duplex Scanning

Duplex scanning is the most promising new technique. It is the combination of ultrasound duplex scanning using a B-mode imager with the pulsed Doppler instrument providing both imaging and flow patterns. Thrombi can be visualized within the veins and the flow observed if the veins remain patent. Duplex scanning allows visualization of venous valves for competency assessment.[2]

Venacavography

Venacavography is the radiographic imaging of the venous system that is obtained by injecting radiopaque contrast into the dorsal pedal area. Hypersensitivity reactions limit its use.

Management of Venous Ulcers

Treatment of venous ulcers is directed toward control of various underlying medical disorders.

Control of Underlying Medical Disorders

Various contributing factors need to be identified and treated. Diabetes mellitus must be controlled because hyperglycemia increases destruction of the microcirculatory system and impairs wound healing. Obesity and increased intra-abdominal conditions must be managed so they do not compromise the venous return to heart.[11] Hypertension must be controlled as it exacerbates capillary pressure and leakage into the interstitium. Nutritional factors such as height, weight, serum total protein, and serum albumin levels needs to be assessed. Dietary supplementation of zinc, vitamin A, vitamin C, and proteins are recommended to promote wound healing. A review of current medications is important as certain medications may impede wound healing. These include corticosteroids and nonsteroidal anti-inflammatory drugs. These drugs may mask infections in chronic wounds and inhibit the inflammation phase of healing in acute wounds.[1]

Reduction of Edema

Edema reduction is achieved by elevation of the legs and compression. In patients with predominant venous ulcers or a mixed etiology, knowledge of the degree of arterial involvement is essential before compression is applied to the limb. *Ankle pressure index* (API) is defined as

$$API = Systolic\ Ankle\ Pressure/Systolic\ Arm\ Pressure$$

A normal API is equal to or greater than one. Compression should not be applied if the API is less than 0.8.

A correctly applied compression bandage supports the superficial veins, helps prevent capillary leakage, and reduces tissue edema. Compressive bandages should be applied when the leg is at its least edematous stage (i.e., first thing in the morning). Intermittent periods of leg elevation and avoidance of prolonged sitting or standing should be advised.

Current compression methods include elastic bandages or elastic stockings, Unna boots or Velcro-bands boots, and intermittent pneumatic compression boots. The ideal pressure for healing to take place is generally around 40 mm Hg at the ankle, reducing over the calf. For patients with severe postphlebitic syndrome with stasis dermatitis and ulceration, some authors advocate the use of heavy rubberized elastic bandages wrapped from the base of the toes to the knee instead of elastic stockings.[3] The elastic compression therapy does not alter the deep venous hemodynamics significantly, although it does reduce tissue edema by preventing leakage from the capillaries.

In 1883, Unna developed a gauge bandage impregnated with zinc oxide, glycerin, water, and gelatin for application over clean uninfected ulcers to promote the formation of granulation tissue without the necessity of daily dressing changes. Unna boots are generally recommended for patients with physical impairments that prohibit daily dressing changes and have been a traditional technique in the treatment of venous stasis ulcers. The Unna boot needs to be changed once a week.[3]

The Velcro-bands boot system consists of series of custom-made buckles that have the advantage of being easy to remove for daily inspection and cleaning of ulcers.

Care of the Wound

Wounds should be cleaned with a noncytotoxic cleaner or normal saline. The use of an antimicrobial cleaner such as povidone-iodine should be avoided in noninfected wounds because these preparations are cytotoxic and impede fibroblast formation. Silver sulfadiazine is frequently used for short-term management of infected ulcers. Another important principle is never to allow open wounds to dry (i.e., use moist dressings). Moist dressings may also relieve pain. Any local infection needs to be controlled with systemic antibiotics. The use of topical antibiotics should be discouraged. Generally, chronic ulcers with their surrounding scar tissues are poorly perfused. Débridement of unhealthy tissue, often followed by skin grafting, may be required for healing.

Eczema

Eczema is a common complication in the management of venous ulcers. Severe eczema with signs of clinical infection is treated with topical corticosteroid ointment.

Surgical Treatment

Approximately 80–85% of venous ulcers heal with medical management. For the remaining 15–20%, surgical intervention is necessary.[1] A full- or split-thickness allograft may be used to promote wound healing. It can be applied either directly to a clean granulating ulcer or the ulcer may be excised and a skin graft applied primarily. Bilayer artificial skin consists of an inner layer of collagen sponge and an outer silicone layer. When applied to a full-thickness wound bed, the fibroblasts and capillaries infiltrate the collagen layer and then connect to a synthetic connective tissue matrix similar to dermis in 2–3 weeks.[1] Months after healing, the silicone layer is peeled off and a split-thickness graft is placed to cover the area. The cosmetic effect of this procedure is equal to or better than traditional grafting technique, although controlled research is warranted. Recurrences are common if nothing is done to treat the diseased veins. The initial operation should include ligation and stripping of the greater saphenous vein and the ligation of incompetent perforators in the region of the ulcer.

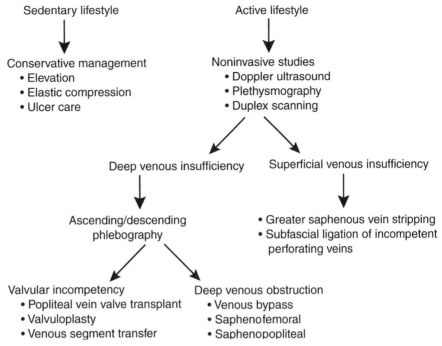

Sedentary lifestyle

Conservative management
• Elevation
• Elastic compression
• Ulcer care

Active lifestyle

Noninvasive studies
• Doppler ultrasound
• Plethysmography
• Duplex scanning

Deep venous insufficiency

Superficial venous insufficiency

Ascending/descending
phlebography

• Greater saphenous vein stripping
• Subfascial ligation of incompetent
  perforating veins

Valvular incompetency
• Popliteal vein valve transplant
• Valvuloplasty
• Venous segment transfer

Deep venous obstruction
• Venous bypass
• Saphenofemoral
• Saphenopopliteal

FIGURE 25.2   *Algorithm for the treatment of chronic venous insufficiency and venous ulcers. (Reprinted with permission from F Sabido, VJ Milazzo, RW Hobson II. Management of the Postphlebitic Syndrome. In WP Ritchie Jr, G Steele Jr, RH Dean [eds], General Surgery. Philadelphia; JB Lippincott, 1995;756.)*

The skin grafting has a postoperative success rate of 50–90%, but approximately 30–50% of ulcers reoccur subsequently.[12] For patients with recalcitrant leg ulcers due to deep venous insufficiency or post thrombosis, shave therapy is an effective surgical method with favorable long- and short-term results. This procedure involves excision of a circumscribed area of lipodermatosclerosis together with the ulceration. The shave therapy can be combined with removal of insufficient superficial or perforating veins. Long-term compression with stockings is necessary because shave therapy does not reduce the pathological reflexes in deep veins.

Paratibial fasciotomy has had good results, but can only be used in ulcers of the medial ankle.[12] When ulceration recurs in spite of these measures, more radical surgical procedures are indicated. The most successful of these is ligation of all the perforating veins. Even after this procedure, there is a recurrence rate of 10%.[12] There has been increasing interest and success in direct venous valve repair or transplantation, because a competent valve in the deep venous system restores a limb to a compensated condition and allows healing of stasis ulceration.

Rarely, after many years, a chronic ulcer may undergo malignant transformation (Marjolin's ulcer). Therefore, intractable ulcers should always be biopsied.

Figure 25.2 reviews the treatment algorithms for chronic venous insufficiency and venous ulcers.[3]

Patient Education

Patients at risk for venous ulcers should be educated about steps they can take to reduce the incidence and recurrence of ulceration. These steps include

- Avoidance of standing or sitting for prolonged periods
- Regular exercise
- Leg elevation at rest
- Balanced diet
- Smoking cessation
- Weight reduction, if necessary

References

1. Rudolph DM. Pathophysiology and management of venous ulcers. J Wound Ostomy Contin Nurs Soc 1998;25:248.
2. Schwartz SI, Shires GT, Spencer FC, Galloway AC. Venous and Lymphatic Disease. In Principles of Surgery. New York: McGraw-Hill, 1998;1014.
3. Sabido F, Milazzo VJ, Hobson RW II. Management of the Postphlebitic Syndrome. In WP Ritchie Jr, G Steele Jr, RH Dean (eds), General Surgery. Philadelphia: JB Lippincott, 1995;749–760.
4. Browse NL, Burnard KG. The cause of venous ulceration. Lancet 1982;2:243.
5. Layer GT, Stacey MC, Burnard KG. Stanozolol and the treatment of venous ulceration: an interim report. Phlebology 1986;1:197.
6. Scott HJ, Coleridge Smith PD, Scuerr JH, et al. A histological study into white blood cells and their association with lipodermatosclerosis and ulceration. Br J Surg 1991;78:210.
7. Widmer LK, Hall T, Kaclin H, et al. Epidemiology and Sociomedical Importance of Peripheral Venous Disease. In JT Hobbs (ed), The Treatment of Venous Disorders. London: MTP Press, 1977;3.
8. Bauer G. A roentgenological and clinical study of the sequelae of thrombosis. Acta Chir Scand 1992;86:1.
9. Rutherford RB, et al. The Noninvasive Management of Chronic Venous Insufficiency. In RB Rutherford (ed), Vascular Surgery. Philadelphia: WB Saunders, 1989;1237.
10. Hobson RW II. Lower Extremity Varicosities. In JL Cameron (ed), Current Surgical Therapy. Philadelphia: BC Decker, 1989;605.
11. Black SB. Venous stasis ulcers: a review. Ostomy Wound Manage 1995;41:525.
12. Schmeller W, Gaber Y, Gehl HB. Shave therapy is a simple, effective treatment of persistent venous leg ulcers. J Am Acad Dermatol 1998;39:232.

26   Wound Care Pain Management

Jack L. Rook and Sergey Bogdan

Chronic wound pain is a clinical problem confronted by practitioners in most medical specialties at one time or another. Chronic wound pain affects millions of Americans, including those with leg ulcers, diabetic ulcers, and pressure ulcers, yet research in this area is extremely limited. The field of pain management has been evolving since the early 1980s. It is now considered much more acceptable to utilize opioid analgesics for chronic nonmalignant pain problems, as compared with even the very recent past. In fact, appropriate pain management is now considered a standard of good medical practice whereas in the past, fears of analgesic overuse and addiction dominated the minds of health care providers. Despite extensive growth in the field of pain medicine, pressure ulcer pain is usually inadequately treated, if managed at all. A literature search for wound care pain management suggests that this area of medicine is truly in its infancy. Further research needs to be conducted to determine the most effective pain management technique for wound and pressure ulcer pain.

To adequately study this area of pain control, more effort must be directed toward pain management in patient care. This includes the systematic steps of assessing the situation, collecting data about the probable cause of the patient's pain, and alleviating the pain as much as possible. One should remember that all pain is real and that it is a personal experience perceived only by the individual. Pain is a complex phenomenon that is universal, but very specific to each individual experience. Numerous factors influence pain perception, including age, sex, personality, emotional state, cognitive status, culture, social background, and previous pain experience.[1,2]

Review of Literature

There is a paucity of literature describing pain management as it relates to wound care. No peer-reviewed, prospective studies on this subject have yet been performed. Dallum and colleagues utilized a cross-sectional study design to document perception of pressure ulcer pain among 132 hospitalized patients at a large, urban medical center. To quantify the intensity of pain, subjects used the Visual Analog Scale (VAS) and the Faces Rating Scale (FRS) (a series of six faces, ranging from a smiling, happy face to a crying, frowning face). The Folstein Mini-Mental State Examination assessed mental status. The presence of depression was evaluated by the Beck Depression Inventory.

The group comprised 44 subjects who were able to respond to the evaluation instruments and 88 subjects (67%) who were unable to respond. The respondents included 48% who scored below 24 on the Folstein Mini-Mental State Examination (indicative of cognitive impairment), and 52% who were found to be cognitively intact. Forty-one percent of the respondents denied pressure ulcer pain and 59% reported pain of some type.

This study concluded that

1. Patients with pressure ulcers experience pain, and many perceive the pain as severe.
2. Despite their experiences of pain, most subjects did not receive analgesics for pressure ulcer pain relief.
3. The often-held belief that the more severe pressure ulcer stages cause less pain because of destruction of sensory nerve endings was not validated. In contrast, subjects with stage IV pressure ulcers had more pain than those with pressure ulcers of lower stage.
4. Two-thirds of the subjects were unable to respond to various questions in the study. However, it should not be concluded that these subjects were free of pain simply because they were unable to express their pain experience.
5. Patients who were cognitively impaired or for whom English was not their first language had an easier time responding to the FRS than to the VAS.
6. The evaluation of pain by means of the VAS or FRS reveals that even cognitively impaired patients express pressure ulcer–related pain when clear and simple evaluation tools are properly used.[3]

An article by Krasner presents a theoretical definition of the chronic wound pain experience and its subcomponents (noncyclic acute wound pain, cyclic acute wound pain, and chronic wound pain). The chronic wound pain experience is defined as the complex, subjective phenomenon of extreme discomfort experienced by a person in response to skin and flesh or tissue injury.

1. Noncyclic acute wound pain is single-episode acute wound pain.
2. Cyclic acute wound pain is periodic acute wound pain that recurs due to repeated treatments or interventions.
3. Chronic wound pain is the persistent pain that occurs without manipulation. It is anticipated that most chronic wound patients experience all three types of pain at some time.

The article also proposes pharmacologic and nonpharmacologic interventions to optimize patient outcomes for each subcomponent.[4]

In a study on the quality of life of patients with leg ulcers, 67% of patients reported severe pain, 20% experienced mild to moderate pain, and more than 50% suffered from itching.[5] The importance of distinguishing between leg ulcers caused by venous versus arterial insufficiency was stressed, as treatment depends upon the underlying etiology of the ulcer. Vascular procedures such as bypass graft or balloon angioplasty would be considered to alleviate the pain associated with impaired perfusion, whereas more conservative measures were used to treat the pain from venous ulcers (leg elevation, compression therapy, walking exercises, and intermittent pneumatic compression therapy). For most patients with venous ulcers, pain decreased significantly within a few weeks after the start of appropriate wound therapy.[6,7]

Holm et al. described the use of topical anesthetics such as lidocaine-prilocaine cream (EMLA) on wounds. Studies have shown that applying it 30 minutes before débridement significantly reduces pain associated with wound care procedures.[8]

Last, the pressure ulcer treatment guidelines have only a few paragraphs on the subject of pressure ulcer pain management.[9,10]

Ascending and Descending Pain Pathways

Why do patients with pressure ulcers suffer from pain? What is there about the ulcer that leads to the perception of pain? To better understand these concepts, it is important for treating personnel to have some knowledge of the pathophysiology and neuroanatomy involved in the transmission and modulation of pain. This necessitates a discussion of ascending pain pathways (painful impulses traveling from the wound, through the peripheral and central nervous system, ultimately to the brain), and a descending pain modulatory (inhibitory) system traveling from the brain to the spinal cord.

The peripheral nerve is made up of different types of nerve fibers, both afferent (towards the spinal cord) and efferent (away from the spinal cord) (Figure 26.1). The afferent fibers include the large A-alpha fibers and the smaller A-delta and C fibers. The large myelinated A-alpha fibers are concerned with transmission of nonpainful (non-nociceptive) stimuli such as light touch and vibration. It is the smaller myelinated A-delta and unmyelinated C fibers that carry pain (nociceptive) information from the periphery into the dorsal horn of the spinal cord.

Nociceptive nerve terminals have been found in all structures that could potentially be involved in a pressure ulcer including skin, dermis, muscle, joints, and bone tissue. Nerve terminals in these structures can relay nociceptive information into the spinal cord via the A-delta and C fibers (Figure 26.2).[11–17]

As the pressure ulcer erodes through the tissues, damaged cells release or synthesize chemicals that are irritative to the nociceptive nerve terminals (potassium, acetylcholine, adenosine triphosphate, bradykinin,

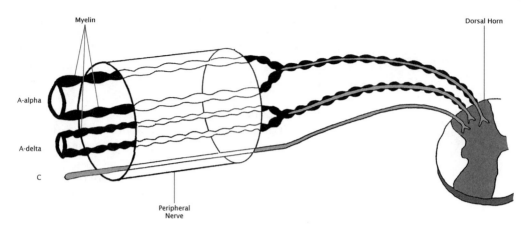

FIGURE 26.1 *Major mixed nerve in cross section, demonstrating the afferent fibers (A-alpha, A-delta, and C fibers). The nociceptive C fibers are unmyelinated. The A-delta and A-alpha fibers are myelinated. These afferent nerve fibers carry both noxious and non-noxious information into the dorsal horn of the spinal cord.*

serotonin, histamine, and prostaglandins). This leads to the phenomenon of transduction whereby chemical stimuli create electrical activity in the sensory nerve endings.[18–24] After transduction comes transmission of the electrical impulse through the nerve fiber into the dorsal horn of the spinal cord (Figure 26.3).

All afferent pain fibers make connections (synapses) with second-order pain transmission cells in the dorsal horn of the spinal cord. The second-order cells transmit the painful impulses toward the brain. The axons from these cells travel across the spinal cord to the anterolateral quadrant and then ascend toward the brain where there are connections with third-order pain transmission cells.[25–28] The third-order cells,

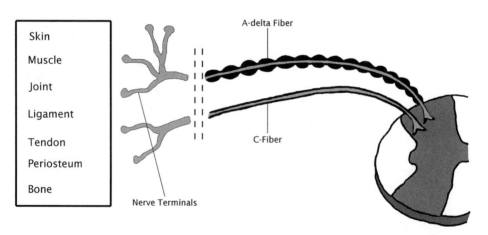

FIGURE 26.2 *Nociceptive nerve terminals of A-delta and C fibers have been found in all structures potentially involved in pressure ulcers.*

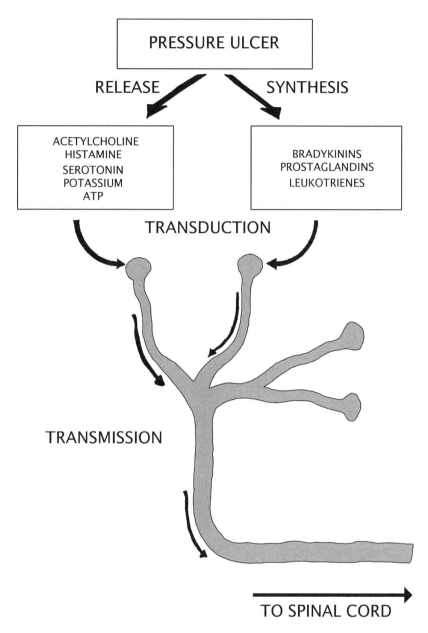

FIGURE 26.3 *Damaged tissue causes the release or synthesis of noxious chemicals. Transduction and transmission follows. (ATP = adenosine triphosphate.)*

located in the thalamus (Figure 26.4), are part of two distinct tracts of nerve fibers which have evolved phylogenetically over time. There is a primitive midline pathway known as the *paleospinothalamic tract* whose third-order cells originate in the medial thalamus and travel to the frontal cortex, limbic system, brain stem, and hypothalamus. The paleospinothalamic tract, being a primitive pathway, is concerned with the emotional response to pain.[25,29,30] A newer evolutionary pathway,

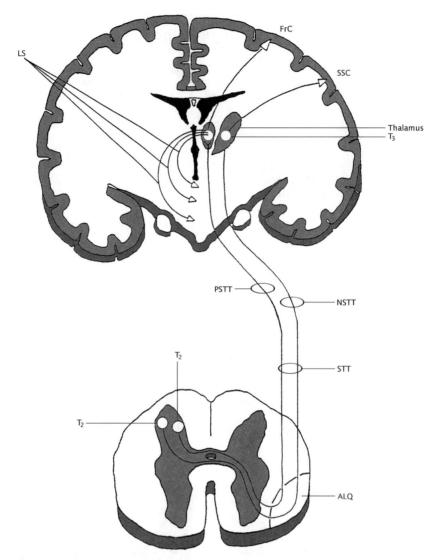

FIGURE 26.4   *Axons from second-order pain transmission cells (T2) cross to the contralateral anterolateral quadrant (ALQ) to form the spinothalamic tract (STT). The STT subsequently forms two distinct tracts as it enters the brain, known as the* paleospinothalamic tract (PSTT), *and the* neospinothalamic tract (NSTT). *These tracts synapse with third-order cells (T3) in the thalamus. The paleospinothalamic tract, which is concerned with the emotional aspects of pain, then has third-order projections to the frontal cortex (FrC) and the limbic system (LS). The neospinothalamic tract travels through the lateral thalamus with dense third-order projections to the somatosensory cortex (SSC). The neospinothalamic tract is concerned with localization of the pain impulses.*

known as the *neospinothalamic tract*, has a more lateral course through the thalamus, with dense projections to the somatosensory cortex. The neospinothalamic tract helps to localize where pain is coming from. It is most active in patients with acute or postoperative pain. On the other hand, activity in the midline paleospinothalamic

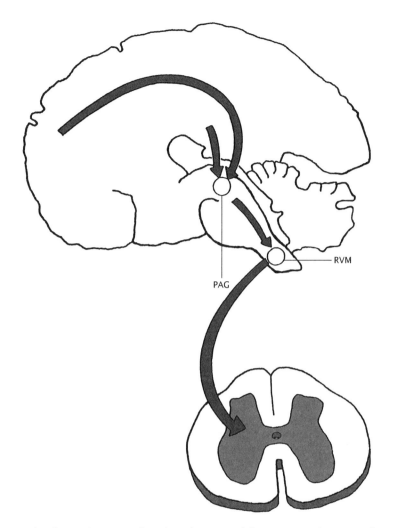

FIGURE 26.5 *The descending opioid mediated pain modulatory system begins in the cortex and interacts with neurons in the brain stem, initially at the periaqueductal gray (PAG) of the pons, with subsequent connections at the rostroventral medulla (RVM). From the rostroventral medulla, the descending system sends fibers to the outer layers of the dorsal horn of the spinal cord. Here, the release of neurotransmitters including norepinephrine, serotonin, and endorphins, cause inhibition of second-order pain transmission cells, thus modulating the ascending pain pathways.*

tract is more common in chronic pain patients producing poorly localized discomfort, depression, anxiety, and sleep disturbance.[25]

There is a descending opioid-mediated pain modulatory system that begins in the cortex and interacts with neurons in the hypothalamus, brain stem, and spinal cord. This descending system is activated by stress, pain, and opioids (both endogenous endorphins and exogenous oral or parenteral narcotics) and is inhibited by anxiety, tension, and depression. Activation of this system causes inhibition of second order pain transmission cells at the spinal cord level (Figure 26.5) by neurotransmitters released in the dorsal horn (norepinephrine, serotonin, and endorphins).[31–45]

An understanding of ascending and descending pain pathways is always helpful in formulating a treatment plan for virtually any type of pain problem—including the pain associated with pressure ulcers. It is always necessary to decrease nociceptive input coming from the wound. However, it is also important to alleviate depression, anxiety, and tension. Opioid analgesia may also prove helpful. Endogenous opioids are usually stimulated through aerobic exercise—not a practical treatment option in patients with pressure or vascular ulcers. A discussion on the use of exogenous opioids is forthcoming. Attempts to increase levels of serotonin and norepinephrine may enhance analgesia. This can be done through a variety of antidepressant medications including the tricyclic antidepressants (amitriptyline, nortriptyline, imipramine, and trazodone), which increase both neurotransmitters, and the newer selective serotonin reuptake inhibitor antidepressants, which selectively increase serotonin levels. Such medications may prove helpful in the management of both depression and certain chronic pain states.

Etiology of Pain in the Pressure Ulcer Patient

There are many potential causes of pain in patients who have pressure ulcers (Table 26.1). The ulcer itself can be painful. As noted previously, damaged tissue liberates noxious chemicals, and there may be synthesis of other nociceptive substances in the damaged area. In addition, as the ulcer erodes through tissue planes, there is destruction of nerve terminals. One of the qualities of peripheral nerves is that they do regenerate. The nociceptive nerve terminals send out immature sprouts of nerve tissue that have been shown to be overly sensitive to stimuli— both noxious and non-noxious.[46] Therefore, the pain elicited by wound dressing changes and surgical débridement is amplified due to this primitive neural tissue.

Infection further irritates these free nerve endings. Bacteria liberate enzymes, which are highly irritative to nerve terminals. If an infection progresses to the point where it infiltrates bone, patients may suffer from the severe pain of osteomyelitis. X-ray changes, positive radionucleotide studies, marked elevation of the sedimentation rate, and elevation of the white blood cell count provide additional evidence of infection. Fever may or may not be associated with this diagnosis.

Wound management, including dressing changes, surgical débridement of wounds, and postoperative pain associated with grafting and flap procedures, can be a severely painful process.

There are other pain-producing problems that can occur in patients prone to pressure ulcers. In the elderly patient, contractures may develop as sequelae of immobility. Attempts to correct the shortened tissue are quite uncomfortable. Other possible pain producers in this patient population are muscle spasm in the region of the ulcer; concomitant orthopedic or rheumatologic abnormalities such as compression fractures, osteoarthritis, rheumatoid arthritis; or other connective tissue disease.

Spasticity can be quite uncomfortable for spinal cord injured patients. In addition, spasticity is typically worse when pressure ulcers are not well

TABLE 26.1   Potential causes of pain in pressure ulcer patients

The ulcer itself
Pressure ulcer treatment
    Wound dressing changes
    Surgical débridement
    Postoperative pain after grafting or flap procedures
Would infection
Concomitant pain generators in the elderly or debilitated patient
    Contractures
    Muscle spasm
    Orthopedic or rheumatologic abnormalities
Pain in spinal cord injury
    Neurogenic pain
    Spasticity
    Autonomic dysreflexia
Claudication with peripheral vascular disease
Diabetic neurogenic pain

treated. In this way, even though the spinal cord injured patients may not perceive the actual ulcer, they may experience discomfort from the spasticity. Additionally, in high thoracic paraplegics and quadriplegics, the phenomenon of autonomic dysreflexia characterized by facial flushing, severe headaches, and elevation of blood pressure can be precipitated by the presence of a poorly treated pressure ulcer. Aggressive treatment of ulcers is essential to minimize these potentially painful complications seen in the spinal cord injured population.[47]

There are pain problems that can occur in ulcer patients with peripheral vascular disease or diabetes. Patients with arterial insufficiency can suffer from the pain of claudication, due to ischemia of major muscle groups in the lower extremities. Chronic ischemia, secondary to peripheral vascular disease, may render even minimal injuries very painful, impedes healing, and predisposes patients to secondary infectious complications.[48,49] In contrast, peripheral neuropathies, such as those associated with diabetes, can render, otherwise, painful injuries painless. Diabetics may also develop a peripheral neuropathy characterized by neuropathic pain that has a burning, shooting, unrelenting nature.

Assessment

The chronic wound pain experience has been described as having either a noncyclic acute component, a cyclic acute component, or a chronic wound pain component. The experience of wound pain is the complex subjective phenomenon of extreme discomfort experienced by a person in response to skin or tissue injury. Noncyclic acute wound pain occurs with intermittent sharp débridement or drain removal. Cyclic acute wound pain occurs with daily dressing changes and turning and repositioning of the patient. Chronic wound pain may occur in some patients who have persistent discomfort without manipulation of the involved tissues.[4]

When performing assessment of these patients, it is necessary to evaluate age, cognitive status, overall physical condition, and type of wound. Ulcers are usually grouped according to cause: arterial, vasculitic, venous, diabetic, or pressure. Ulcers can be categorized by location as well. Pressure and diabetic ulcers are usually over pressure sensitive areas whereas arterial, vasculitic, and venous ulcers are usually distal and relatively shallow. It is also important to monitor liver and kidney functioning, as all medications prescribed for pain management are metabolized in these organs.

With advancing age, the skin becomes thinner, drier, more prone to swelling, and easily bruised. Thus, direct contact between adhesive material and the skin should be minimized so as not to permit new sites of ulceration to develop.

When the patient has cognitive dysfunction, it is imperative to observe the patient carefully during dressing changes and repositioning to look for indications of discomfort. Changes in blood pressure and heart rate may correlate with discomfort; however, a lack of change in vital signs does not necessarily correlate with a lack of pain. Lack of expression or response from the patient is not an indicator that pain does not exist; the clinician should constantly assess and treat the pain. Because pain may be evoked or may be especially acute during dressing change and débridement, the caregiver should be careful to prevent such discomfort and make efforts to relieve it.

For patients who are cognitively intact, their report of discomfort is the hallmark of pain assessment. Questionnaires are available that utilize VAS and functional numeric scales that may prove helpful. The VAS, a 10-cm line anchored at the ends with the terms *no pain* or *pain as bad as you can imagine*, can be used to analyze worst, least, and average daily pain for patients with chronic wound pain. It can also be used to analyze the degree of pain during dressing changes or surgical débridement. The VAS can be repeated after pain management has been instituted (Figure 26.6A). Functional numeric scales, zero to ten scales anchored at the ends by *does not interfere* and *completely interferes*, may also provide useful information. A variety of functions can be assessed (general activity, mood, ability to walk, pursue vocational or avocational pursuits, relate with others, sleep, engage in basic activities of daily living, and enjoy life) using this measurement tool (Figure 26.6B).

As mentioned earlier, the FRS may be a more appropriate assessment tool for patients who are cognitively impaired (Figure 26.6C).[3]

Treatment

The management of ulcer pain requires a combination of conservative measures, medications, and appropriate wound care (Table 26.2). Some high-technology options are available (for example, implantation of morphine pumps and spinal cord stimulators) that may be appropriate to manage pain in select cases.

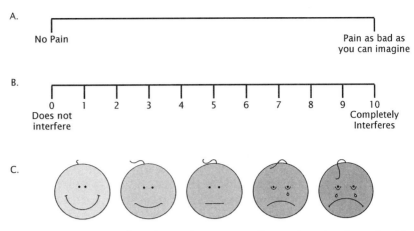

FIGURE 26.6 *(A) The Visual Analog Scale is a 10-cm line anchored at the ends with the terms* no pain *or* pain as bad as you can imagine; *(B) functional numeric scales are 0–10 scales anchored at the ends by* does not interfere *and* completely interferes. *A variety of functions can be assessed using this scale format; (C) the Faces Rating Scale may be a more appropriate assessment tool for patients who are cognitively impaired.*

TABLE 26.2   The management of pressure ulcer pain

Wound dressings
Physical and occupational therapy
   Modalities to relieve pain and spasm
   Modalities for wound cleansing
   Positioning and seating
   Adaptive equipment
Transcutaneous electrical nerve stimulation
Alternative therapies
Pharmacologic management
   Nonopioid analgesics
      Nonsteroidal anti-inflammatory drugs
      Acetaminophen (Tylenol)
      Muscle relaxants
   Adjuvant medications
      Tricyclic antidepressants
   Anticonvulsants
      Carbamazepine (Tegretol)
      Phenytoin (Dilantin)
      Valproic acid (Depakote)
      Clonazepam (Klonopin)
      Gabapentin (Neurontin)
   Mexiletine hydrochloride (Mexitil)
   Clonidine (Catapres)
   Opioid analgesics (see Table 26.5)
Wound care
Epidural analgesia
Morphine pump implantation
Spinal cord stimulation

Wound Dressings

Ulcers are often painful, and treatment may be influenced by whether or not a particular dressing causes discomfort. One of the aims of treatment should be to make dressing changes as painless, comfortable, and gentle as possible, and for this reason nonadherent dressings are preferred. There are several types of wound dressings that can be considered for elderly patients to diminish pain and hasten healing. The goal is to maintain a moist environment at the surface of the wound to reduce necrosis, prevent wound desiccation, stimulate growth factor production and release, activate enzymes, lower wound pH, stimulate angiogenesis, inhibit bacterial proliferation, and stimulate fibroblast, keratinocyte, and endothelial cell proliferation.

A wound dressing can be described as active, interactive, or passive. An active dressing creates a favorable local environment for healing. An interactive dressing (alginates, foams, hydro gels, hydrofibers, graft skin) not only provides ideal conditions for wound healing, but also plays an active part in wound management. An interactive dressing may cleanse and débride necrotic wounds or promote granulation and re-epithelialization. If a cleansing débriding-type dressing is applied to a clean granulating ulcer, there is no interactive effect. Dressings that have only a protective function, such as nonadhesive dressings, gauze, and wound contact material, are considered to be passive. Primary wound contact material, such as nonmedicated tulle dressings (e.g., paraffin-gauze dressings), is nonallergenic, inexpensive, and has low adherence, and thus may cause less pain during dressing changes.[50]

Wet-to-dry saline dressings are used to débride wounds, but have several disadvantages. Such dressings can denude new epithelium and macerate the skin surrounding the ulcer. This can lead to new erosion and ulceration and increase the risk of candidal infections in the surrounding skin. These dressings are generally recommended only in certain situations (in a deep ulcer where bone and tendon are involved).[51]

Moisture-retaining and occlusive dressings (DuoDerm, OpSite, and hydrocolloids) keep the wound surface hydrated. It is unclear whether those dressings that are completely impermeable to both gas and liquids are better than semipermeable ones, which allow only gas into the wound. The occlusive dressing also has a lower infection rate than nonocclusive dressings and mobilizes the body's own resources for wound healing by retaining the moist wound conditions.[52]

Another modality, time-outs during the dressing changes, gives the patient increased control and helps to reduce pain. The patient should be taught that he or she can call a time-out during dressing changes whenever the pain becomes intolerable. This works well, either with self-dressing changes or with patient assistance with dressing changes.[53]

Physical and Occupational Therapy

Physical and occupational therapy can prove very helpful to the pressure ulcer pain patient. Appropriate modalities such as hot packs, cold packs, and massage can be applied to lessen any reactive muscle spasm in the area of ulceration. Caution must be used with any heating modality if the ulcer is due to peripheral vascular disease, as elevated temperature in the area of the wound can increase the metabolic demands of surrounding tissues, which can worsen the ulcer and possibly lead to amputation. Stretching exercises may help to improve contractures that have developed as a result of immobility. Ultraviolet therapy and whirlpool can be used to cleanse wounds. For patients with peripheral vascular disease, treatment includes a walking program to help stimulate collateral circulation in the lower extremities. Therapists can also provide care regarding positioning, seating devices, and adaptive equipment, which minimizes pressure to the ulcer. The goals of physical and occupational therapy are to decrease muscle spasm, contractures, and pain, and to aid in débridement, cleansing, and prevention of wounds.

Transcutaneous Electrical Nerve Stimulation

The use of transcutaneous electrical nerve stimulation (TENS) has become a helpful adjunct for treatment of many different acute and chronic painful conditions. Melzack and Wall's gate control hypothesis explains TENS's pathophysiologic efficacy. Melzack and Wall proposed that large-diameter myelinated primary afferents exert an inhibitory effect on dorsal horn pain transmission neurons,[46,54] and that selective stimulation of such afferent fibers would alleviate pain. The large diameter afferents are easy to activate with externally applied low-threshold electrical stimuli. In contrast, unmyelinated nociceptive afferent fibers are less sensitive and not activated with low-level electrical stimulation.

Advantages of TENS are as follows: it is a relatively inexpensive form of pain control if used in the long-term; it may help decrease oral analgesic requirements; it puts the patient in a position of control over his or her pain; the onset of pain relief is almost immediate; and occasionally, a few minutes of stimulation provide several hours of sustained analgesia.[55,56]

Disadvantages of TENS include the potential awkwardness of the TENS wire electrodes, skin irritation by electrode adhesive, and the possibility that the effectiveness of TENS may wear off over time.[57]

There are a variety of commercial stimulators available, and it is critical that the person demonstrating TENS have complete knowledge of the various units, appropriate locations for electrical pads, and the most appropriate settings for intensity and frequency.

Alternative Therapies

Many nonconventional therapies have been tried to improve wound healing and decrease pain.

Electromagnetic Therapy
One study found a significant reduction in pain intensity in patients with long-standing venous ulcers who were treated with electromagnetic therapy. Long-standing venous ulcers that were resistant to routine therapy

improved in terms of ulcer healing and pain. However, further work must determine the optimal treatment, dose, timing, and endurance of electromagnetic therapy.[58]

Acupuncture and Therapeutic Touch

In addition to acupuncture, some alternative and complementary medicine treatments may also offer benefits to patients with wound-related pain. However, studies report mixed results of therapeutic touch with full-thickness wounds. One of these studies states that it is particularly helpful in speeding wound healing, removing infection, and decreasing discomfort and pain in people with minor to serious wounds.[59] Controlled attention and distraction may use either auditory music or foci of attention. Concentration on an external focus promotes muscular relaxation and distraction from painful stimuli by altering the pain threshold. Approximately one-half of the patients experience a benefit in pain reduction using this modality; the other half distinctly dislikes it.

Controlled Attention and Distraction Hypnosis

Another technique of induction of the dissociative state through focus is hypnosis. Well-controlled studies of hypnosis with clinical populations are virtually nonexistent. It has been shown in several reports that hypnotized patients reported a lower pain rating during dressing changes, as compared with those who received information and attention from a psychologist.[60] The control group reported the most pain. A trained individual is needed for this modality, but the patient can also be trained in self-hypnosis. The nursing staff can be trained to facilitate the induction of hypnosis once the patient has learned the technique. Hypnosis also has been demonstrated to prevent and treat anxiety and depression as well as to allow patients to experience more control.[61]

Prayer

Prayer is defined by Dossey as communication with the transcendent or absolute. A feeling of genuine caring or compassion for the recipient is common to most forms of prayer. No objective effects on wound healing have been shown with prayer, but some subjective improvement has been observed.[62]

Relaxation

Relaxation may be achieved by numerous self-care techniques, such as breathing exercises, autogenic training, yoga, tai chi, meditation, progressive relaxation, and others. The physiologic responses, including decreased heart rate and metabolism, have been shown to be helpful in treatment of wound pain and chronic pain, as well as anxiety, depression, insomnia, and other conditions. The most effective method is simple physical relaxation. No specific literature indicates an effect on wound healing. However, deep breathing exercises may decrease the discomfort of dressing changes.[62]

Biofeedback

Biofeedback is a technique that uses physiologic parameters of body functions, such as skin temperature, heart rate and blood pressure to pro-

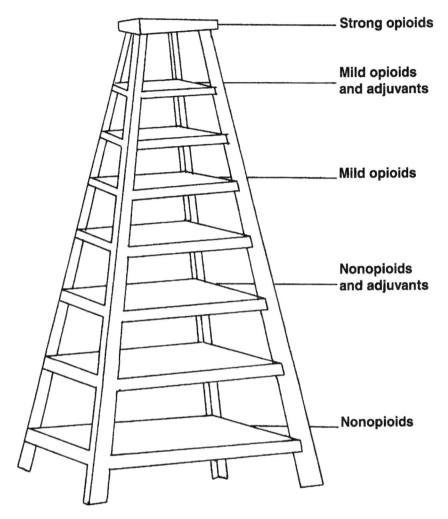

Strong opioids

Mild opioids and adjuvants

Mild opioids

Nonopioids and adjuvants

Nonopioids

FIGURE 26.7   *The analgesic ladder. (Reprinted with permission from A Cassvan, LD Weiss, JM Weiss, et al. Cumulative Trauma Disorders. Boston: Butterworth–Heinemann, 1997;196.)*

vide objective feedback to the patient regarding the effectiveness of relaxation exercises. This technique can be very helpful in teaching patients to control muscle tone or regional blood flow, which also can help to diminish pain.

Pharmacologic Management

Appropriate medication management for acute and chronic pain relies on the concept of the analgesic dosing ladder (Figure 26.7). According to this scheme, nonopioid analgesics are tried first followed by a progression to stronger medications. Adjuvant medications (medications that enhance the properties of traditional analgesics) are utilized to potentiate the respective nonopioid or opioid analgesics through each step of the analgesic ladder.[63]

TABLE 26.3 Common muscle relaxants

Trade	Generic
Flexeril	Cyclobenzaprine 10 mg
Lioresal	Baclofen 10 or 20 mg
Norflex	Orphenadrine citrate
Norgesic	Orphenadrine citrate 25 mg/aspirin 385 mg/caffeine 30 mg
Norgesic Forte	Orphenadrine citrate 50 mg/aspirin 770 mg/caffeine 60 mg
Parafon Forte DSC	Chlorzoxazone
Robaxin	Methocarbamol 500 mg
Robaxin-750	Methocarbamol 750 mg
Skelaxin	Metaxalone 400 mg
Soma	Carisoprodol 350 mg
Soma Compound	Carisoprodol 200 mg/aspirin 325 mg
Valium	Diazepam

Nonopioid Analgesics

Nonopioid analgesics can be tried first. These include aspirin and the other nonsteroidal anti-inflammatory drugs, acetaminophen (Tylenol), and muscle relaxants. One of the anti-inflammatories, ketorolac tromethamine (Toradol), is available in a parenteral (injectable) form, and it does provide fairly potent analgesia. Muscle relaxants may prove helpful if there is associated reactive muscle spasm. Muscle relaxants are generally indicated for short-term use in treatment of acute muscle spasm, but some, such as cyclobenzaprine hydrochloride (Flexeril) and baclofen (Lioresal), may be appropriate for long-term use in patients with chronic myofascial pain and spasm.[64–66] There are many other muscle relaxants available (Table 26.3). The chronic use of Valium should be avoided as it is sedating, may worsen depression, and is potentially habit-forming.

Adjuvant Medications

A variety of adjuvant medications are available that enhance the properties of traditional analgesics. For example, tricyclic antidepressants (TCAs) are believed to have both analgesic and adjuvant qualities.[67,68] Antihistamines have adjuvant qualities and are also somewhat sedating. They may prove effective in promoting better-quality sleep in patients who have chronic pain.[69] Caffeine is frequently added to traditional analgesics to enhance their potency.

TCAs have assumed an important role in the treatment of patients with chronic pain.[70–79] TCAs have three potential useful effects for the chronic pain patient including analgesia, sedation, and antidepressant actions. However, the TCAs relieve pain and help promote sleep at lower dosages, at lower plasma levels, and in a shorter period of time than normally required for treatment of depression. For example, chronic pain patients often benefit from low-dose amitriptyline (Elavil) (10–75 mg) with analgesic and hypnotic properties seen within days. On the other hand, the severely depressed patient requires higher doses (100–150 mg), and several weeks usually go by before a therapeutic effect is realized.[80]

TABLE 26.4 Tricyclic antidepressants

Tricyclic antidepressants	Usual daily dose (mg)
Amitriptyline HCl (Elavil)	75–150
Desipramine HCl (Norpramin)	75–200
Doxepin HCl (Adapin, Sinequan)	75–150
Imipramine HCl (Tofranil)	50–200
Nortriptyline HCl (Pamelor)	75–100
Trazodone HCl (Desyrel)	150–200

Of the TCAs (Table 26.4), amitriptyline and imipramine are the most sedating. Trazodone is also quite sedating, although it is not a true TCA in its structure. TCAs are thought to block the presynaptic reuptake of norepinephrine and serotonin, thereby making more available to exert its various effects (analgesia, sedation, and antidepressant actions).

Anticonvulsants, Mexiletine, and Clonidine

Anticonvulsants, mexiletine, and clonidine are frequently helpful in diabetic ulcer patients with associated neurogenic pain due to peripheral neuropathy. Clinical features of neurogenic pain include pain out of proportion to what would be expected given the clinical examination, burning or shooting pain, and physical findings consistent nerve irritation (positive Tinel signs, allodynia, hyperalgesia).

Anticonvulsants   The usefulness of anticonvulsants has only been established for the treatment of neuropathic pains that have a paroxysmal component. Paroxysmal pains do occur with diabetic neuropathy. There is also evidence that nonlancinating neuropathic pains may also respond to anticonvulsants.[81–87] The precise mechanism for anticonvulsant pain relief is not completely understood. It is felt that damaged nerves have demyelinated patches of primary afferent axons that become ectopic sites of impulse generation. The demyelinated regions are sites of ephaptic spread, and pain triggered from the periphery is due to the short-circuiting of impulses from non-nociceptive to nociceptive afferents at the site of damage (Figure 26.8). The anticonvulsants are specifically valuable for neuropathic pain because they have been shown to reduce the ectopic discharges emanating from damaged peripheral nerves.[80,88–90]

Carbamazepine (Tegretol) is currently the first line drug for the treatment of lancinating neuropathic pain. This medication needs to be started at the lowest possible dosage and titrated appropriately until there is a therapeutic effect. Therapy is begun with a dosage as little as 100 mg per day. This can be increased progressively until pain relief is obtained or signs of toxicity appear. For most patients, relief is obtained at plasma concentrations between 5 and 10 µg/ml.[91] In a given patient, there is a very sharp threshold for plasma level required to obtain relief. Therefore, to fully determine effectiveness of the drug when doing a trial with carbamazepine, dosage should

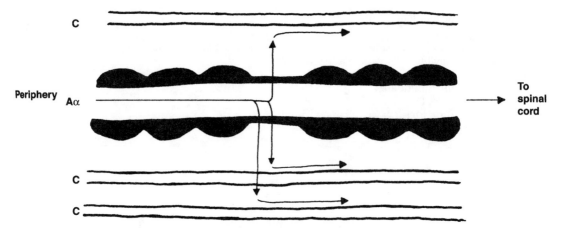

FIGURE 26.8   *Ephaptic transmission: The demyelinated regions are sites of ephaptic spread. Pain is triggered from the periphery by a short-circuiting of impulses from non-nociceptive to nociceptive afferents at the site of damage. (C = unmyelinated C-nociceptive afferent fiber; Aα = myelinated non-nociceptive A-alpha fiber.) (Reprinted with permission from A Cassvan, LD Weiss, JM Weiss, et al. Cumulative Trauma Disorders. Boston: Butterworth–Heinemann, 1997;55.)*

be titrated upwards until there is a positive response or the development of side effects.

The most common dose-related side effects are sedation, ataxia, vertigo, blurry vision, nausea, and vomiting. A mild leukopenia occurs in about 10% of patients, and in rare cases there can be irreversible aplastic anemia. Regular monitoring of hematologic and liver functions is recommended.

Other anticonvulsants available include phenytoin (Dilantin), valproic acid (Depakote), clonazepam (Klonopin), and gabapentin (Neurontin). These drugs should also be titrated upwards slowly until they prove effective or the patient develops significant side effects. Dilantin dose should start at 100 mg per day, and can be increased to 400 mg per day. Therapeutic blood levels are usually 10–20 µg/ml. Common adverse reactions include nystagmus, ataxia, slurred speech, decreased coordination, mental confusion, dizziness, insomnia, nervousness, and headache. It is recommended that serum drug levels, liver functions, and hematologic profiles be checked regularly.

Clonazepam (Klonopin) dosage can start at 0.5 mg two to three times per day and titrated upwards based on clinical response. As with other benzodiazepines, sedation, a principal side effect, could be a problem during the day. However, with a half-life of 18–30 hours, it is possible that the majority of the dosages can be given at night, which also promotes better-quality sleep.

Valproate (Depakote) should be started at a dose of 125–250 mg three to four times per day. Dosages should be increased gradually to a maximum of 1–2 g per day. Optimum effectiveness may occur with serum levels 50–100 µg/ml. Major untoward reactions include nausea and gastrointestinal upset, sedation, platelet dysfunction, hair loss, tremor, and hepatotoxicity. Contraindications include childhood (relative contraindication), pregnancy, and significant hepatic disease. It is recommended that hematologic and liver function studies be checked before and during treatment. Blood level monitoring of the drug should be carried out periodically.[80,82,92]

Gabapentin (Neurontin), one of the newer anticonvulsants is now recommended as a first line treatment for various types of neurogenic pain. Dosage should begin at 300 mg per day, with a maximum of 1,800 mg in three divided doses. Major untoward side effects include somnolence, fatigue, dizziness, and ataxia.[93]

Mexiletine hydrochloride (mexitil)   Mexiletine hydrochloride (Mexitil) is an orally active antiarrhythmic agent that is structurally similar to lidocaine. It may prove helpful in the treatment of neurogenic pain when more traditional modalities and medications fail to provide relief of symptoms.[94] Mexiletine, like lidocaine, inhibits the inward sodium current of neural membranes, thus reducing the rate of rise of the action potential and interfering with neural impulse transmission. It may prove useful in patients who clinically appear to have irritated peripheral nerves, damaged nerves, or neuromas.

Mexiletine is well absorbed from the gastrointestinal tract. Peak blood levels are reached in 2–3 hours, and half-life is 10–12 hours. The most common adverse reactions to mexiletine are reversible upper gastrointestinal distress and central nervous system effects (light-headedness, tremor, and coordination difficulties), which can often be avoided by administration with food and careful dose titration. The dosage of mexiletine must be individualized on the basis of response and tolerance, both of which are dose related. Administration with food or antacid is recommended. Dosage can begin as low as 150 mg, one to two times per day, with gradual titration every few days to a maximum dose of 1,200 mg per day. Mexiletine is contraindicated in the presence of second or third degree arteriovascular block.[95–97]

Clonidine (catapres)   Clonidine (Catapres) is an antihypertensive agent with pain-relieving qualities. In chronic painful conditions, clonidine has an antinociceptive action at the spinal cord level.[98–103] Clonidine is often sedating, and can be initiated as a nighttime dose as low as 0.1 mg. If tolerated, it can be given as a b.i.d., t.i.d., or as a higher nighttime dosage. It is also available as patches (TTS-1, TTS-2, and TTS-3) that can be changed weekly, providing for steady drug levels and greater convenience. The most frequent adverse reactions include dry mouth, daytime drowsiness, dizziness, constipation, and sedation. Clonidine may be a helpful medication in the treatment of neurogenic pain, myofascial pain, withdrawal from addictive substances, and sleep disturbances associated with chronic pain. It is a nonaddictive drug that can enhance the potency of traditional analgesics including opioids.

Opioid Analgesia

The use of narcotics for chronic benign pain (also known as *chronic nonmalignant pain*) is still a somewhat controversial issue. However, appropriate management of acute and chronic pain has become a standard of good medical practice over the past few years, and the prescription of opioid analgesics has become more widespread. Nevertheless, for every physician who believes that narcotic analgesics are indicated for those patients with chronic pain, objective pathology, and failure of conservative and sometimes even surgical intervention, there are still numerous opponents (medical personnel and lay people) who feel that such management is detrimental to the patient and society. The principal reasons for this opposition are

1. Knowledge of opioid pharmacology is often lacking in the medical community (among physicians, nurses, and pharmacists).
2. The risks of opioid toxicity and the development of addiction are typically overestimated.[104]
3. Important terminologies with respect to opioid use (for example, *addiction, tolerance, dependence,* and *pseudoaddiction*) are poorly understood terms.

Addiction, a psychosocial phenomenon, differs from tolerance and dependence, which are pharmacological and biological properties of opioid analgesics. It must be understood that a patient can be tolerant to and dependent on an opioid without being addicted to it.

Addiction, or *psychological dependence,* has been defined as a behavioral pattern of drug use, characterized by overwhelming or compulsive use of a drug, the securing of its supply, and the high tendency to relapse after withdrawal.[105] An American Medical Association task force described addiction as a chronic disorder characterized by "the compulsive use of a substance resulting in physical, psychological, or social harm to the user and continued use despite that harm."[106]

Addiction needs to be differentiated from pseudoaddiction, which is an iatrogenic syndrome characterized by abnormal behaviors that develop as a consequence of inadequate pain management.[107] Addiction and pseudoaddiction are behavioral phenomena. Tolerance and dependence are biological sequelae of the pharmacologic properties of opioids. Tolerance can be defined as the need for higher doses of an opioid over time to maintain the same analgesic effect. Physical dependence is a pharmacologic property of the opioids characterized by the occurrence of an abstinence syndrome (withdrawal syndrome) after abrupt discontinuation of the drug or administration of an antagonist.[105,106,108]

Although there are no statutory limitations on the treatment of pain with opioid drugs,[109] many physicians perceive an unacceptable degree of personal risk involved in the prescription of such medications to patients with nonmalignant pain. Such perceived risks have a powerful conscious and subconscious effect on the prescribing habits of virtually all physicians. After taking a history, opioid therapy should be considered if a physician feels that the patient has a serious problem with objective pathology to account for the pain.

Opioids are available in various strengths, ranging from mild to moderate to very strong preparations. They are available in oral, transdermal, sublingual, and parenteral forms. Some medications have sustained-release derivatives that enable patients to take fewer tablets during the day, thereby enhancing compliance.

Morphine remains the standard against which other opioid analgesics are measured. Morphine is a purified alkaloid obtained from opium. Many semisynthetic derivatives are made by relatively simple modifications of the morphine molecule.[110] Morphine is available for oral, rectal, intramuscular, intravenous, sublingual, epidural, and intrathecal administration.

With all opioids, including morphine, the effect of a given dose is less after oral than parenteral administration, due to variable but significant first pass metabolism in the liver. For example, 60 mg of oral morphine are required to achieve similar blood levels to 10 mg of an intramuscular, intravenous, sublingual, or subcutaneous dose. After oral or parenteral administration of morphine, its duration of analgesic action lasts approximately 4–6 hours. The drug's half-life is 2 hours, and depending on the situation, its analgesic potency may be insufficient to control pain after only 2–3 hours. Therefore, patients treated with oral or parenteral morphine may require regular and frequent doses to maintain adequate analgesia.[110]

Fortunately, morphine is available as a slow-release oral preparation. Sustained-release morphine sulfate (MSSR) is available in 15-, 30-, 60-, 100-, and 200-mg tablets. Duration of action is in the range of 8–12 hours, so b.i.d. to t.i.d. dosing is possible. A dosage of 60 mg of MSSR b.i.d. would be the equivalent of taking 20 mg of oral morphine every 4 hours (six doses per day). Certainly, b.i.d. dosing is much more convenient for a patient.

Some key features of MSSR, its sustained-release derivative, and other opioid preparations can be found in Table 26.5. Each drug has different features with respect to analgesic potency (categorized as either mild, intermediate, or strong), duration of action, routes of administration, metabolism, combinations with nonopioid analgesics, receptors stimulated, side effects, and toxicities.

Oral opioids are the preferred route of treatment in ambulatory patients and in patients undergoing procedures related to pressure ulcer management. However, for postoperative patients and those requiring aggressive débridement of their wounds, parenteral opiates may provide better analgesia. For patients with chronic ulcer pain, opioid analgesics should be administered by the clock and by mouth, if possible. Regularly scheduled dosing prevents rapid drop-off of drug levels with breakthrough pain.

The pharmacologic effects of opioids are based on their ability to bind to stereospecific opioid receptors. The greater the binding ability (affinity), the more potent the analgesic qualities of the drug. Three major categories of opioid receptors have been described, designated mu, kappa, and delta. The mu and kappa receptors are concerned with analgesia. The consequences of stimulating delta opioid receptors in humans are uncertain.[111–114] Opioids affect the central nervous system (including analgesia, sedation, euphoria, decreased hypothalamic hormone secretion, pupillary changes, depression of respiratory drive, suppression of cough, and effects on the nausea and vomiting centers in the brain stem), cardiovascular system, and gastrointestinal tract.[115–117]

The relief of pain is felt to occur because of activation of the opioid-mediated descending pain inhibitory pathways. At the spinal cord level, there is also a direct inhibition of second-order pain transmission cells, because of opioid binding with kappa receptors in the dorsal horn grey matter.[40–45]

TABLE 26.5   Common opioid analgesics

Mild opioids
    Propoxyphene hydrochloride (HCl)
    Propoxyphene napsylate
        Brand names: Darvon (propoxyphene HCl), Darvon Compound-65 (propoxyphene HCl, aspirin, caffeine), Darvon-N (propoxyphene napsylate 100 mg), Darvocet-N (propoxyphene napsylate [50 mg, 100 mg], acetaminophen 650 mg)
        Routes of administration: PO
        Duration of action: 4–6 hrs
        Metabolism: liver and kidney
    Codeine
        Brand names: Tylenol #2 (15 mg codeine phosphate, 300 mg acetaminophen), Tylenol #3 (30 mg codeine phosphate, 300 mg acetaminophen), Tylenol #4 (60 mg codeine phosphate, 300 mg acetaminophen)
        Routes of administration: PO, IM
        Duration of action: 4–6 hrs
        Metabolism: liver and kidney
        Advantages
            High oral to parenteral potency (in terms of total analgesia, codeine is about 60% as potent when given orally as when it is injected intramuscularly)
            Abuse potential is lower than that of morphine
            Suppresses cough (with dosages as low as 10–20 mg)
        Disadvantages
            Short duration of action necessitates frequent dosing
            Dosage is limited by its combination with Tylenol; maximum dosage should be about 12 per day because of the Tylenol
    Pentazocine HCl
        Brand names: Talwin (pentazocine lactate), Talwin Compound (pentazocine HCl, aspirin 325 mg), Talwin NX (pentazocine hydrochloride and naloxone hydrochloride), Talacen (pentazocine HCl, acetaminophen 650 mg)
        Routes of administration: IM, SC, PO
        Duration of action: 4–7 hrs
        Metabolism: liver and kidney
        Advantages
            Less abuse potential than other opioids
            The addition of naloxone (opioid receptor antagonist) in Talwin NX dissuades against parenteral abuse of the drug
        Disadvantages
            In higher dosages, pentazocine increases heart rate and blood pressure; it is therefore contraindicated in patients with coronary artery disease and hypertension
            Pentazocine is irritating to subcutaneous and muscle tissues, and repeated injections over long periods of time result in fibrosis and possible contractures
    Hydrocodone bitartrate
        Brand names: Anexsia 5/500 (hydrocodone 5 mg, acetaminophen 500 mg), Anexsia 7.5/650 (hydrocodone 7.5 mg, acetaminophen 650 mg), Lorcet 10/650 (hydrocodone 10 mg, acetaminophen 650 mg), Lortab 2.5, 5, or 7.5/500 (hydrocodone 2.5, 5, or 7.5 mg and acetaminophen 500 mg), Vicodin (hydrocodone 5 mg, acetaminophen 500 mg), Vicodin ES (hydrocodone 7.5 mg, acetaminophen 750 mg), Vicodin HP (hydrocodone 10 mg, acetaminophen 660 mg), Norco (hydrocodone 10 mg, acetaminophen 325 mg)
        Routes of administration: PO
        Dose: 5–10 mg (1–2 tablets)
        Duration of action: 4–5 hrs
        Metabolism: liver and kidney
        Advantages
            Antitussive qualities
        Disadvantages
            Dosage limited by presence of Tylenol; dosage varies depending on preparation; Tylenol consumption should not exceed 4 g/day
            Short duration of action

TABLE 26.5 continued

Intermediate opioids
   Oxycodone HCl
      Brand names: Percodan (oxycodone 5 mg, aspirin 325 mg), Percocet (oxycodone 5 mg, Tylenol 325 mg),
         OxyContin (sustained-release oxycodone in 10-, 20-, 40-, 80-mg tablets), Tylox (oxycodone 5 mg,
         Tylenol 500 mg), Oxy IR (oxycodone 5 mg)
      Dosage: 5–10 mg every 4–6 hrs for derivatives with Tylenol or aspirin; Oxy IR has no ceiling dose;
         OxyContin 10-80 mg PO 2–3 times per day
      Duration of action: 4–5 hrs for all except OxyContin (6–12 hrs)
      Metabolism: liver and kidney
      Advantages
         OxyContin has longer half-life for more convenient dosing; no ceiling dose
      Disadvantages
         With most preparations (except Oxy IR and OxyContin), the dosage is limited by Tylenol or
            aspirin (i.e., maximum of 8–12 tablets per day)
Strong opioids
   Morphine sulfate
      Brand names: MS Contin, Oramorph SR, Roxanol, MSIR
      Duration of action: 6–12 hrs for MSSR; 2–4 hrs for MSIR
      Metabolism: metabolized in the liver and excreted in the kidneys; small amounts of morphine
         persist in the feces and urine for several days after the last dose
      Advantages
         Sustained analgesia with less frequent dosing (MSSR)
      Disadvantages
         Side effects (nausea, vomiting, and constipation), and cost (MSSR)
   Methadone HCl
      Brand names: Dolophine, Methadone
      Routes of administration: IM, PO
      Duration of action: 4–24 hrs
      Metabolism: biotransformation in the liver; metabolites are excreted through the kidney and bile
      Advantages
         Inexpensive
         Long duration of action
         Often well tolerated with good analgesia and few side effects
         Efficacy by the oral route
         Because of its long duration of action, it is useful in treatment of addiction and detoxification
      Disadvantages
         Needs to be titrated slowly until optimal dosage is reached; because of its long half-life, repeated
            doses may build up with increased sedation and confusion after a few days
         In the United States, special controls on methadone have been enacted in an effort to prevent its
            unregulated large-scale use in the treatment of opioid addiction
         Patients and physicians frequently do not want to use methadone because of its connotations
            with the addict population, despite its analgesic potency
   Hydromorphone HCl
      Brand Name: Dilaudid
      Routes of administration: PO (2-, 4-, and 8-mg tabs), rectal (3 mg), IM, SC
      Duration of action: 4–6 hrs
      Metabolism: liver and kidney
      Advantages
         Good, short-term analgesia
      Disadvantages
         Short duration of action
   Meperidine HCl
      Brand name: Demerol, Mepergan (meperidine 50 mg/Phenergan 25 mg)
      Routes of administration: IM, IV, SC, PO
      Duration of action: 4–6 hrs
      Metabolism: liver and kidney

continued

TABLE 26.5   continued

Disadvantages
  Poor oral absorption (the oral to parenteral potency ratio is lower that than of codeine)
  Short duration of action
  Large doses repeated at short intervals can produce tremors, muscle twitches, hyperactive reflexes,
    and convulsions; these excitatory symptoms are due to the accumulation of normeperidine, a
    breakdown product of Demerol which has a half-life of 15–20 hrs and is a central nervous
    system excitant
  Because normeperidine is eliminated by both kidney and liver, decreased renal or hepatic func-
    tion increases the likelihood of such toxicity
Levorphanol tartrate
  Brand names: Levo-Dromoran
  Routes of administration: IM, IV, SC, PO (2-mg tabs)
  Duration of action: 6–8 hrs
  Metabolism: liver and kidney
  Advantages
    Clinical reports suggest that it produces less nausea and vomiting than morphine in
      sensitive patients
    Long duration of action
  Disadvantages
    Repeated administration at short intervals, may lead to accumulation of drug in plasma
Fentanyl
  Brand names: Sublimaze, Duragesic transdermal system
  Routes of administration: IM, IV, epidural, intrathecal, transdermal, (Duragesic patches: 25, 50, 75,
    and 100 µg/hr).
  Metabolism: liver and kidney
  Duration of action: Duragesic patches last 72 hrs, IM, IV, or epidural/intrathecal administration
    only lasts 1–2 hrs
  Advantages
    Steady serum levels for prolonged periods with each patch
    Fentanyl is estimated to be 80 times as potent as morphine as an analgesic
    Its lipophilic qualities make it useful for transdermal application, and, when used with epidural or
      intrathecal routes, it does not migrate as far in the cerebrospinal fluid as morphine, and provides
      potent analgesia for shorter periods
  Disadvantages
    Cost of the transdermal patches
    Not available in oral forms[97]

The mechanism by which opioids produce euphoria, tranquility, and other alterations of mood is not entirely clear. It is felt that mu opioids activate dopaminergic neurons that project to the nucleus accumbens, resulting in opioid-induced euphoria.[118,119]

Morphine acts in the hypothalamus to inhibit the release of gonadotropin-releasing hormone and corticotropin-releasing factor, thus decreasing circulating concentrations of luteinizing hormone, follicle stimulating hormone, and adrenocorticotropic hormone. As a result of decreased pituitary trophic hormones, plasma testosterone and cortisol concentrations decline. In females, the menstrual cycle may be disrupted. However, with chronic administration, tolerance develops to the effect of opioids on the hypothalamic-releasing factors, resulting in normalization of menstrual cycles in women and circulating testosterone in men.[120,121]

Morphine and most mu- and kappa-opioid agonists cause pupillary constriction (meiosis) by an excitatory action on the nucleus of the oculomotor nerve. A pathognomic sign of opioid toxicity or overdosage is pin-point pupils.[110]

Morphine-like opioids depress respiration by a direct inhibitory effect on brain stem respiratory centers. Therapeutic doses of opioids depress all phases of respiratory activity (rate, minute volume, and tidal exchange) and may also produce irregular breathing. In humans, death from opioid poisoning is nearly always due to respiratory arrest.[115] Morphine and related opioids also depress the cough reflex, at least in part by a direct effect on a cough center in the medulla.[110]

Nausea and vomiting produced by morphine and other mu-agonist opioids are unpleasant but common side effects that result from the drugs' direct stimulation of the emesis center in the medulla. Some individuals never vomit after morphine, whereas others do so each time the drug is administered. The nausea and vomiting are worse if the patient is ambulatory, suggesting a vestibular component.[110] In addition to the central actions, opioids decrease gastric motility, leading to abdominal bloating, discomfort, and increased risk of vomiting.

Therapeutic doses of morphine-like opioids produce peripheral arteriolar and venous dilatation. In some patients, orthostatic hypotension and fainting may occur with changes of position.[110] Opioids may have profound effects on the gastrointestinal tract. In the stomach, relatively low doses of morphine decrease gastric motility, thereby prolonging gastric emptying time. Progressive gastric distension can further aggravate the centrally induced nausea and can increase the likelihood of esophageal reflux. Prolonged gastric emptying may retard absorption of orally administered medications.[122]

In the small intestine, morphine diminishes biliary, pancreatic, and intestinal secretions and delays digestion of food. The viscosity of bowel contents increases as water is more completely absorbed and intestinal secretions are decreased. This contributes to the problem of constipation.[123]

In the large intestine, four processes contribute to opioid-induced constipation: (1) propulsive peristaltic waves are diminished or abolished in the colon; (2) the resulting delay in the passage of feces causes considerable desiccation which further retards its advance through the colon; (3) anal sphincter tone is greatly augmented; (4) and the reflex anal sphincter relaxation response to rectal distension is reduced.[110,124]

Opioids would not be considered beneficial if the side effect profile outweighed the most important beneficial effect, analgesia (Table 26.6). Potential side effects include mood changes, nausea and vomiting, sedation, subtle cognitive impairment, respiratory depression, constipation, and urinary retention.

Almost all opioids produce adverse reactions, but those that do occur are generally manageable and nonhazardous.[125] Dangerous reactions such as respiratory depression occur rarely if at all in the literature on opioids and chronic nonmalignant pain. The pain itself seems to have a stimulating effect on medullary centers for respiration. Nevertheless, this potential complication should be kept in mind, particularly with elderly patients who have respiratory compromise (chronic obstructive pulmonary disease, asthma, pneumonia, congestive heart failure, or

TABLE 26.6 The physiologic effects of opioids

Central nervous system effects
  Analgesia
  Sedation
  Euphoria, tranquility, alterations of mood
  Dysphoria
  Subtle cognitive impairment
  Decreased hypothalamic hormone secretion
  Pupillary changes (meiosis)
  Depressed respiratory drive
  Cough suppression
  Stimulation of medullary emesis center
Cardiovascular system
  Peripheral arteriolar and venous dilation
Gastrointestinal tract
  Prolonged gastric emptying
  Decreased biliary, pancreatic, and intestinal secretions
  Constipation
Urinary retention

pneumonectomy patients). In such cases, opioids should be titrated slowly, with serial checking of arterial blood gases or pulse oxymetry. Sleep studies might be helpful in looking for the development of abnormal respiratory patterns, sleep apnea, and decreased oxygen saturation during sleep.

A combination of other adverse reactions such as fatigue, nausea, vomiting, and dizziness may also occur in the initial phase of opioid therapy. However, these effects often subside during the course of therapy.[125] In the case of persistent nausea, one of the following suggestions might prove helpful:

- Wait a few weeks after initiation of treatment to see if tolerance develops to this side effect.
- Switch to a different opioid which may be better tolerated.
- The regular use of low-dose metoclopramide (Reglan) may help promote gastric emptying if gastroparesis is contributing to the problem.
- H$_2$ blockers may prove helpful.
- Administration of the opioid in combination with promethazine (Phenergan) or hydroxyzine (Vistaril) decreases nausea, and these medications have the added effect of potentiating opioid analgesics.

Prevention of constipation is obligatory for patients managed on chronic opioids. This is one common side effect that patients usually do not become tolerant to.[125] Treatment measures would include adding fiber to the diet, stool softeners, and laxatives.

There is great concern that opioids could produce changes in cognition that may hamper rehabilitation and cause a deterioration of functional status. However, patients seem to have a rather rapid development of tolerance to the subtle cognitive impairment produced by opioid drugs. Clinical experience in the management of these patients suggests that chronic opioid administration is usually compatible with normal cognitive and psychological functioning. Nonetheless, it is true that occasional patients report persistent mental clouding sufficient to impair function.[126,127]

According to the literature, only a very small percentage of patients have developed abuse problems when using opioids for chronic, nonmalignant pain. In a national survey of more than 10,000 burn patients without a history of drug abuse who were administered opioids for burn pain, no cases of addiction were identified.[128]

Wound Care

It is essential to keep wounds as clean as possible, both for optimal healing and to minimize pain. This requires appropriate dressing changes, antibiotics, use of whirlpool and ultraviolet therapy, and if necessary, surgical débridement.

Epidural Analgesia

For patients who require painful débridement of pelvic or lower extremity ulcers in a hospital setting, it may be helpful to call in an anesthesiologist to assist in pain management. The anesthesiologist can insert an epidural catheter for infusion of a low-dose anesthetic. Low-dose anesthetics provide both analgesia and improvement of blood flow to the wound (by inactivating sympathetic nerve fibers that control blood vessel tone). The epidural catheter can be left in for prolonged periods of time so that intermittent bolus injections of the anesthetic can be utilized throughout care of the wound.

Morphine Pump Implantation

Some patients who suffer from intractable chronic wound pain have tried and failed all reasonable forms of conservative treatment including the use of opioids. These patients may be candidates for one of the high-technology modalities currently available for pain management— insertion of a morphine pump or spinal cord stimulator. With both devices, patients can undergo percutaneous trials to determine their helpfulness before surgical implantation is attempted.

Since the discovery of opioid receptors in the outer layers of the spinal cord, the intrathecal space has become a popular route for application of exogenous opioid drugs. This technique may provide potent analgesia to the suffering patient, usually with few systemic side effects. This analgesic technique may be extremely helpful for select chronic wound patients with severe pain who are intolerant of oral opioid analgesics. The intrathecal morphine could also relieve pain associated with ischemia and possibly diabetic neurogenic pain.

Potential candidates should have failed all reasonable forms of treatment. Trials with adequate doses of oral opioids should be attempted before opioid pump implantation. However, some patients are unable to achieve adequate analgesia via the oral route, as side effects to traditional analgesics and the opioids (especially sedation, confusion, and other forms of cognitive impairment) make oral administration impractical. Use of the spinal route can be

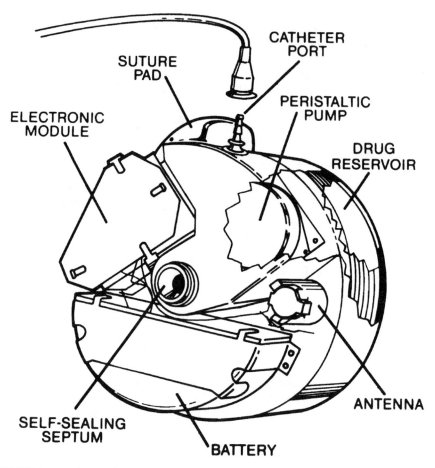

FIGURE 26.9 *The Medtronic SynchroMed infusion pump. (Courtesy of Medtronic, Inc., Minneapolis, MN.)*

justified only if it results in greater pain relief than conventional routes with less troublesome or fewer unwanted effects.

Once an appropriate candidate for morphine pump implantation has been identified, a trial of intrathecal opioids via spinal injection can be performed by an anesthesiologist. The patient should be observed for analgesic response, side effects, and complications. If the patient has a favorable analgesic response, he or she may wish to proceed with infusion pump placement. Each system consists of several parts, which are surgically implanted into the patient's body: an infusion pump, a catheter, and a filling port (Figure 26.9). The device is surgically implanted, usually by a neurosurgeon. Initially, a subcutaneous pocket is made into which the reservoir portion of the pump is inserted. Then, a tunnel is created leading from the pump to the spinal canal. A catheter inserted through the tunnel connects the pump with the intrathecal space. Once the catheter and pump are in place, the wounds are

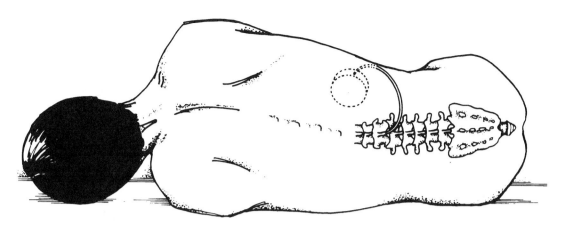

FIGURE 26.10 *The surgically implanted morphine infusion pump. (Courtesy of Medtronic, Inc., Minneapolis, MN.)*

closed (Figure 26.10). Initially, frequent postoperative follow-up for titration of flow rate is recommended. After that, return visits may vary from weekly to monthly for refill of the pump reservoir.[129–133]

Spinal Cord Stimulation

A new technique was developed in 1967 for the management of chronic intractable pain, utilizing radio frequency–induced electrical stimulation of the spinal cord via implanted electrodes placed over the dorsal columns.[134] The term *spinal cord stimulation* (SCS) came to be used to describe this technique. As SCS is a costly procedure, patients must be carefully selected. If rigid criteria for selection are adhered to, 60–80% efficacy can be expected with spinal neuroaugmentation.[135–139] Permanent implantation is only considered if trial stimulation provides significant pain relief. The trial stimulation electrode is placed via needle into the epidural space. Patience is required for proper positioning of the electrode, as the electrically induced paresthesias need to cover the painful dermatomes. After a 10-day trial, the patient should be able to determine if he or she wishes to proceed with permanent implantation. Permanent implantation requires a surgical procedure whereby the SCS electrical pulse generator is implanted into a subcutaneous pocket and hooked up to the appropriately placed epidural electrode (Figures 26.11 and 26.12).[140,141]

There is general agreement that, when applied to appropriate patients by trained practitioners, realistic goals of treatment include

- 60–70% efficacy
- 50–75% pain relief when efficacious
- Reduction in narcotic or analgesic intake
- Improvement in activity levels and quality of life[135–139,142]

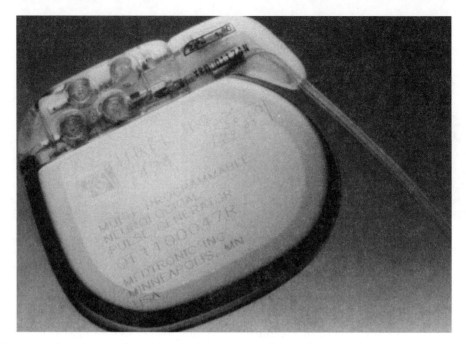

FIGURE 26.11   *The spinal cord stimulator pulse generator. The Medtronic Itrel II pulse generator delivers electrical impulses via an insulated lead electrode. (Courtesy of Medronic, Inc., Minneapolis, MN.)*

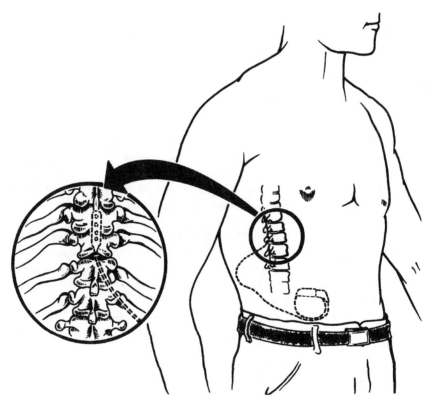

FIGURE 26.12   *The Medtronic Itrel implantable spinal cord stimulation system has a completely internalized pulse generator and one quadripolar lead. (Courtesy of Medtronic, Inc., Minneapolis, MN.)*

SCS has become an easily implemented, low-morbidity technique for treatment of properly selected intractable pain patients. SCS may be appropriate for selected patients with intractable pain problems related to chronic ulcers, neurogenic pain secondary to peripheral neuropathy, and pain associated with peripheral vascular disease (claudication, ischemic ulcers). For patients with vascular disease or ischemic ulcers, this modality has been shown to relieve pain and improve blood flow.[143–147] Applications for SCS continue to expand with improvements in technology and with more widespread understanding and acceptance of the methods.

Pain in Specific Ulcer Types

Venous Ulcers

Venous ulcers are frequently associated with pain, immobility, social isolation, and embarrassment. Pain is considered by many patients to be the worst aspect of having an ulcer, but the majority of health care professionals do not routinely assess for pain. Although the patient may live with his or her ulcer for many years, reduction of anxiety and depression has been reported after ulcer healing and pain reduction.[148] Pain as a feature in venous leg ulcers is constantly neglected in medical literature.

Two types of pain are associated with venous leg ulcers: nociceptive, where the stimulus and the response are directly related; and neuropathic, where there is no direct relationship between stimulus and response.[149] Both types may be relieved by conventional analgesia up to and including opioids. Patients who do not obtain relief from these analgesics can be offered other agents, such as antidepressants and anticonvulsants. Some of the patients may respond to sympathectomy. Because venous hypertension is relieved and blood flow to the ulcer is increased by leg elevation and positioning, these should be recommended as part of the treatment program.

Infection in any chronic venous wound, thought to be a cause of ulcer pain despite little evidence of the absolute bacterial count in venous ulcers, correlates with both pain and healing.[58] Even though there is no conclusive evidence that antibiotics increase rates of ulcer healing, prescription of antibiotics has been associated with relief of pain.

Pain may also be caused by allergies, inappropriate dressings, or may be multifactorial. Accurate assessment helps identify the most likely cause of pain and helps in its successful treatment. The type and pattern of analgesia administered affect the adequacy of pain management. The medical staff should consider the timing of analgesia to provide effective pain control and should review the type of dressing being used. Hydrocolloids and foam dressings can be useful as they are less traumatic when removed than other kinds of dressings.[148] Using a pain management tool helps to monitor the success of pain control measures. Once the cause has been established, steps should be taken to try to reduce pain to a tolerable level.

Arterial Ulcers

In contrast to venous ulcers, the key to treatment of arterial ulcers is improvement in the vascular perfusion to the affected area. An ischemic ulcer may be managed conservatively, provided it does not cause severe pain or progressive gangrene. In most patients, the ulcer is progressive, generally increasing in size and causing severe rest pain or gangrene. Surgical revascularization is the mainstay of treatment although a radiologist may perform placement of a stent or angioplasty. The nonsurgical options to reduce pain by treatment of the ulcer alone have not proven to be effective. However, such options as prostaglandins and wound dressing changes may be indicated when surgical therapy is impossible. With an adequate blood supply re-established, most arterial ulcers progress to healing, with concomitant diminished pain, unless there are complicating factors.[150,151] Amputation may be necessary for a nonhealing ulcer or chronic pain.

Burns

A disruption of the integrity of the skin, especially with burns, can lead to hypothermia and a substantial loss of fluids, electrolytes, and protein. This drainage from the skin surface can also leak medications, accounting in part for the high doses of narcotics, antibiotics, and other medications required by burn patients. When managing pain in these patients, the clinician should keep in mind that immeasurable, insensible losses may lead to a requirement for very large doses of analgesic medications, which usually need to be titrated. With burn wounds, it is easier and more therapeutic to control pain preemptively than it is to limit and manage pain once it is established. Inadequate pain control can lead to anticipatory anxiety that exacerbates the perception of pain, and so creates a need for higher doses of analgesia, decreases the effectiveness of physical and occupational therapies and prolonging hospitalization.

A number of additional secondary sources of pain in burns should be differentiated, such as pain from fractures, ulcers, tubes, splints, central venous catheters, muscle spasms, pressure ulcers, and wound-related pain (caused by exposed bare nerve surfaces). Wound covering by bandages or skin allografts is often used to diminish wound-related pain. Monitoring fluctuating pain levels and evaluating treatment efficacy are extremely important, because the burn pain follows a nonlinear reduction over time, unlike the pain seen with most other injuries. Therefore, the pain management plan must be flexible and constantly reevaluated. No caretaker is as effective as the patient in evaluating pain medication requirements. Caretakers tend to undermedicate, secondary to fear of respiratory depression or addiction.[152]

References

1. Clinical Practice Guideline, No. 15: Treatment of Pressure Ulcers. Rockville, MD: US Department of Health and Human Services, 1998;30–31.

2. McCaffery M. Nursing Management of the Patient with Pain (2d ed). Philadelphia: JB Lippincott, 1979.
3. Dallam L, Smyth C, Jackson BS, et al. Pressure ulcer pain: assessment and quantification. J Wound Ostomy Cont Nurs 1995;22:211.
4. Krasner D. The chronic wound pain experience: a conceptual model. Ostomy Wound Manage 1995;41:20.
5. Phillips T, Stanton B, Provan A, et al. A study of the impact of leg ulcers on quality of life: financial, social, and psychologic implications. J Am Acad Dermatol 1994;31:49.
6. van Rijswijk, L. Relieving pain during ulcer healing. Am J Nurs 1995;95:28.
7. Ennis WJ, Meneses P. Leg ulcers: a practical approach to the leg ulcer patients. Ostomy Wound Manage 1995;41(7A):52S.
8. Holm J, Andren B, Grafford K. Pain control in the surgical débridement of leg ulcers by the use of a topical lidocaine-prilocaine cream, EMLA. Acta Derm Venereol Suppl (Stockh) 1990;70:132.
9. Bergstrom N, Bennett MA, Carlson CE, et al. Treatment of Pressure Ulcers. Clinical Practice Guideline, No. 15; Rockville, MD: Agency for Health Care Policy and Research. AHCPR Publication No. 95-0652, 1994.
10. Acute Pain Management Guideline Panel. Acute Pain Management: Operative or Medical Procedures and Trauma. Clinical Practice Guideline, No. 1; Rockville, MD: Agency for Health Care Policy and Research. AHCPR Publication No. 92-0032, 1992.
11. Bessou P, Perl ER. Response of cutaneous sensory units with unmyelinated fibers to noxious stimuli. J Neurophysiol 1969;32:1025.
12. Beitel RE, Dubner R. Response of unmyelinated (C) polymodal nociceptors to thermal stimuli applied to monkey's face. J Neurophysiol 1976;39:1160.
13. LaMotte RH, Campbell JN. Comparison of responses of warm and nociceptive C-fiber afferents in monkey with human judgments of thermal pain. J Neurophysiol 1978;41:509.
14. Campbell JN, Meyer RA. Primary Afferents and Hyperalgesia. In TL Yaksh (ed), Spinal Afferent Processing. New York: Plenum Press, 1:86:59–81.
15. Freeman MAR, Wyke B. The innervation of the knee joint: An anatomical and histological study in the cat. J Anat 1967;101:505.
16. Langford LA, Schmidt RF. Afferent and efferent axons in the medial and posterior articular nerves of the cat. Anat Rec 1983;206:71.
17. Stacey JJ. Free nerve endings in skeletal muscle of the cat. J Anat 1969;105:231.
18. Juan H, Lembeck F. Action of peptides and other algesic agents on paravascular pain receptors of the isolated perfused rabbit ear. Naunyn-Schmiedebergs Arch Pharmocol 1974;283:151.
19. Perl ER. Sensitization of Nociceptors and its Relation to Sensation. In JJ Bonica, D Albe-Fessard (eds), Advances in Pain Research and Therapy (Vol. 1). New York: Raven, 1976;17–28.
20. Beck PW, Handwerker HO. Bradykinin and serotonin effects on various types of cutaneous nerve fibers. Pflugers Arch 1974;347:209.
21. Bisgaard H, Kristensen JK. Leukotriene B_4 produces hyperalgesia in humans. Prostaglandins 1985;30:791.
22. Burgess PR, Perl ER. Cutaneous Mechanoreceptors and Nociceptors.

In A Iggo (ed), Handbook of Sensory Physiology (Vol.2): Somatosensory System. Berlin: Springer, 1973;29.

23. Lembeck F. Sir Thomas Lewis's nocisensor system, histamine and substance P-containing primary afferent nerves. Trends in Neurosci 1983;6:106.

24. Levine JD, Lau W, Kwiat G, Goetzl EJ. Leukotriene B$_4$ produces hyperalgesia that is dependent on polymorphonuclear leukocytes. Science 1984;225:743.

25. Fields HL. Pain Pathways in the Central Nervous System. In HL Fields (ed), Pain. New York: McGraw-Hill, 1987;41–78.

26. Willis WD, Kenshalo DR Jr, Leonard RB. The cells of origin of the primate spinothalamic tract. J Comp Neurol 1979;88:543.

27. Willis WD, Trevino DL, Coulter JD, Maunz RA. Responses of primate spinothalamic tract neurons to natural stimulation of hindlimb. J Neurophysiol 1974;37:358.

28. Albe-Fessard D, Berkley KJ, Kruger L, et al. Diencephalic mechanisms of pain sensation. Brain Res Rev 1985;9:217.

29. Kaufman EFS, Rosenquist AC. Efferent projections of the thalamic intralaminar nuclei in the cat. Brain Res 1985;335:257.

30. Melzack R, Casey KL. Sensory, Motivational, and Central Control Determinants of Pain: A New Conceptual Model. In D Kenshalo (ed), The Skin Senses. Springfield, IL: Thomas, 1968;423–439.

31. Fields HL, Heinricher MM. Anatomy and physiology of a nociceptive modulatory system. Philos Trans R Soc Lond B Biol Sci 1985;308:361.

32. Fields HL, Basbaum AI, Clanton CH, Anderson SD. Nucleus raphe magnus inhibition of spinal cord dorsal horn neurons. Brain Res 1977;126:441.

33. Westlund KN, Bowker RM, Ziegler MG, Coulter JD. Descending Noradrenergic Projections and Their Spinal Terminations. In HGJM Kuypers, GF Martin (eds), Descending Pathways to the Spinal Cord. Progress in Brain Research Series, 1982;57:219–238.

34. Westlund KN, Bowker RM, Ziegler MG, Coulter JD. Origins and terminations of descending noradrenergic projections into the spinal cord of the monkey. Brain Res 1984;292:1.

35. Reddy SVR, Yakah TL. Spinal noradrenergic terminal system mediates antinociception. Brain Res 1980;189:391.

36. Belcher G, Ryall RW, Schaffner R. The differential effects of 5-hydroxytryptamine, noradrenaline, and raphe stimulation on nociceptive and non-nociceptive dorsal horn interneurons in the cat. Brain Res 1978;151:307.

37. Duggan AW. Pharmacology of descending control systems. Philos Trans R Soc Lond B Biol Sci 1985;308:375.

38. Dahlstrom A, Fuxe K. Evidence for the existence of monoamine neurons in the central nervous system. II. Experimental demonstration of monamines in the cell bodies of brain stem neurons. Acta Physiol Scand Suppl 1964;232:1.

39. Jordan LM, Kenshalo DR, Martin RF, et al. Depression of primate spinothalamic tract neurons by iontophoretic application of 5-hydroxytryptamine. Pain 1978;5:135.

40. Fields HL. Central Nervous System Mechanisms for Control of Pain Trans-

mission. In HL Fields (ed), Pain. New York: McGraw-Hill, 1987;99–132.

41. Glazer EJ, Basbaum AI. Axons which take up (^{3}H) serotonin are presynaptic to enkephalin immunoreactive neurons in cat dorsal horn. Brain Res 1984;298:389.

42. Ruda MA. Opiates and pain pathways: demonstration of enkephalin synapses on dorsal horn projection neurons. Science 1982;215:1523.

43. Fields HL, Emson PC, Leigh BK, et al. Multiple opiate receptor sites on primary afferent fibers. Nature 1980;284:351.

44. Hiller JM, Simon EJ, Crain SM, Peterson ER. Opiate receptors in culture of fetal mouse dorsal root ganglia (DRG) and spinal cord: predominance in DRG neurites. Brain Res 1978;45:396.

45. Mudge AW, Leeman SE, Fischbach GD. Enkephalin inhibits release of substance P from sensory neurons in culture and decreases action potential duration. Proc Natl Acad Sci U S A 1979;76:526.

46. Fields HL. Painful Dysfunction of the Nervous System. In HL Fields (ed), Pain. New York: McGraw-Hill, 1987;133–170.

47. Staas WE, Formal CS, Gershkoff AM, et al. Rehabilitation of the Spinal Cord–Injured Patient. In JA DeLisa (ed), Rehabilitation Medicine—Principles and Practice. Philadelphia: JB Lippincott, 1988;635–659.

48. Campbell JN, Meyer RA. Primary Afferents and Hyperalgesia. In TL Yaksh (ed), Spinal Afferent Processing. New York: Plenum Press, 1986;59–81.

49. Burgess PR, Perl ER. Cutaneous Mechanoreceptors and Nociceptors. In A Iggo (ed), Handbook of Sensory Physiology (Vol. 2). Berlin: Springer, 1973;29–78.

50. Hansson C. Interactive wound dressings: a practical guide to their use in older patients. J Drugs Aging 1997;11(4):271.

51. Hansson C, Faergeman J, Swanbeck G. Fungal infections occurring under bandages in leg ulcer patients. Acta Derm Venereol 1987;67:341.

52. Eaglstein WH. Occlusive dressings. J Dermatol Surg Oncol 1993;19:716.

53. McCaffery M. Nursing approaches to non-pharmacological pain control. Int J Nurs Stud 1990;27(1):1.

54. Melzack R, Wall PD. Pain mechanisms: a new theory. Science 1965;150:971.

55. Fields HL. Nondrug Methods for Pain Control. In HL Fields (ed), Pain. New York: McGraw-Hill, 1987;307–334.

56. Meyer GA, Fields HL. Causalgia treated by selective large fibre stimulation of peripheral nerve. Brain 1972;95:163.

57. Woolf CJ. Transcutaneous Electrical Nerve Stimulation. In PD Wall, R Melzack (eds), Textbook of Pain. Edinburgh: Churchill Livingstone, 1984;884–896.

58. Alinovi A, Bassissi P, Pini M. Systemic administration of antibiotics in the management of venous ulcers. J Am Acad Dermatol 1986;15:186.

59. Alternative Medicine: Expanding Medical Horizons: A Report to the National Institutes of Health of Alternative Medical Systems and Practices in the United States. Washington, DC: US Government Printing Office, NIH Publication No. 94-066, 1994.

60. Patterson DR, Burns GL, Everett JJ, Marvin JA. Hypnosis for the treatment of burn pain. J Consult Clin Psychol 1992;60(5):713.

61. Van der Does AJ, Van Dyck R. Does hypnosis contribute to the care of

burn patients? Review of the evidence. Gen Hosp Psychiatr 1989;1192:119.

62. Dossey L. Healing Words: The Power of Prayer and the Practice of Medicine. San Francisco: HarperCollins, 1993.

63. World Health Organization. 1986 Cancer Pain Relief. Geneva: World Health Organization, 1986.

64. Bennett R, Gutter RA, Campbell SM, Andrews RP. A comparison of cyclobenzaprine and placebo in the management of fibrositis: a double blind study. Arthritis Rheum 1988;31:1535.

65. Hamaty D, Valentine JL, Howard R, Howard CW. The plasma endorphin, prostaglandin, and catecholamine profile of patients treated with cyclobenzaprine and placebo: a 5-month study. J Rheumatol 1989;16(Suppl 19):164.

66. Reynolds W, Moldofsky H. The effects of cyclobenzaprine on sleep physiology and symptoms in FMS. J Rheumatol 1991;18(3):452.

67. Atkinson JH Jr, Kremer EF, Garfin SR. Psychopharmacological agents in the treatment of pain. J Bone Joint Surg 1985;67:337.

68. Walsh TD. Antidepressants in chronic pain. Clin Neuropharmacol 1983;6:271.

69. Rumore MM, Schlichting DA. Clinical efficacy of antihistaminics as analgesics. Pain 1986;25:7.

70. Couch JR, Hassanein RS. Amitriptyline in migraine prophylaxis. Arch Neurol 1979;21:263.

71. Gomersall JD, Stuart A. Amitriptyline in migraine prophylaxis. J Neurol Neurosurg Psychiatry 1973;36:684.

72. Diamond S, Baltes BJ. Chronic tension headache treated with amitriptyline—a double blind study. Headache 1971;11:110.

73. Lance JW, Curran DA. Treatment of chronic tension headache. Lancet 1964;1:1236.

74. Watson CP, Evans RJ, Reed K, et al. Amitriptyline versus placebo in postherpectic neuralgia. Neurology 1982;32:671.

75. Gomez-Perez FJ, Rull JA, Dies H, Guillermo J. Nortriptyline and fluphenazine in the symptomatic treatment of diabetic neuropathy. A double-blind cross-over study. Pain 1985;23:395.

76. Kvinesdal B, Molin J, Froland A, Gram LF. Imipramine treatment of painful diabetic neuropathy. JAMA 1984;251:1727.

77. Turkington RW. Depression masquerading as diabetic neuropathy. JAMA 1980;243:1147.

78. Gringas M. A clinical trial of Tofranil in rheumatic pain in general practice. J Int Med Res 1976;4:41.

79. Scott WAM. The relief of pain with an antidepressant in arthritis. Practitioner 1969;202:802.

80. Fields HL. Anticonvulsants, Psychotropics, and Antihistamine Drugs in Pain Management. In HL Fields (ed), Pain. New York: McGraw-Hill, 1987;285–306.

81. Blom S. Tic douloureux treatment with new anticonvulsant. Arch Neurol 1963;9:285.

82. Maciewicz R, Bouckoms A, Martin JB. Drug therapy of neuropathic pain. Clin J Pain 1985;1:39.

83. Dunsker SB, Mayfield FH. Carbamazepine in the treatment of the flashing pain syndrome. J Neurosurg 1976;45:49.

84. Espir MLE, Millac P. Treatment of paroxysmal disorders in multiple sclerosis with carbamazepine (Tegretol). J Neurol Neurosurg Psychiatry 1970;33:528.

85. Fields HL, Raskin NH. Anticonvulsants and Pain. In HL Klawans (ed), Clinical Neuropharmacology. New York: Raven, 1976;173–184.

86. Shibasaki H, Kuroiwa Y. Painful tonic seizure in multiple sclerosis. Arch Neurol 1975;30:47.

87. Rull JA, Quibrera R, Gonzalez-Millan H, Castaneda OL. Symptomatic treatment of peripheral diabetic neuropathy with carbamazepine (Tegretol): double blind crossover trial. Diabetologia 1969;5:215.

88. Wall PD. Changes in Damaged Nerves and Their Sensory Consequences. In JJ Bonica, JC Liebeskind, D Albe-Fessard (eds), Advances in Pain Research and Therapy (Vol. 3). New York: Raven, 1979;39–52.

89. Yaari Y, Devor M. Phenytoin suppresses spontaneous ectopic discharge in rat sciatic nerve neuromas. Neurosci Lett 1985;58:117.

90. Burchiel KJ. Carbamazepine inhibits spontaneous activity in experimental neuromas. Exp Neurol 1988;102:249.

91. Tomson T, Tybring G, Bertilsson L, et al. Carbamazepine therapy in trigeminal neuralgia, clinical effects in relation to plasma concentration. Arch Neurol 1980;37:699.

92. Rall TW, Schleifer LS. Drugs Effective in the Treatment of the Epilepsies. In AG Gilman, A Gilman, LS Gilman, et al. (eds), The Pharmacological Basis of Therapeutics. New York: Macmillan, 1985;446–472.

93. Backonja M, Beydoun A, Edwards KR, et al. Gabapentin for the symptomatic treatment of painful neuropathy in patients with diabetes mellitus. JAMA 1998;280:1831.

94. Davis RW. Phantom sensation, phantom pain, and stump pain. Arch Phys Med Rehabil 1993;74:79.

95. Chabal C, Russell LC, Burchiel KJ. The effect of intravenous lidocaine, tocainide, and mexiletine on spontaneously active fibers originating in rat sciatic neuromas. Pain 1989a;38:333.

96. Dejgaard A, Petersen P, Kastrup J. Mexiletine for the treatment of chronic painful diabetic neuropathy. Lancet 1988;29:9.

97. Physician's Desk Reference (48th ed). Montvale, NJ: Medical Economics Data Production Company, 1994;616–619.

98. Fleetwood-Walker S, Mitchell R, Hope PJ, et al. An alpha$_2$-receptor mediates the selective inhibition by noradrenaline of nociceptive responses of identified dorsal horn neurones. Brain Res 1985;334:243.

99. Yaksh TL, Reddy SVR. Studies in the primate on the analgesic effects associated with intrathecal actions of opiates, adrenergic agonists, and baclofen. Anesthesiology 1981;54:451.

100. Wong KC, Franz DN, Tseng J. Clinical pharmacology of alpha$_2$-agonist and beta-adrenergic blocker. Acta Anaesthesiol Sin 1989;27:357.

101. Spaulding TC, Fielding S, Venafro II, Lal H. Antinociceptive activity of clonidine and its potentiation of morphine analgesia. Eur J Pharmacol 1979;58:19.

102. Zemlan FP, Corrigan SA, Pfaff DW. Noradrenergic and serotonergic mediation of spinal analgesia mechanisms. Eur J Pharmacol 1980;61:111.

103. Reddy SVR, Maderdrut JL, Yaksh TL. Spinal cord pharmacology of adrenergic agonist-mediated antinociception. J Pharm Exp Ther 1980;213:525.
104. Portenoy RK. Chronic opioid therapy in nonmalignant pain. J Pain Symptom Manage 1990;5(1):S46.
105. Jaffe JH. Drug Addiction and Drug Abuse. In AG Gilman, LS Goodman, TW Rall, F Murad (eds), The Pharmacological Basis of Therapeutics (7th ed). New York: Macmillan, 1985;532–581.
106. Rinaldi RC, Steindler EM, Wilford BB, Goodwin D. Clarification and standardization of substance abuse terminology. JAMA 1988;259:555.
107. Weissman DE, Haddox JD. Opioid pseudoaddiction—an iatrogenic syndrome. Pain 1989;36:363.
108. Dole VP. Narcotic addiction, physical dependence, and relapse. N Engl J Med 1972;286:988.
109. Haislip GR. Impact of Drug Abuse on Legitimate Drug Use. In CS Hill, WS Fields (eds), Advances in Pain Research and Therapy (Vol. 2): Drug Treatment of Cancer Pain in a Drug-Oriented Society. New York: Raven, 1989:205–211.
110. Jaffe JH, Martin WR. Opioid Analgesic and Antagonists. In AG Gilman, LS Goodman, TW Rall, F Murad (eds), The Pharmacological Basis of Therapeutics. New York: Macmillan, 1990;485–521.
111. Martin WR, Eades CG, Thompson JA, et al. The effects of morphine and nalorphine-like drugs in nondependent and morphine-dependent chronic spinal dog. J Pharmacol Exp Ther 1976;197:517.
112. Pfeiffer A, Brantl V, Herz A, Emrich HM. Psychotomimesis mediated by κ-opiate receptors. Science 1986;233:774.
113. Millan MJ. Multiple opioid systems and pain. Pain 1986;27:303.
114. Heyman JS, Vaught JL, Raffa RB, Porreca F. Can supraspinal delta-opioid receptors mediate antinociception? Trends Pharmacol Sci 1988;9:134.
115. Martin WR. Pharmacology of opioids. Pharmacol Rev 1984;35:283.
116. Martin WR, Sloan JW. Neuropharmacology and Neurochemistry of Subjective Effects, Analgesia, Tolerance, and Dependence Produced by Narcotic Analgesics. In WR Martin (ed), Handbook of Experimental Pharmacology (Vol. 45/I), Drug Addiction I: Morphine, Sedative/Hypnotic and Alcohol Dependence. New York: Springer, 1977.
117. Duggan AW, North RA. Electrophysiology of opioids. Pharmacol Rev 1983;35:219.
118. Wise RA, Bozarth MA. A psychomotor stimulation theory of addiction. Psychol Rev 1987;94:469.
119. Koob GF, Bloom FE. Cellular and molecular mechanisms of drug dependence. Science 1988;242:715.
120. Howlett TA, Rees LH. Endogenous opioid peptides and hypothalamo-pituitary function. Annu Rev Physiol 1986;48:527.
121. Grossman A. Opioids and stress in man. J Endocrinol 1988;119:377.
122. Duthie DJR, Nimmo WS. Adverse effects of opioid analgesic drugs. Br J Anaesth 1987;59:61.
123. Dooley CP, Saad C, Valenzuela JE. Studies of the role of opioids in control of human pancreatic secretion. Dig Dis Sci 1988;33:598.

124. Manara L, Bianchetti A. The central and peripheral influences of opioids on gastrointestinal propulsion. Annu Rev Pharmacol Toxicol 1985;25:249.
125. Zenz M, Strumpf M, Tryba M. Long-term oral opioid therapy in patients with chronic non-malignant pain. J Pain Symptom Manage 1992;7:69.
126. Portenoy RK. Chronic opioid therapy in non-malignant pain. J Pain Symp Manage 1990;5:S46.
127. Bruera E, Macmillan K, Hanson JA, MacDonald RN. The cognitive effects of the administration of narcotic analgesics in patients with cancer pain. Pain 1989;39:13.
128. Perry S, Heidrich G. Management of pain during débridement: a survey of US burn units. Pain 1982;13:267.
129. Penn RD, Price JA. Chronic intrathecal morphine for intractable pain. J Neurosurg 1987;67:182.
130. The Synchro Med Infusion System—Patient Information. Ease of Pain, Ease of Mind. Minneapolis, MN: Medtronic, 1990.
131. Auld AW, Maki-Jokela A, Murdoch DM. Intraspinal narcotic analgesia in the treatment of chronic pain. Spine 1985;10:777.
132. Coombs SW, Saunders RL, Gaylor MS. Continuous epidural analgesia via implanted morphine reservoir. Lancet 1981;2:425.
133. Coombs DW, Saunders RL, Gaylor M, Pageau MG. Epidural narcotic infusion reservoir: implantation technique and efficiency. Anesthesiology 1982;56:469.
134. Shealy CN, Mortimer JT, Reswich J. Electrical inhibition of pain by stimulation of the dorsal column: preliminary clinical reports. Anesth Analg 1967;46:489.
135. Spiegelmann R, Friedman WA. Spinal cord stimulation: a contemporary series. Neurosurgery 1991;28:65.
136. DeLaPorte C, Siegfried J. Lumbosacral spinal fibrosis (spinal arachnoiditis). Spine 1983;8:593.
137. Kumar K, et al. Epidural spinal cord stimulation for relief of chronic pain. Pain Clin 1986;1(2).
138. Meglio M, Cioni B, Rossi GF, et al. SCS in management of chronic pain: a nine-year experience. J Neurosurg 1989;70:519.
139. Racz G, McCarran RF, Talboys P, et al. Percutaneous dorsal column stimulator for chronic pain control. Spine 1989;41(1):1.
140. Robb LG, Spector G, Robb M. Spinal Cord Stimulation Neuroaugmentation of the Dorsal Columns for Pain Relief. In RS Weiner (ed), Innovations in Pain Management—A Practical Guide for Clinicians. Orlando, FL: Paul M. Deutsch Press, 1993;33–41.
141. North RB, Kidd DH, Zahurak M, et al. Spinal cord stimulation for chronic, intractable pain: experience over two decades. Neurosurgery 1993;32:384.
142. Spinal Cord Stimulation—Background and Efficacy. Minneapolis, MN: Medtronic, 1991.
143. Erickson DL. Percutaneous trial of stimulation for patient selection for implantable stimulating devices. J Neurosurg 1975;43:440.
144. Hoppenstein R. Percutaneous implantation of chronic spinal cord

electrodes for control of intractable pain: preliminary report. Surg Neurol 1975;4:195.

145. Hosobuchi Y, Adams JE, Weinstein PR. Preliminary percutaneous dorsal column stimulation prior to permanent implantation. J Neurosurg 1972;37:242.

146. North RB, Fischell TA, Long DM. Chronic stimulation via percutaneously inserted epidural electrodes. Neurosurgery 1977;1:215.

147. Zumpano BJ, Saunders RL. Percutaneous epidural dorsal column stimulation. J Neurosurg 1978;46:459.

148. Moffatt CJ, Oldroyd M. A pioneering service to the community: the Riverside leg ulcer project. Prof Nurse 1994;9:486.

149. Mersky H, Bogduk N. Classification of Chronic Pain. Seattle: IASP Press, 1994.

150. Taylor LM, Porter JM. Natural History and Nonoperative Treatment of Chronic Lower Extremity Ischemia. In WS Moore (ed), Vascular Surgery: A Comprehensive Review. Philadelphia: WB Saunders, 1993;223–234.

151. Holloway GA. Arterial ulcers: assessment and diagnosis. J Ostomy Wound Manage 1996;42(3):46.

152. Hamil RJ, Rowlington J. Pain Management for the Patient with Burns or Integument Failure. Handbook of Critical Care Pain Management. New York: McGraw-Hill, 1994.

III | **Therapeutic Positioning**

Section Editor: Deborah D. Hagler

27   Therapeutic Positioning

Deborah D. Hagler and Sara E. Kennedy

> The major determinant of pressure ulcer development is not how sick the patient is, but how good the caregiver is.
>   Kenneth Olshansky, M.D.[1]

Imagine an older woman with a history of multiple cerebrovascular accidents (CVAs). She is sitting in a facility-owned wheelchair of unknown ancestry. The wheelchair is far too big and she is slumping to the right side. The hammock shape of the slung upholstery brings her femurs into internal rotation and adduction, and her feet fall into plantar flexion without the support of footrests. Fatigued, her head flexes forward on her chest. Her oxygen saturation remains a tenuous 91 and she has difficulty swallowing. Her primary visual input is the faded blue and white of her gown. Her right shoulder has subluxed and hangs without support between the seat and the armrest.

The staff notices red areas that do not blanch to the touch on her thoracic spine and coccyx when she is later helped to the bed.

Imagine further that the picture of this woman is now ten years in the future. Left untreated, her "positioning" would lead to abnormal tone influences, painful, fixed contractures, and high risk of loss of skin integrity. Further, she would experience gradually decreasing abilities to engage with the environment and people around her, growing sensory deprivation, weight loss, and increased dependence in feeding and all functional mobility. It is not unlikely that this cascade of events would lead to death due to nonhealing wounds over her bony prominences.

Therapeutic positioning is the dynamic process of addressing all of these problems, from postural alignment to tissue load management, from positioning to allow function to normalizing tone, from the management and prevention of joint contractures to reducing pain and improving sitting tolerance. Therapeutic positioning is a modality of treatment that enlists the skills of all the rehabilitation professionals, including occupational and physical therapists, speech-language pathologists, rehabilitation nurses, dietary services staff, and, often, technology suppliers. Each must work closely with the patient and family to thoroughly evaluate problem areas and develop a treatment plan to reduce all risk factors to wellness. This chapter introduces benefits of therapeutic positioning, the role of the health care team, key concepts necessary to any therapeutic positioning plan, and case studies to illustrate these concepts.

Benefits of Therapeutic Positioning

Although it is difficult to delineate the number of individuals affected by a lack of therapeutic positioning, a variety of data exist that illuminate the need for more education and networking in this area of patient treatment. The Agency for Health Care Policy and Research (AHCPR) lists therapeutic positioning as the first choice of intervention when a pressure ulcer is identified. The AHCPR found pressure ulcers to vary between studies but noted incidence as high as 29.5% among the general hospital population.[2] Some populations, such as individuals with spinal cord injury, elderly orthopedic patients, and critical care patients face an even higher incidence of pressure ulcers. All of these populations could benefit from assessment and treatment of positioning problems.

Therapeutic positioning can positively influence such conditions as joint contractures, problems with falling, unintended weight loss, and facilitate independence in self-care and wheelchair propulsion. State health care departments survey these and other factors in nursing facilities on both percentage and individual bases. In the overall population of a facility, the following figures are "red flags" for initiating a restorative nursing program[3]:

- More than 35% of residents are incontinent
- More than 20% of residents are dependent on wheelchairs
- More than 15% of residents are fed by staff
- More than 5% of residents have restraints
- More than 10% of residents use catheters
- More than 6% of residents have skin breakdown

Facilities are obligated by federal regulations to see that residents' abilities in activities of daily living do not diminish unless circumstances of the individual's clinical condition clearly show that diminution was unavoidable.[3] Therapeutic positioning is a critical modality to utilize in preserving and improving the postural alignment, functional skills, and mobility of residents in extended care facilities. If 20% of residents can acceptably be dependent on wheelchairs, then certainly all of those residents require seating modifications for pressure distribution and reduction or postural support. Many of those residents who do not use wheelchairs full time could also benefit from modifications in their bedside chair or dining room chair to improve such activities as sit-to-stand or to relieve pressure on a kyphotic thoracic spine.

Therapeutic positioning can also assist in reducing the length of bedrest and improving body alignment when in bed. The risks of prolonged bedrest, so often prescribed for pressure ulcers, are well documented in health care literature.[4] Bedrest reduces respiratory movement, impairs oxygen and carbon dioxide exchange, impairs movement of secretions, increases risk of aspiration pneumonia, and accelerates catabolic activity thereby resulting in a rapid breakdown of cells and protein deficiency. Bedrest stimulates the parasympathetic nervous system, resulting in gastric complaints, constipation, diarrhea, decreased gastric flow, and increased glucose intolerance. The sequelae of progressive weakness, joint contractures, and alteration in sleep and arousal cycles are the most visible signs of bedrest. Positioning can allow for therapeutic sitting time to increase tolerance in the upright posture. Appropriate positioning in bed, such as three-quarter side-lying or use of the lower extremity positioning device, can improve alignment, relieve pressure over bony prominences, and assist in the management of joint contractures.

Role of the Health Care Team

Whose responsibility is positioning? It is unfair to assign this 24-hour process to any one team member. Facilities with the lowest incidence of contractures, falls, and acquired pressure ulcers have one thing in common—therapeutic positioning is on everyone's job description.[5] While not every member of the team has the skills to evaluate and identify causative factors and treat for them, all members of the health care team should be able to identify patients under their care with poor functional positioning and risk for decreased skin integrity, and further be able to access the appropriate professionals immediately. According to the National Pressure Ulcer Advisory Panel, the cost of treating a pressure ulcer averages $125,000,[6] while the cost of a course of therapy to assess, provide appropriate support surfaces and aids to postural alignment, and educate the staff and patient on all aspects of the problem is a small fraction of this amount.

While one professional may spearhead the treatment plan in providing therapeutic positioning, attempting to address problems in an isolated manner cannot be successful. Suppose the physical therapist decides that a developing pressure ulcer must be treated with an alternative support surface and places this under the patient with good results. This same patient wheels into the dining room and finds that his or her knees no longer fit under the table and he or she must eat from a side position. Perhaps an occupational therapist determines that a patient needs a solid seat insert to improve the base of support in pelvic positioning and installs one, and then the spouse finds that they can no longer fold the chair to place in the back seat for the traditional Sunday drive. Certainly, examples of failed teamworking grow more complicated than this, but these examples serve to illustrate the need to work with all members of the team before deciding on a treatment plan whenever possible.

To assist beginning staff in the development of a therapeutic positioning program, the following delineation of roles is proposed. Obviously, a nurse or therapist sometimes works alone by necessity, but then at least the sole practitioner knows the kind of questions that must be asked and the sort of help that may be requested.

A physical therapist assesses the patient using the body systems approach, examining the integumentary, cardiovascular, cardiorespiratory, genitourinary, gastrointestinal, neuromuscular, and musculoskeletal systems. With the overall function of the systems in mind, the therapist looks specifically at the following areas, among others:

- Patient and family goals
- Postural alignment
- Integration of reflexes and muscle tone
- Muscle strength
- Range of motion: especially hip, knee, ankle
- Balance
- Head control
- Transitional movements
- Sensation
- Gait or other mobility
- Skin integrity
- Footwear
- Existing support surfaces
- Fixed versus flexible deformities

The physical therapist contributes a unique in-depth knowledge of mobility, from what is possible to what is compromised and why. Any independent movement of the patient contributes greatly to overall function, pressure reduction, and maintenance of mobility. When possible, goals to increase possibilities for independent movement are critical to the success of any positioning plan.

An occupational therapist (OT) uses an occupational performance approach once components are assessed. In addition to the concerns mentioned above, the OT provides unique contributions to the team in assessing the patient's skills in the following areas:

- Psychosocial
- Cognitive
- Perceptual
- Activities of daily living
- Continence
- Functional mobility within daily routines
- Upper extremity function and fine motor skills
- Activity tolerance
- Family and staff education needs

The OT sets goals to promote purposeful activity and maximize the patient's independence to the fullest possible extent. A patient may require adaptive equipment to achieve a stable base of support at the trunk to free the extremities from a primary balance role and enable the performance of fine motor tasks and vocational skills. Patients who can assume even the simplest task have an improved quality of life. Even individuals who require some setup and supervision to feed themselves are at far less risk for pressure ulcers than those who must be fed by staff.[7] The OT's use of therapeutic positioning as a treatment modality can provide far-reaching effects in the course of caring for a patient in any environment.

The speech-language pathologist provides critical information including an assessment of cognitive and communication strengths and deficit areas and optimal positioning for the following:

- Swallowing
- Respiration
- Speech production
- Access of communication assistive devices

The influence of the head and neck position on swallowing is well documented but not always integrated into the process of positioning an individual in the chair and bed. Swallowing is a 24-hour-a-day activity of daily living, so positioning to support the optimum anatomical position is critical. Usually the chin-tuck position, with the cervical spine slightly flexed and the head in midline, is the safest position to avoid aspiration of solids or liquids into the lungs. Speech-language pathologists can conduct a video-swallow study for those at risk of aspiration and can determine at that time the most appropriate position. This vital information must then be integrated into the patient's positioning program. In addition, therapeutic positioning can increase a patient's tolerance for self feeding, chewing, and swallowing, thus increasing their opportunity for good caloric intake to promote healing. A speech-language pathologist can be invaluable in determining methods to communicate with a patient who has cognitive or speech impairments as well. Any patient who can assume responsibility for all or part of their own program achieves a much greater outcome than those who must rely on caregivers for all needs. Nutrition as a critical factor in wound healing is well documented,[7] and a speech-language pathologist can be key in maximizing nutritional intake.

Another objective for the speech-language pathologist is to improve breath support for understandable speech. For example, an individual has a fixed thoracic kyphosis and is seated in a chair that has a 90-degree seat-to-back angle; gravity pulls the shoulders and head toward the floor. This position compromises respiratory function, reducing the vital capacity of the lungs and therefore volume and duration of voicing. This individual also tends to hyperextend the cervical spine to get eye contact with others, further increasing risk of aspiration of food into the trachea. (Accommodation for a fixed kyphosis is discussed later in the chapter.) In summary, the abilities to chew, swallow, interact with the environment, and speak with audible volume are influenced by positioning of the individual in a chair or bed. The speech-language pathologist is the appropriate professional to assess these functions in relation to positioning.

Nursing professionals play a crucial role in therapeutic positioning. The nurse can be considered a "first responder" in a patient's care and must be cognizant of risk factors related to positioning. Current nursing education literature finds that nursing responsibility includes the areas of assessment of and reporting on deficits in self-care; movement and mobility; risks to skin integrity; and deficits in sensory functions, eating and swallowing, respiratory and circulatory systems, bowel and bladder functions, cognition, communication and behavioral patterns, sensation, perception, and pain patterns.[5] Given the breadth of this level of responsibility, it is to the nurse's and patient's benefit that other professionals are included in problem solving as soon as deficits are noted. The nursing staff has a 24-hour perspective on patient care and therefore can systematically examine, detect, and communicate any changes in skin appearance, the functional outcomes of positioning, real-life experience with self-care and mobility tasks, and can assist tremendously in patient and family education and follow-through. Nurses gather valuable information regarding nutritional intake and observing symptoms of pain, fatigue, and weakness.

Technology suppliers offer a wide range of available products, funding information, and often, skilled problem solving to the health care team. Even the most experienced therapists have difficulty keeping up with new products as rapidly as they are introduced in this expanding market. Communication with suppliers is best done through a knowledgeable therapist who can articulate the principles of positioning and the needs of the particular patient with the supplier. This avoids the one-brand-serves-all approach that can occur whenever vendors work by commission. Resources such as the AHCPR *Clinical Practice Guideline* for pressure ulcers and an algorithm to assist in determining the optimal support surface are helpful in guiding the therapist in the decision process.[2]

Depending on the patient's circumstances, there are other valuable members of the positioning team. Maintenance may repair wheelchairs, keep track of inventory and spare parts, remove wheels from beds to assist in chair to bed transfers, and provide a host of experience and tools to assist the health care professional. Housekeeping can be invaluable in locating missing pieces of equipment, providing appropriate laundering care for covers and cushions, and even identifying patients who may benefit from positioning as they go about their daily work. Relationship building with all of these coworkers facilitates the success of any therapy program attempted in a facility.

The successful use of therapeutic positioning as a modality requires a transdisciplinary approach. The transdisciplinary team not only works together for common goals, but works across discipline lines by teaching each other skills for use with current and future patients. Positioning is very often a complex process of reducing risk factors and maximizing function that challenges all members of the team. While the concept of postural alignment is well known throughout the health care disciplines, the long-term benefit of positioning and the critical knowledge of how to intervene is by no means a standard part of physician, nursing, or therapy training. Instead, health care professionals learn techniques through teaming with mentors, through specialty course work, from technology suppliers, and unfortunately, through trial and error with patients. From pediatrics to geriatrics, therapeutic positioning is a treatment modality shared mostly through individual contacts. Because of this scarcity of objective resource material, health care practitioners rely more often on their own circle of peers and colleagues, their problem solving abilities, and the response of patients in treatment.

Therapeutic Positioning Concepts

There are many concepts commonly referred to in this treatment modality that require some further understanding. This section discusses these concepts in more detail before addressing the anatomical and neurologic basis of positioning.

Tissue Load Management

Tissue load management refers to the mechanical forces of interface pressure, shearing, and friction on the external and internal surfaces of the body.

Interface Pressure
Interface pressure is the perpendicular force exerted on the individual by the support surface itself. The support surfaces include the bed, the chair, shoes, clothing, orthotics, and even wrinkles in the linens. Interface pressure can be measured in millimeters of mercury (mm Hg), using either a hand-held pressure evaluator or a computerized mapping system placed between the surface and the body. In a healthy individual, the capillary closing pressure of the arterioles is 25–32 mm Hg. For the venules the pressure is much lower at 12 mm Hg.[8] For individuals with compromised vascular function, such as geriatric patients with peripheral vascular disease, arteriole capillary closing pressure has been found as low as 12 mm Hg. With continuous pressure at levels above 12–32 mm Hg, blood flow to the tissues stops, causing tissue injury and death. When measuring interface pressure, the critical measurement is pressure over the bony prominences, for these areas cannot withstand sustained high pressures. Muscular, soft-tissue areas can sustain higher pressures because pressure is distributed over a larger area. Therefore, a key principle in therapeutic positioning is to transfer weight bearing from the bony prominences to larger, muscular weight-bearing areas and to limit sustained pressure over bony prominences through regular weight shifting, pressure reduction, and pressure relieving support surfaces.

Shearing Forces
Shearing forces are generated when the skin adheres to the contact surface and the subcutaneous tissue slides in the opposite direction. For example, shearing forces occur when a patient slides down in bed or slides forward in the wheelchair seat. The bony prominences move down while the covering skin of the muscle and subcutaneous tissue adheres to

the support surface and doesn't move with the body. Shearing forces tear, stretch, and compress tissue and blood vessels causing damage and death to tissue. It is important to note that interface pressure is required for shearing to take place. If interface pressure is eliminated, shearing is a nonfactor. If shearing, in turn, is eliminated, twice the interface pressure can be tolerated without injury. Shearing often results in ulcers that are irregularly shaped and undermined along the fascial planes. Prevention of shearing forces involves careful caregiver education in turning, positioning, and transferring patients; the correct selection of support surfaces; and reduction or elimination of interface pressure.

Friction

Friction occurs when an area of skin is rubbed or moved across a coarse surface repeatedly, causing damage to the epidermis, sometimes even extending to the dermis. This most often occurs when a patient has abnormal repetitive movements secondary to central nervous system (CNS) pathology. Friction can also occur when an individual is in an agitated or anxious state or when sensation is impaired or absent. Ulcers caused from friction often appear as fluid-filled blisters or denuded, reddened skin. When interface pressures' friction is eliminated, these superficial ulcers usually resolve rapidly. Friction cannot occur where there is no repeated contact with the skin. Elbow and heel ulcers caused by repeated rubbing on the linens are common examples of problems caused by friction. Protective lubricants and sealants can also provide some protection from friction. Often, all three factors of tissue load management combine to some degree in the genesis of a pressure ulcer and must be assessed and eliminated to remove pressure and allow healing.

Temperature and Moisture

Tissue load management also involves factors of temperature and moisture. When determining which support surfaces to use for an individual, the management of temperature and moisture must be considered. Every degree of elevation in temperature corresponds with an increase in the metabolic demand placed on that particular area of skin. Metabolic demands should be stabilized in an area of skin already compromised by a wound. Increased temperature and moisture also impair the adherence of wound dressings. Excessive heat and moisture contribute to maceration of the affected skin. Maceration refers to the softening of tissue by soaking until the connective fibers are dissolved.[9] Maceration leads to white, very soft skin prone to injury from pressure. Attending to this factor can improve the speed of wound healing and prevent injury to the surrounding skin.

Moisture management includes the control of all moisture affecting the skin, including bodily fluids from bowel and bladder, perspiration, and wound drainage or exudate. Healing wounds require a carefully managed moist environment, whereas too much moisture impedes healing, promotes bacterial growth, and is itself a risk to skin integrity. Many incontinent patients can respond to behavioral techniques to restore a measure of bladder and bowel control. Intervention with an appropriate containment device as well as cleansing, moisturizing, and protecting skin with appropriate skin care products are also appropriate management techniques. Perspiration must be controlled through the utilization of clothing, covers, liners, and other materials in the support surfaces that allow air exchange and breathability. Some individuals are at particular risk for skin breakdown due to perspiration alone, and these patients especially benefit from newer surfaces that maximize air exchange and ventilation.

Wound exudate is another critical factor in moisture management. Primary and secondary dressings are used to promote a moist environment—neither too wet nor too dry. Wound exudate not properly managed causes macerated and occasionally denuded skin. Strikethrough of wound exudate becomes an easy transport for bacteria into the open wound environment.

All of these concepts: forces of interface pressure, shearing, friction, and factors of temperature and moisture are critical considerations when assessing and treating tissue load management, and must be included within the realm of therapeutic positioning.

Anatomic Basis of Positioning

The anatomic basis of positioning begins with a discussion of "normal" positioning. In normal subjects, the human body follows a predictable pattern in sitting and recumbent positions. In sitting, the ears start a vertical line extending through the shoulders and the hip when viewed from the side. The spine retains its natural curvature at the cervical and lumbar level. Viewed from the front, the shoulders are symmetrical and balanced equally over the trunk and level pelvis. The pelvis assumes a neutral rotation and neutral or anterior tilt depending on the activity of the trunk.

Have the patient sit on a firm surface with knees at 90 degrees and feet supported to observe for pelvic symmetry in sitting. The anterior superior iliac spines (ASIS) should be nearly level with the posterior superior iliac spines (PSIS), so that the pelvis resembles a shallow bowl of water with the liquid horizontal to the floor. Sitting with a posterior tilt reduces the hip flexion to less than 90 degrees and increases pressure on the sacrum. Sitting with an anterior tilt is rare, but pitches the body forward, increasing pressure on the ischial tuberosities (ITs) thereby causing some difficulty with maintaining the center of gravity over the base of support.

Any pelvic obliquity will appear during this observation and must be determined to be either fixed or flexible. Flexible deformities should be positioned for gentle correction; while accommodation and support are given to fixed deformities to reduce worsening of the joint range. It is also imperative to examine and evaluate for flexibility of the pelvis anteriorly and posteriorly for asymmetries in pelvic rotation and to determine if fixed or flexible. Pelvic and spinal mobility can best be determined with the patient supine on a firm surface. Fixed and flexible pelvic and spinal deformities and asymmetries commonly require custom-molded seat and back supports fitted solely for the individual to accommodate fixed deformities and to gently correct flexible deformities. Patients with high tone and fixed abnormalities often find that these customized supports provide more freedom of movement than being strapped into a poorly supporting chair. Periodic reassessment of these supports should be a routine facet of the successful positioning program. Patients with significant weight, height, and tonal changes may require remolding of supports.

The femurs are neutral, with hip, knee, and ankle flexion at 90 degrees. In this position, the weight of the body is distributed over the largest area in sitting. Weight is shifted off the poorly protected ischials and sacrum and onto the well-protected and much longer femurs. This shift follows the principle that a higher pressure can be sustained and sustained for longer periods when distributed over a larger area.[10] An accurate measure of true hip flexion is necessary for proper positioning. With the patient supine on a firm surface, palpate the ASIS during slow, passive hip flexion. True hip flexion stops at the point where the ASIS begins to move posteriorly, thereby achieving increased range due to pelvic movement instead of the hip joint. Attempting to force a range-limited hip joint into a position of 90-degree flexion by positioning the patient in a chair to a 90-degree seat-to-back angle only causes the body to accommodate elsewhere, often in a posterior pelvic tilt or trunk asymmetry to gain more motion and comfort.

The rib cage is free to move and the abdominal organs have both room and alignment for proper function. The center of gravity helps keep the body safely in the chair and facilitates thoracic spine extensors to maintain the upright posture. The postural muscles exhibit a minimum of tension allowing the individual to sit for longer periods without strain.

Positioning affects the safety and ease of many functions including communication, environmental interaction, and eating and swallowing by providing improved postural stability. To illustrate, consider the effects of positioning on eating and swallowing

- Allows for slight trunk flexion required for swallowing
- Increases swallow efficiency and decreases reflux by facilitating an "open chest" position
- Allows for slight chin-tuck and forward neck flexion during swallowing
- Avoids chin to chest posturing that makes chewing difficult and causes the individual to move food against gravity
- Avoids cervical hyperextension (this commonly occurs when a patient with marked kyphosis attempts to achieve eye contact horizontally, thus opening trachea during swallowing)
- Supports the trunk in a symmetrical position versus lateral leaning
- Increases proximal stability for upper extremity hand to mouth function

The back height can aid in managing weakness through proper sizing. For example, back height should reach no higher than approximately 1 in. below the inferior angle of the scapula for an individual who can self-propel, but should extend higher for patients who are dependent for balance or mobility. Standard wheelchairs offer no support to normal spinal curvatures, particularly the lumbar spine. Even new, the typical upholstery quickly assumes a hammock shape that encourages thoracic kyphosis

TABLE 27.1   Wheelchair measurements

Seat width: width across hips at widest point plus no more than 2 in.

Seat depth: posterior hip to popliteal crease of knee at 90-degrees flexion, minus 2–3 in. Add thickness of seat back insert if applicable.

Seat height for self-propulsion: popliteal crease to heel of shoe with knee at 90-degrees flexion; incorporate seat cushion, drop seat if indicated.

Back height: seat to 1 in. below inferior angle of scapula for most upper extremity propellers. Add mid-scapula to top of shoulder for full back height, for those requiring additional trunk support.

Armrest height: seat to elbow with shoulder adducted and elbow flexed at 90 degrees plus 1 in. and cushion thickness.

Foot plate depth: foot plate should extend beyond the metatarsal heads. Choice often limited by the wheelchair manufacturer.

Headrest height: top of shoulder occiput to extend to top of head.

A standard wheelchair has 18-in. seat width, 16-in. seat depth, 19.75-in. seat height from floor, and 10-in. arm height.

and sacral sitting with increased pressure and shear over the sacrum. See Table 27.1 for a guide to wheelchair measurements.

Slight alterations of wheelchair-seating configuration put different demands on the postural control mechanism. Sitting with knees higher than femurs causes increased trunk flexion and sacral sitting as the body attempts to distribute weight more equally. Conversely, when knees are positioned lower than hips, increased trunk extension appears and circulation can be impaired mid femur. This position is sometimes used in therapy to activate trunk extensors, but clearly it would not be a position of choice long term.

A seat width that is too wide leads to leaning toward a support surface such as the armrests or a shifting of the hips to one side and can worsen trunk asymmetries. If optimal sizing is not possible, therapists can compensate by filling the extra space with hip guides or using flared back cushions, or both. Too little seat width contributes to poor independent weight shifting, friction and pressure on the lateral thighs and rib cage, and potentially impaired sit-to-stand position change. Armrests that are too high encourage shallow upper chest breathing, neck stiffness, and reduced shoulder range of motion over time, and the patient may not use the armrest and may fall into thoracic kyphosis. Armrests that are too low increase the weight taken by the ITs and contribute to trunk instability and fatigue; the patient may lean to one side or slide forward on the seat to access armrests that are too low.

Footrests positioned under the seat, resulting in less than a 90-degree angle at the knees, thereby causing the lower legs and feet to flex under the body, reduce the turning space, increase the "tipping" ability of the wheelchair, and reduce the base of support. Wheelchair athletes often desire this position during sports but it is unsuitable for the average user.

Neurologic Basis of Positioning

The neurologic basis of positioning begins with an understanding of abnormal muscle tone and postural reflex mechanisms. These dynamic factors can change during the course of a patient's disability, making positioning an exacting challenge. Fixed deformities and contractures will result if abnormal muscle tone is not managed consistently over time. Therapeutic positioning is a modality that can inhibit abnormal reflux patterns and muscle tone and can facilitate normalized tone. Therapeutic positioning, combined with consistent passive and active range-of-motion exercises, can stop the development of contractures and deformities. Range-of-motion exercises alone will not prevent the development of life-threatening contractures.

Muscle tone is classified as high, low, or mixed—hypertonicity, hypotonicity, rigidity, or fluctuating. High tone can range from mild, wherein full range is possible; to severe, when movement is very difficult and contractures appear. Hypertonia is characterized by decreased mobility, increased abnormal reflexes, and decreased ability to initiate movement. Hypotonia is a decrease in ability to resist gravity with poor cocontraction around joints and a reduction in reflex activity. Rigidity is a classification of tone in which joints resist movement in two or more directions. Fluctuating tone occurs when the individual with CNS dysfunction loses the ability to modulate movement that as noted occurs in choreiform or athetoid motion. Assessment of tone involves close observation in a variety of positions, joint range assessment, positions at rest, and response to inhibition and facilitation techniques.

Muscle tone responds to environmental and even emotional changes. Tone is increased by sympathetic nervous system activation such as the "fight or flight" response, and is related only to the individual's perception of stress, whether physical or emotional. Therefore, a patient afraid of falling exhibits signs of high muscle tone in an ill-fitting wheelchair, even if there is little chance of falling. Conversely, the parasympathetic nervous system reduces muscle tone when it is active, slowing the heart beat, lowering blood pressure, and deepening respiration. Observing for signs of these responses can assist the therapist in designing the most appropriate seating and positioning plan.

Reflexes are normally integrated into the neuromuscular system early in life and only appear in periods of great stress unless upper motor neuron lesions occur.[11] These reflexes are activated by body positions, which must be considered and contained if a patient with CNS dysfunction is positioned appropriately. The tonic neck reflexes in particular cause difficulties with positioning. See Table 27.2 for more information on tonic neck reflexes. While these are the most commonly seen primitive reflexes, certainly there are many other primitive reflexes that can affect positioning. The reader is directed to neurodevelopmental treatment resources for more discussion.

Abnormalities of tone and the presence of primitive reflexes directly alter the ability of an individual to control posture at all times and in all situations. Postural control must be evaluated to adequately assess how much support is needed in sitting and lying positions without oversupporting the body. As stability in a posture precedes mobility and motor control, supporting the body in a stable posture is key to furthering motor control goals.[12] When the body is adequately supported, move-

TABLE 27.2   Tonic neck reflexes

Reflex	Description	Positioning interventions
Symmetric tonic neck reflex	Neck extension causes upper extremity extension, lower extremity flexion Neck flexion causes upper extremity flexion and lower extremity extension	Avoid elevation of head of bed with neck flexion through use of pillows (use firm head positioning cushion) Support neck and head in neutral in sitting Provide adequate support for proximal stability and weak extremities symmetrically Utilize supported side-lying position Pelvic positioning belt may be necessary at beginning stages
Asymmetric tonic neck reflex	Head turning causes extension in limbs on the face side of the body and flexion in limbs on the occipital side	Provide excellent proximal stability Support weak upper extremity Achieve neutral head positioning Alternate side-lying with supported supine positioning
Tonic labyrinthine reflex	Originates in the otoliths of the ear when head position is altered. Neck extension causes an increase in extensor tone throughout the body in all positions, neck flexion increases flexor tone throughout.	Support neck from hyperextension in supine and sitting Increase segmentation of body through side-lying positioning Pelvic positioning belt may be necessary when in wheelchair until reflex integrates

ment requires less effort and strain, movement is more selective, and primitive movement patterns are more easily overcome. The more opportunity an individual has to experience normal movement patterns, the more automatic and refined those movements become. The reverse is also true. For example, a patient with unilateral neglect who habitually looks away from the affected side experiences increasing flexor tone in the involved arm and leg, may assume a sitting posture primarily weight bearing on the "uninvolved" hip, and eventually experience fixed contractures making transfers and self-care impossible. Table 27.3 illustrates the cycle of poor positioning with neurologically involved patients.

Particularly in acute care, the scope of a patient's medical and rehabilitative challenges can cause the health care team to discount any minor problems with positioning. This situation should encourage health care professionals to treat positioning problems more thoroughly, especially considering the commonly fragmented continuum of care that patients can experience.

Assessment

Identification of functional problems is the first step in designing the treatment plan to address any positioning problem. Treatment of these problems can only proceed with the identification of the most likely

TABLE 27.3 Progression of poor positioning

Physical stress
Fear—emotional stress
Increased sympathetic arousal
Increased tone
Poor isolation of movement
Decreased segmentation of trunk
Increased dependence on synergistic movement
Decreased rotational component in any movement
Decreased responsiveness to postural changes
Postural insecurity
Inability to develop antigravity muscles
Increased presence of primitive reflexes
Increased dependence on environment
Fixed joint contractures
High risk for skin integrity problems
Pain in routine movements
Inability to sit
Increased contractures with bed rest
Compromised cardiovascular, respiratory, digestive functions
Death

underlying cause of the functional clinical picture. To illustrate: a patient may be sliding forward in a wheelchair for a variety of reasons including the influence of primitive reflexes, extensor tone, lack of true hip flexion, attempts to reach the floor for limited self-propulsion, excessive pressures or pain over the ITs, too-low foot support, or even a slipping seat cushion. Attempting to correct the positioning problem without defining the underlying cause(s) leads to a poor outcome and a waste of a precious resource: time.

Assessment begins by examining the patient on a firm surface to detect deviations in joint range of motion, pelvic and spinal mobility, pathological reflexes and tone, muscle strength, body type, functional abilities, movement patterns, and sensory deficits. Examination and evaluation of the patient's skin condition is also imperative, noting and specifically describing the location, size, depth, color, and presence of necrotic and granulation tissue, fascial undermining, tunneling, color and amount of exudate, condition of surrounding skin, date of onset, current treatment regimen, and most importantly, the cause of the wound (i.e., pressure, trauma, friction, etc.). Assessment then proceeds with a close observation of posture in the seated and recumbent positions, noting preferred positions. The clinician notes deviations from normal postural alignment, the presence of any structural deformities, and contractures. Beginning to work more actively with the patient, the clinician notes movement patterns, flexibility, and function as well as sensation, pain, and the pattern of a typical day. The clinician determines the body type and an estimation of pressure distribution. Body types as related to positioning are as follows:

- "Spiky-bony"; or very sharp, protruding bones easily palpated
- "Flat-bony"; greater surface area to absorb pressure

- "Heavy-bony"; similar to "flat-bony" but larger skeletal mass exerting higher interface pressures

Obesity increases risks due to the very poor vascularization of fatty tissue. Additionally, soft-tissue changes rapidly due to atrophy or weight loss so "adequate soft-tissue" cannot be considered a safety net for positioning.

The clinician estimates pressure distribution through knowledge of most common pressure ulcer sites and typical occurrence rates.[13]

Supine

- Occiput 1%
- Scapula 5%
- Elbow 9%
- Spine 2%
- Sacrum or coccyx 16%
- Heels 18%

Side-Lying

- Ear and parietal area <1%
- Shoulder <1%
- Iliac crest 2%
- Trochanter 15%
- Knee 5%
- Lateral malleolus 10%
- Foot <1%

Seated

- Ischial tuberosities 12%
- Sacrum—incidence unavailable

Interface pressure readings are best taken with a pressure meter to gain objectivity. Hand-held meters and pressure mapping devices are both available. Without these measuring devices, specific areas of increased pressure cannot be accurately identified until the pressure ulcer begins to form. Also, pressure meters allow the clinician to accurately interpret the result of therapeutic intervention in a measurable, repeatable manner. Any pressure reading below 11 mm Hg can be considered safe if skin is intact. Pressure should be eliminated over wounds for optimal healing. Patients who can independently weight shift to relieve pressure and have adequate sensation and cognition may do so before pressures are critical and can safely sustain higher-pressure readings, but staying under the upper end of the 12–32 mm Hg range is prudent.

Interface pressure should be measured over all the bony prominences listed and under any unusual bony protuberance. Pressures should also be taken under splints, orthotics, or other devices as determined by the

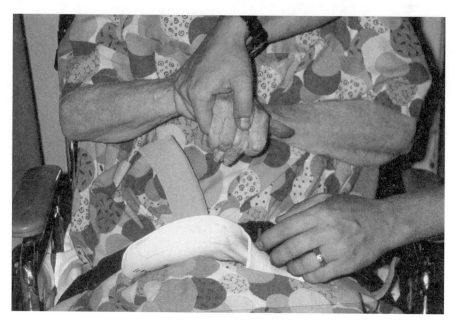

FIGURE 27.1 *Inhibition techniques are used before donning the hand splint designed to reduce wrist and hand contractures.*

clinician (Figures 27.1, 27.2, and 27.3). Interface pressure should be measured in all positions, in the bed and the chair. Pressures should also be taken using the layers of incontinent padding or sheets typically used. The sensor of the hand-held meter should be placed on the patient's skin to obtain the most accurate reading. These readings can be an invaluable tool in enlisting the support of the patient, family, and daily caregivers in

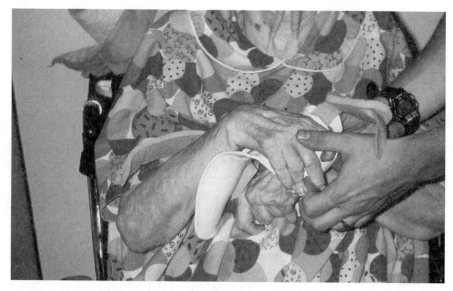

FIGURE 27.2 *The splint is placed on the patient without increasing flexor tone.*

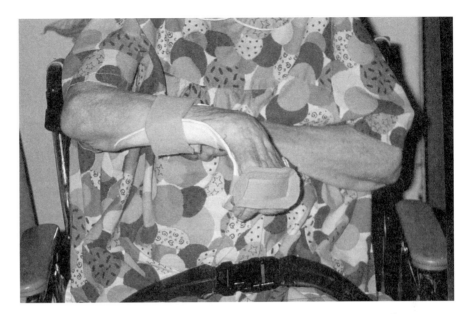

FIGURE 27.3   *Pressures are measured with the splint in place, in a variety of positions.*

keeping such padding to a bare minimum as padding only reduces the efficacy of any support surface.

Pressures must be taken with the head of the bed elevated to the patient's preferred position to demonstrate the often-extreme pressure placed on the sacrum. This objective reading will assist in educating staff and family members about the relationship of head elevation and interface pressure over the sacrum, thereby increasing compliance in utilizing the lowest head elevation tolerated. Therapists can use manual readings to supplement the meter readings so that they have some tactile skill in this estimation for screening purposes without the meter. The assessment process proceeds to include other fact finding necessary to the patient's specific situation before goals can be identified and a treatment plan established. See the Therapeutic Positioning System (TPS) seating and bed evaluations for examples of the assessment process (Figure 27.4).[14]

Treatment

In the one-dimensional world of language, it is only possible to discuss one major positioning problem at a time. Certainly positioning problems are not limited to a specific area of the body in isolation. To assist in the understanding of the treatment process, consult Table 27.4 for a discussion of common positioning problems, possible underlying causes, and suggested interventions. The novice clinician is encouraged to alter only one or two positioning aspects at a time to allow for careful observation of intervention results. Beginning at the pelvis is recommended, using neurodevelopmental principles as a basis. Photographs can be another aid in developing an accurate and thorough treatment plan, affording the clinician an opportunity to study subtle changes in postural alignment in

Therapeutic Positioning System™ Seating Evaluation

Page 1 of 2
Order # TSEF
5/96

Name ______________________ Primary Diagnosis ______________________

Date ______________________ Secondary Diagnosis ______________________

Reason for Referral ______________________

1. Current Seating

☐ Wheelchair—Type ______________ ☐ Standard ☐ Narrow ☐ Other ______________

☐ Recliner Gerichair ☐ Other ______________

	Yes	No	Comments:
Armrests	☐	☐	
Legrests	☐	☐	
Good Condition	☐	☐	
Appropriate Size	☐	☐	
Current Positioning Devices	☐	☐	

2. Postural Alignment in Chair

Picture:

Head ______________________

Neck ______________________

Shoulders ______________________

Arms ______________________

Trunk ______________________

Hips ______________________

Knees ______________________

Feet ______________________

3. Functional Status

	WFL	Imp.	Comments:
ROM—Upper Extremities	☐	☐	
Lower Extremities	☐	☐	
Strength—Head/Neck	☐	☐	
Trunk	☐	☐	
UEs	☐	☐	
LEs	☐	☐	
Muscle Tone	☐	☐	
Reflex Integration	☐	☐	
Sensation	☐	☐	
Perception	☐	☐	

	Yes	No	Comments:
Alert	☐	☐	
Oriented	☐	☐	
Communication Needs	☐	☐	

	Dep.	Assist.	Ind.	Comments:
Mobility	☐	☐	☐	
Transfers	☐	☐	☐	
Feeding	☐	☐	☐	
Self-care	☐	☐	☐	

Time per day/Activities in chair ______________________

Resource & Training Center

101 North Cascade, Suite 210 • Colorado Springs, CO 80903
(719) 578-5957 (800) 395-6465 FAX (719) 578-8678

FIGURE 27.4 *Therapeutic Positioning System seating and bed evaluation.*

Seating Evaluation (continued)

4. Initial Pressure Readings
Right Ischial Tuberosity _____ mm/Hg _____ _____ mm/Hg
Left Ischial Tuberosity _____ mm/Hg _____ _____ mm/Hg
Coccyx _____ mm/Hg _____ _____ mm/Hg

5. Skin Integrity
Pressure Areas: ☐ Yes ☐ No

Location:				
Stage:				
Size:				

6. Anticipated Equipment/Supply Needs:
_____
_____
_____

7. Restraint Reduction Considerations:
_____
_____
_____

8. Additional Assessment Information:
_____
_____
_____

9. Equipment Issued/Treatment Performed:
_____
_____
_____

10. Final Pressure Readings
Right Ischial Tuberosity _____ mm/Hg _____ _____ mm/Hg
Left Ischial Tuberosity _____ mm/Hg _____ _____ mm/Hg
Coccyx _____ mm/Hg _____ _____ mm/Hg

11. Final Postural Alignment   Picture:
Head_____
Neck_____
Shoulders_____
Arms_____
Trunk_____
Hips_____
Knees_____
Feet_____

12. Long Range Discharge Plans
Date Off A_____
Supply Needs _____
Equipment Needs _____
Date of D/C to Home_____
Supply Needs _____
Equipment Needs _____
Follow-up Considerations _____

13. Additional Needs:
_____
_____
_____

FIGURE 27.4   *Continued.*

Therapeutic Positioning System™
Bed Evaluation
(Addendum to Seating Evaluation)

Name _____ Primary Diagnosis _____

Date _____ Secondary Diagnosis _____

Reason for Referral _____

1. Current Mattress/Bed

☐ Standard ☐ Standard Plus Eggcrate ☐ Low Platform ☐ Trapeze ☐ Full Side Rails ☐ Half Side Rails

☐ Mattress Replacement (Type)_____ ☐ Mattress Overlay (Type) _____

☐ Other_____

2. Postural Alignment in Bed   Picture:

☐ Supine ☐ Right Side-lying ☐ Left Side-lying

Head/Neck _____

Shoulders _____

UEs _____

Trunk _____

Hips _____

LEs _____

Feet _____

3. Functional Status

Bed Mobility: ☐ Dep. ☐ Assist. ☐ Ind.

Time Spent in Bed _____

Activities in Bed _____

Turning Schedule: ☐ Yes ☐ No

4. Initial Pressure Readings

Supine

_____ _____ mm/Hg   _____ _____ mm/Hg
_____ _____ mm/Hg   _____ _____ mm/Hg
_____ _____ mm/Hg   _____ _____ mm/Hg

Right Side-lying

_____ _____ mm/Hg   _____ _____ mm/Hg
_____ _____ mm/Hg   _____ _____ mm/Hg
_____ _____ mm/Hg   _____ _____ mm/Hg

Left Side-lying

_____ _____ mm/Hg   _____ _____ mm/Hg
_____ _____ mm/Hg   _____ _____ mm/Hg
_____ _____ mm/Hg   _____ _____ mm/Hg

5. Anticipated Needs:

_____
_____
_____
_____
_____
_____

Resource & Training Center

101 North Cascade, Suite 210 • Colorado Springs, CO 80903
(719) 578-5957   (800) 395-6465   FAX (719) 578-8678

FIGURE 27.4 *Continued.*

Bed Evaluation (continued)

6. Restraint Reduction Considerations:

_____
_____
_____
_____
_____

7. Supplies Issued/Treatment Performed:

_____
_____
_____
_____
_____

8. Final Pressure Readings

Supine

_____ _____ mm/Hg		_____ _____ mm/Hg	
_____ _____ mm/Hg		_____ _____ mm/Hg	
_____ _____ mm/Hg		_____ _____ mm/Hg	

Right Side-lying

_____ _____ mm/Hg		_____ _____ mm/Hg	
_____ _____ mm/Hg		_____ _____ mm/Hg	
_____ _____ mm/Hg		_____ _____ mm/Hg	

Left Side-lying

_____ _____ mm/Hg		_____ _____ mm/Hg	
_____ _____ mm/Hg		_____ _____ mm/Hg	
_____ _____ mm/Hg		_____ _____ mm/Hg	

9. Final Postural Alignment   **Picture:**

☐ Supine   ☐ Right Side-lying   ☐ Left Side-lying

Head/Neck _____

Shoulders _____

UEs _____

Trunk _____

Hips _____

LEs _____

Feet _____

10. Long Range Discharge Plans

Date Off A_____

   Supply Needs _____

   Equipment Needs_____

Date of D/C to Home_____

   Supply Needs _____

   Equipment Needs_____

Follow-up Considerations_____

11. Additional Needs:

_____
_____
_____
_____
_____
_____

FIGURE 27.4   _Continued._

TABLE 27.4   Quick reference to positioning problems

Functional problem	Possible causes	Intervention
Head position instability	Muscle imbalance Weakness Kyphosis Torticollis	Head support with increase of seat-to-back angle Static stretching provided through positioning in bed Limit sitting time to tolerance
Neck hyperextension	High extensor tone Muscle weakness Rigidity	Head support to facilitate slight flexion Reduction of tone throughout the body Solid back support
Neck forward flexion	Kyphosis Excessive use of pillows Muscle weakness Fatigue	Determine optimal sitting tolerance Increase seat to back angle if kyphotic Static stretch through positioning supine with decreasing flexion
Trunk flexed laterally	Scoliosis Pain response Neurologic sequelae Unilateral neglect Fatigue Seat too wide	Determine optimal sitting tolerance Assess for and support pelvic obliquity Assess for true hip flexion measure Lateral support Static positioning in side-lying for trunk lengthening Decrease seat width or use hip guide to accomodate fixed deformity
Kyphosis	Worsened by fatigue Compression fracture Psychosocial withdrawal	Increase seat-to-back angle to accomodate fixed deformity Allow gravity to open up upper trunk in sitting, supine Reduce neck flexion forward pull
Scoliosis	Pain response Lack of hip or knee flexion Poor positioning over time Structural deformity	Careful assessment of obliquities, accomodate fixed or correct flexible deformity Custom molded seat and back to support Accomodate fixed spinal deformity or correct flexible deformity
Less than 90-degree hip flexion	Pain response over time Tone abnormality Poor positioning over time Prior hip surgery	Increase seat to back angle Supine positioning schedule with support
Less than 90-degree knee flexion	Poor positioning over time Abnormal tone Pain response over time	Calf support at 80% of range Positioning in bed with static stretch and gravity with lower extremity positioning device
"Windswept" laterally	Probable scoliosis Unsupported lower extremity contractures May lack true hip flexion unilaterally Seat width too wide	Support any postural abnormality in trunk or pelvis Lateral support to femur at 80% of tolerated range Ankle straps if tolerated Narrower chair or hip guides
External rotation of hip	Post hip surgery Hip weakness Possible obliquities Scoliosis	Support leg length discrepancy, hip flexion asymmetry Hip guides and trochanter roll Possibly foot-drop splint with derotation component
Adduction of hips	Influence of abnormal tone Muscle tightness Protective reaction Modesty (females)	Increase flexion at hips if possible Check optimal seat depth for better stability Abductor wedge in sitting Full lower extremity positioning device in bed

TABLE 27.4   continued

Functional problem	Possible causes	Intervention
Ankle plantar flexion	Abnormal extensor tone Habitual positioning in supine Muscle weakness/imbalance Neurologic deficit Use of high heels Poor weight bearing and/or foot support	Foot-drop splint Sheet cradle in bed Provide weight bearing to toleration in sitting (utilize extra-depth foot pedals or foot support) Adjust angle of foot plate to accommodate and increase weight-bearing surface (for fixed deformity)
Pressure on heels	Knee flexion contractures Prolonged positioning in supine Friction caused by repetitive movement Immobility	Suspend heels with heel lift boots Support knee contractures Reduce friction through fabric/support surface selection Eliminate pressure on heels in all positions (sitting and supine)
Skin tears on lower extremities	Restless behavior Neurologic disorders causing repetitive movement Sharp areas on wheelchair and injuries with transfers	Footrest Hinge covers and foot pedal covers Cover all protruding parts Reduce effects of friction with appropriate nonskid fabric Encourage shoes and socks
Shoulder elevation	Armrests too high Pulmonary disorders Sympathetic nervous system response Scoliosis	Adjust armrest height Provide increased arm support if needed
Shoulder adduction and internal rotation	Abnormal tone Pain response Response to low body temperature Self-comfort	Customized arm wedge to bring arm away from the body Dress warmly Further assess cause of pain
Upper extremity edema	Shoulder-hand syndrome Postmastectomy Injury Cellulitis Immobility Lack of support	Elevation of forearm, wrist, hand Support wrist extension Facilitate active movement Utilize compression garment and/or padded lap tray

a less stressful setting than at bedside. (Photographs also aid in demonstrating functional progress and providing education.)

The goals of all positioning treatments are

- To reduce risk factors for skin breakdown
- Promote functional gain
- Improve psychosocial functioning (better awareness of the environment, improved ability to communicate)
- Improve physiologic functioning (increased vital capacity, improved swallowing function, etc.)

Observation of these areas assists in reaching long-term goals. A thorough, clinically reasoned assessment makes treatment planning for such a complex set of problems possible and cannot be overemphasized. Also, thorough examination and evaluation of the skin, particularly over weight-bearing bony prominences, should be performed at least every 24 hours to detect any changes that may indicate excessive interface pressure, friction, shearing, or moisture. This is to ensure that quick problem solving is accomplished. The therapeutic positioning case studies offered at the end of this chapter should also assist the understanding of the treatment planning process.

A variety of tools exist to assist the therapist in the selection of the appropriate support surface.[2] The ideal support surface provides the following characteristics[15]:

- Reduces and relieves pressure under bony prominences
- Controls pressure gradient in tissue
- Provides stability
- Facilitates weight shifts
- Facilitates transfers
- Controls temperature at interface
- Controls moisture at skin surface
- Lightweight
- Low cost
- Durable

The clinician must use clinical reasoning to prioritize these characteristics when dealing with a specific situation. In addition, extrinsic factors such as the patient's living arrangement, financial status, amount of time in bed or seated, caregiver abilities, and prognosis have a direct bearing on successful support surface selection. Many times a trial of surfaces is needed before final selection.

Certain tools are needed in this complex assessment and treatment process, including

- Interface pressure evaluator: measures the pressure exerted by the support surface on the bony prominences.
- Goniometer: measures joint range of motion and existing contractures and measures angles on chair or bed (e.g., head elevation in bed, seat-to-back angle).
- Tape measure: used to measure femur length to determine presence of pelvic rotation, knee to floor length, seat width, back height, armrest height, span of ITs, existing chair size, mattress size, and dimensions of other positioning equipment, width of doorways, turning radius, etc.
- Tool box containing a variety of tools used in adjusting new and existing positioning devices, beds, and wheelchairs: Phillips and slot screwdrivers including a power screwdriver, Exacto knife, Allen wrenches, crescent wrenches, hammer, small flashlight for illumination inside contractures, or needed in poorly lit rooms.
- Sensory evaluation kit: to test for pain or temperature, light touch, deep pressure.
- Draw sheet to assess spinal or pelvic mobility.
- Duct tape: always useful in temporary repairs, including disabling adjustable height elevating leg rests when patient is at risk for skin tears.
- Seating and bed assessment forms, wound assessment form, patient education forms.

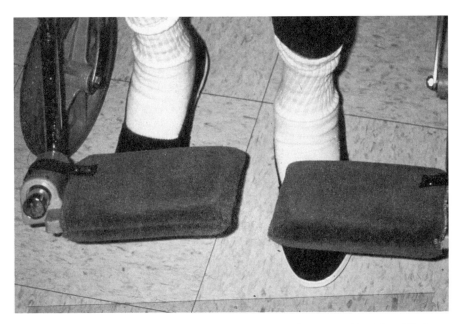

FIGURE 27.5   *Foot pedal covers allow this patient to foot propel inside while leaving foot pedals immediately available when going longer distances.*

- Scissors.
- Gloves.
- Gait belt for use with transfers.
- Wax pencil to mark the spinous processes, ASIS, PSIS, inferior angle of the scapula, and so on when assessing a patient's relationship to a support surface.

Many joint measurements require the firm support of a mat table. A variety of wheelchair sizes as well as commercially available and customizable support surfaces are essential to problem solving and the prescriptive process of positioning.

New equipment proliferates in the positioning field at a fast pace. While it is beyond the scope of this chapter to go into detail about all that is available, certain pieces warrant introduction. Many elderly people are at risk for skin tears and other injuries to skin. Reasons for this higher risk include loss of protective sensation and loss of motor control. The clinician must take special care that contact with sharp surfaces is minimized. Often foot pedals and elevating leg-rest hinges cause injury when in contact with fragile skin. These can be covered with foot pedal and hinge covers. Covering the metal in this way also protects caregivers from injury while setting up for transfers. Properly fitting and supportive shoes are an often overlooked intervention to protect the skin of the feet as well (Figures 27.5, 27.6, and 27.7). Other protective measures include replacing torn upholstery on armrests, seat, and back upholstery; padding table and chair legs if appropriate; and padding bed rails.

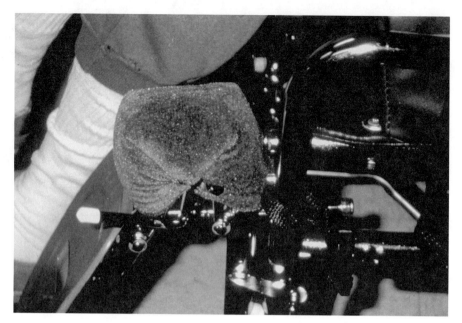

FIGURE 27.6   *Hinge covers shown on these elevating leg rests protect the patient and caregivers from injury during transfers but do not interfere with chair operation.*

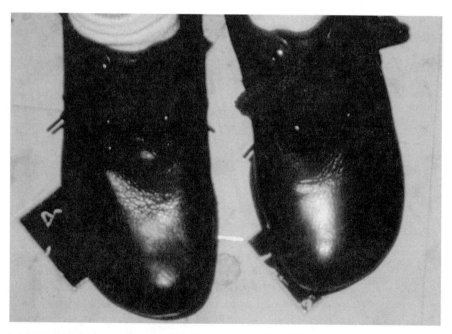

FIGURE 27.7   *Supportive, properly fitting shoes should be encouraged with all patients who can wear shoes.*

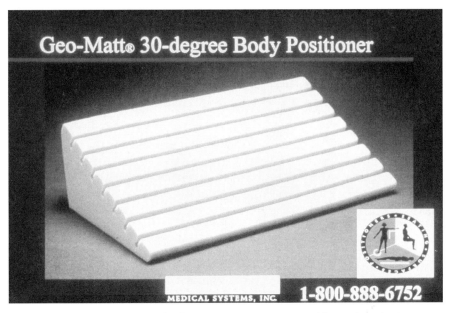

FIGURE 27.8   *The 30-degree body positioner. (Courtesy of Span-America.)*

Bed positioning presents a unique set of challenges. Pillows are neither firm enough nor shaped adequately to assist a patient in achieving and maintaining the side-lying position, particularly under the influence of abnormal tone. Full side-lying itself places too much pressure on the trochanter on the weight-bearing side of the body. Slightly reclining backward from weight bearing directly on the trochanter is called *three-quarter side-lying* or *30-degree side-lying*. The three-quarter side-lying position is critical in eliminating pressure over the IT, sacrum, and coccyx. Without support, however, gravity pulls patients either into full side-lying or falling back into supine. Prone positioning would be beneficial for many patients but unfortunately is tolerated by few, and beds are often not conducive to assuming a prone position. Bed wedges (one example is shown in Figure 27.8) are constructed of high-density foam strong enough to support the patient in 30-degree side-lying. A patient is shown in Figure 27.9 in three-quarter side-lying position with body aligners along her spine. Pillows add to the comfort and support of extremities.

Specialty beds are widely available and well advertised. Replacement mattresses are less well known but can be a better choice for home or institutional purchase for a long-term need (Figure 27.10). A replacement mattress is the same size as a standard hospital mattress, and the firm foam borders and topper in the construction allow for sitting safely on the edge of the bed and do not impair bed mobility. Pressure reduction is achieved with the longitudinal air cylinders under the foam topper. Bed mobility and independent transfers out of bed are generally sacrificed when using a powered specialty bed. Overlays are often chosen when funding is an obstacle, but all overlays raise the height of the bed and can make chair-to-bed transfers and bed mobility more difficult.

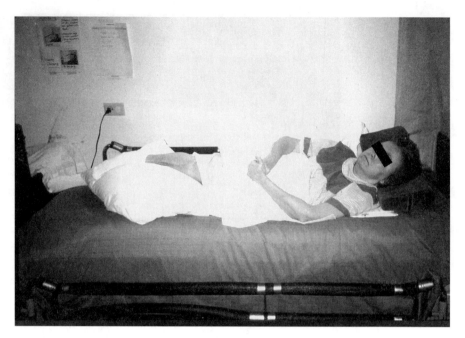

FIGURE 27.9   *A patient positioned three-quarter side-lying with body aligners from Positioning Solutions along her spine.*

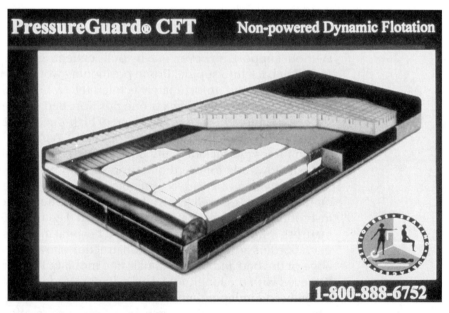

FIGURE 27.10   *The PressureGuard CFT is one example of a mattress replacement. This mattress offers some customization to meet individual needs for pressure reduction. (Courtesy of Span-America.)*

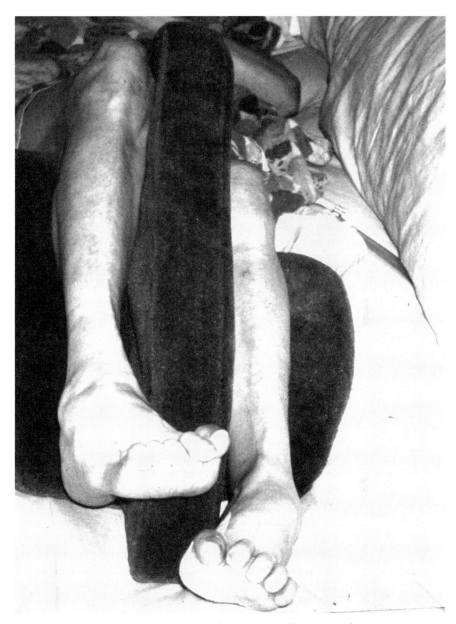

FIGURE 27.11   *The lower extremity bed positioner. This patient has strong tone in the hip adductors and knee flexors, resulting in a stage 1 pressure area at the medial knee. (Courtesy of Positioning Solutions.)*

While careful attention to alignment and prevention of further contracture may be attended to in the sitting position, bed positioning can be often neglected. A patient may spend from one-third to one-half of the day in bed, so using this time for inhibition of abnormal muscle tone, gentle static stretching, and using gravity to assist in the prevention and correction of acquired deformities dramatically increases the effectiveness of the treatment plan. For patients with hip adduction or hip or knee flexion contractures, the lower extremity bed positioner can support these joints out of the position of deformity for a steady, sustained stretch (Figure 27.11). This equip-

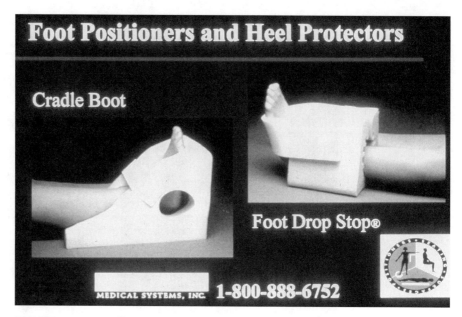

FIGURE 27.12   *Cradle Boot and Foot Drop Stop. (Courtesy of Span-America.)*

ment can also be helpful for patients with hypotonia, who may tend to assume hip abduction in the supine position.

Bed overlays, replacement mattresses, and specialty beds do not eliminate pressure on the bony prominence of the heels automatically. Interface pressure on the heels should be eliminated in the "at-risk" patient. The Heellift Boot, Foot Drop Stop, or the Cradle Boot (Figure 27.12) are examples of pressure eliminating devices. All of these devices attempt to distribute weight bearing along the soft tissue of the calf and away from the posterior heel. Care should be taken to examine the Achilles' tendon for any signs of excessive pressure. Be cautious of using devices made of plastic or other nonconforming material, as patients that have been immobile often have Achilles' tendons that have fibrosed and are bone-like and cannot tolerate high interface pressures. Introduction of another layer between heel and mattress must be avoided, particularly with the "at-risk" foot, as this layer only hides the problem and increases interface pressure. Wounds are especially difficult to heal in this area due to the poorly vascularized tissue and the immediate proximity of bone to the skin surface. Amputation is often necessary, so prevention of ulceration is critical.[16] The clinician would be wise to have several of these devices on hand, as the affected patient's skin integrity probably cannot wait for supply ordering.

Education

Therapeutic positioning plans are only as successful as the follow-through of patients, families, and caregivers. With this in mind, therapists must provide education from the outset to maximize functional outcomes. The most successful plans can be carried out as part of the patient's daily routine with easy to use equipment.

Whenever possible, enroll the rest of the health care team, including the patient and family, in the decisions about equipment, schedules, and purpose. This greatly assists in achieving follow-through and investment among the most important people—the consumer and the day-to-day caregivers. Using equipment that remains attached to the chair versus equipment that must be attached daily makes the use of equipment routine. Often patients have specific likes and dislikes regarding fabric choices, color, and timing of use of positioning devices. Respect these. For example, an adult male with muscular dystrophy participated actively in the design of a head support to maintain his neck in alignment with his trunk, to support his neck from excessive left rotation due to a muscle imbalance, and to allow pain-free sleeping in this supported position. He chose colors, decided on the placement of straps, and participated actively in the problem solving for keeping the support in place even when he used his bed ladder to reposition himself. This level of investment led to the successful integration of this piece of equipment into his daily routine, whereas other devices piled up in the family's garage.

If utilizing splinting, time the wearing schedule with some other routine in the patient's life, such as the nursing turning schedule, prompted voiding opportunities, or rest periods.

Document the placement and purpose of all equipment and send copies to every likely person involved, especially in a nursing facility. A picture can do this with less effort, with or without the individual present, as regulations permit in the particular situation. A tag attached permanently to the bed or wheelchair, detailing equipment currently in use can be invaluable to the often-transient staff of many care facilities. Documentation is critical to the process of restraint tracking and reduction in an extended care facility.[17] When using a restraint in positioning, clearly illustrate

- Problems leading to the intervention
- How the device enables safety and a higher level of function or mobility
- What alternatives were trialed and failed
- What occurs without the device
- When the device should be used
- When pressure relief in the form of restraint removal occurs
- Future plans for reducing the restraint
- How the restraint is the least restrictive option

If a patient can remove a restraint independently, it is not considered a restraint at all, but documentation of this ability remains critical.

A treatment modality of this complexity is by definition a dynamic process. As an individual changes over time, the positioning goals change as well. Positioning devices and support surfaces need to be reassessed, modified, and even replaced to match the individual's changing status and needs. Those patients with neurologic involvement and pathologic reflex involvement, abnormal movement patterns, and altered sensations usually require the longest duration of intervention. Ascertaining reflex-inhibiting, tone-reducing postures and movements and facilitating appropriate postural control takes more time than accommodating for a fixed contracture or allowing for heel strike for a patient who would benefit from self-propulsion in a wheelchair. Also, some individuals may take 3–4 months to stabilize in their new positioning and should be followed at a reduced level to ensure a good outcome.

A system must be in place to ensure that patients are reassessed at regular intervals so that any problems can be identified and systematically addressed. Some patients require intervention because they have improved and need fewer postural supports and can even upgrade goals to improve mobility. Others benefit from modifications to their program because of disease process progression, weight loss, or other complicating factors. In long-term care facilities, this regularly scheduled follow-up is often coordinated with care planning. In assisted living environments, positioning screenings can be carried out as part of routine health clinics. When seen on an outpatient basis, follow-up is more difficult but remains critical, as the following case studies illustrate. A reasonable time period for reassessing positioning using open-celled foam is 6–8 months due to the lifespan of the foam itself. Closed cell foam devices can stretch the time between reassessments, but consider the clinical picture of the patient before deciding on a future date. Weight loss or gain of more than 5 lb may necessitate a change in support surfaces. Positioning can be compared to dynamic splinting: a therapist closely observes for changes and rarely stops therapy entirely while the patient is still using the device. Too much postural support for an individual beginning to increase in independent mobility is just as dangerous as too little support for the dependent patient. In any case, a therapist should expect change and teach the consumer and family to expect this as well.

Therapeutic Positioning Case Studies

The first case study illustrates the problem with intervention occurring too late in the progression of problems related to the poor management of tonal abnormalities discussed earlier. An 82-year-old man with a history of multiple CVAs had been admitted into a long-term care facility. He demonstrated pathologic reflexes and extremely high tone in synergistic patterns. He was incontinent of bowel and bladder and used a catheter. At the time of admission he was able to participate in some limited activities of daily living and used smoking as a primary leisure activity. He was unable to effectively weight shift for pressure relief. Thus, before the development of problems, he was a clear candidate for pressure ulcers due to poor management of abnormal tone; difficulty in achieving pressure relief; frequent irritation from wetness, perspiration, and stool on the skin; and risk of shearing due to frequent need to be moved up in bed.

He developed a pressure ulcer on the left IT and physician's orders eventually stopped this patient from sitting in a wheelchair. In Figure

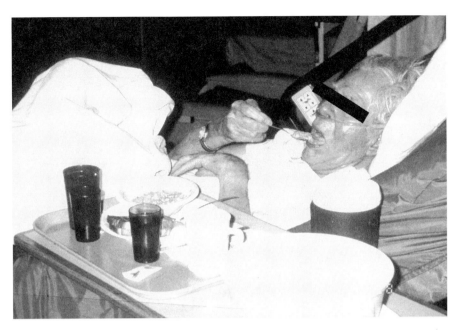

FIGURE 27.13   *Patient attempting to eat in bed.*

27.13, he is pictured attempting to eat in bed. Due to the poor positioning for eating and swallowing, he coughed throughout the meal and often could not complete self-feeding because of exhaustion. Whereas the recommended serum albumin level in the general diet is 3.5 g/dl, his albumin level was 2.0 and falling, worsening the possibilities of not only healing this ulcer, but of survival.

As the health care team believed that sitting was causing the pressure ulcer on the left IT, he was allowed to "sit" only in the geriatric recliner chair with a Roho cushion, shown in Figure 27.14. With prolonged positioning in these supine positions, flexor tone in the lower extremities increased so that his heels eventually approximated his buttocks in a fixed contracture. Restorative nursing was repeatedly called in for range-of-motion programs, but increasing pain and tightness made this excruciating and pointless. The patient's knee range-of-motion alone took more than 30 minutes to allow for movement away from the IT, but rebounded immediately after stopping the passive exercise, without positioning to reinforce tone reduction. Figures 27.15 and 27.16 illustrate the progression of the knee range-of-motion contracture and the difficulty in increasing range. Note the ineffectiveness of soft, unstructured supports such as bed pillows in making any impact on contractures. The patient even lost the available range needed to "sit" in the geriatric recliner chair and so was confined to bed only, with the leg contractures continuing to worsen.

Therapy had been requested earlier in the course of the patient's stay but denied because "the patient cannot sit." This should have alerted the health care team that this patient was in acute danger of worsening contractures. Treating the inability to sit in itself would have been an appro-

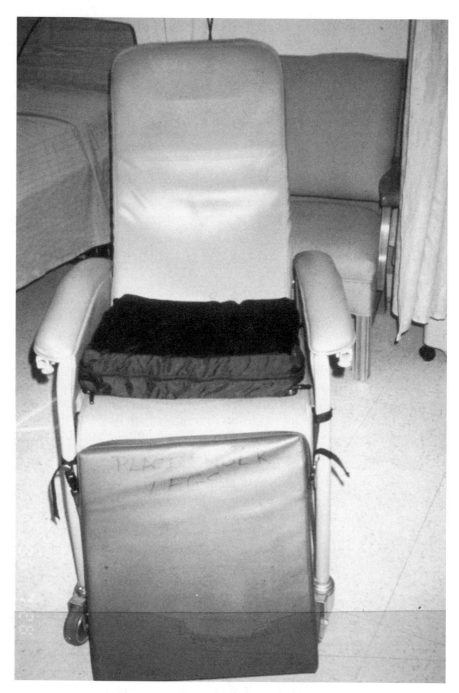

FIGURE 27.14   *Geriatric reclining chair with a Roho cushion.*

priate action. Therapy was eventually approved very late in the patient's progression of problems, long after restorative nursing had abandoned the range-of-motion program as too painful and traumatic for the patient.

Even hygiene activities were extremely difficult and painful. Circulation to the lower extremities was severely compromised due to the tightness of

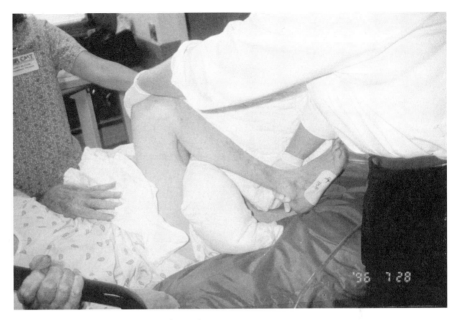

FIGURE 27.15   *Knee range-of-motion contracture.*

the knee contractures, eventually contributing to a wound along the lateral border of the foot shown in Figure 27.17. Had intervention addressed the true causes of the original pressure ulcer on the left IT (Figure 27.18), this patient would certainly have had a more favorable outcome.

Skilled intervention was critical in the following areas:

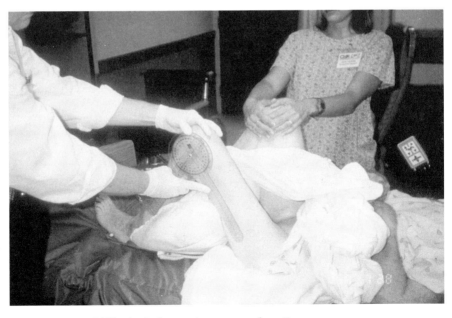

FIGURE 27.16   *Difficulty in increasing range-of-motion.*

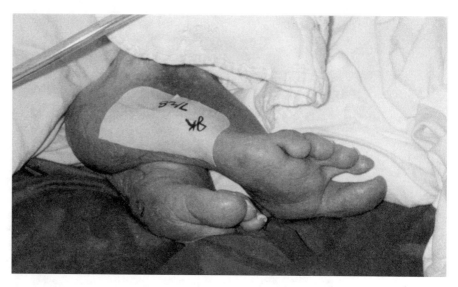

FIGURE 27.17   *A wound along the lateral border of the foot.*

- Careful interface pressure assessment of all weight-bearing bony prominences, especially those where a pressure ulcer exists
- Management of tone before it became so difficult to address
- Development of a realistic range-of-motion program utilizing tone reduction techniques and appropriate medication and instructing restorative nursing when such a program was feasible
- Therapeutic positioning to lengthen soft tissue and reduce the rebound effect following range; education for all staff and family

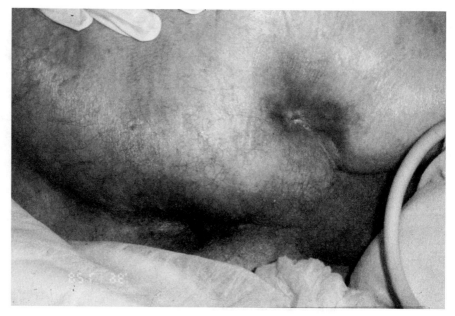

FIGURE 27.18   *Pressure ulcer on the left ischial tuberosity.*

- Development of a therapeutic sitting program which removed pressure from the ITs and reduced pressure over other bony prominences
- Facilitate the use of pain medication in conjunction with the physical management of this complex patient

Unfortunately, this patient died of aspiration pneumonia several days after therapy was initiated.

In this painful example, intervention occurred too late in the course of treatment and tone management was essentially ignored. This patient demonstrated many of the risk factors for pressure ulcer development before the onset of the actual ulcer. Even at that point, further sequelae in this cascade of events could have been avoided with a therapeutic sitting program; especially avoiding bed rest in supine; focusing on tone management; utilizing a bed leg-positioning device to encourage gentle tissue lengthening when in bed; activities to promote functional mobility; and family training. The health care team also assumed that a specialty bed and a Roho cushion would take care of the pressure problems. No support surface on its own can solve all pressure problems, but instead must be used in conjunction with therapeutic positioning and with assessment and careful follow-up to ensure efficacy.

The failure to recognize the long-term effects of abnormal tone rests on the entire health care team in this example, from acute care to the long-term care facility. Patients who do not demonstrate progress in the customary areas noted on the Functional Independence Measure or other outcome criteria are at high risk for this lack of meaningful intervention in positioning. With some attention early on to achieving a stable sitting position, this patient would never have been assigned to the bed rest that eventually made his condition irreversible. Indeed, attention to proximal stability is at the heart of many respected treatment philosophies in rehabilitation of the patient with CVA. Without that proximal stability, fine motor abilities cannot emerge, and a true picture of potential in activities of daily living lies hidden. Certainly range-of-motion exercises are never enough to counteract severe tonal influences.

The second case study illustrates positioning on an ongoing basis for an individual with cerebral palsy, mental retardation, and a seizure disorder. This patient is a long-term resident of an extended care facility and was 45 years old at the time of this case study. He had chronic challenges with abnormal tonal influences, achieving upright alignment, worsening contractures, and problems with skin integrity. A therapy screening also determined that the staff noted increasing frustration with self-feeding and leisure activities. From the screening, therapists noted worsening flexion contractures in the left upper extremity, making dressing and hygiene difficult and placing the patient at risk for a loss of skin integrity. Extension contractures and windsweeping at the hips were increasing as well. In Figure 27.19 the patient is viewed from the side. Note the significant hip and knee extension, causing the base of support to be moved from the ITs to the sacrum and coccyx. He cannot achieve a midline posture, with the trunk seen pushing to the left and the hips windsweeping to the right. Hips are adducted and internally rotated. Hip guides are in

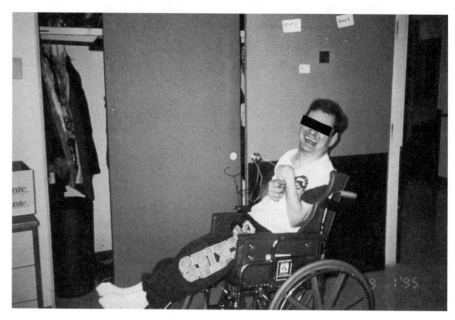

FIGURE 27.19   *Patient viewed from the side.*

place, but are not adequate on their own to assist in reducing windsweeping, as the problem is more proximal in nature. The patient did not have foot protection or lower extremity support and couldn't tolerate any stabilization of the feet. This patient attended a day program and community outings with the legs extended in just this manner, at high risk for injury to himself and others. Severe extensor tone and strong spasms were present throughout but particularly in the cervical spine and hip and knee extensors. He had recurrent coccygeal breakdown. A spiky bony skeletal structure also contributed to breakdown. Weight distribution over the soft tissue of the thighs could not be reliably achieved due to tonal influences. Although the problems were progressing, this patient had exhibited these same issues for many, many years.

Risk factors and critical problems included management of abnormal tone, problems with shearing as he slid forward on any support surface, friction, and the ongoing challenge of bladder incontinence to skin integrity.

Upon assessment, the patient was found rotated in the chair in compensation for a lack of true 90-degree hip flexion. An antithrust cushion alone was not adequate to facilitate positioning. A drop back attached to the wheelchair accommodated for this lack of hip flexion, greatly reducing the tonal abnormalities throughout the body. The drop back created the necessary "tilt in space" orientation to allow gravity to assist the patient in maintaining a more upright posture without triggering the intense extensor tone activity. Figure 27.20 demonstrates the significant change of positioning with the antithrust cushion and drop back to break up the patient's severe extensor tone.

A trial using both a footrest and calf support with foot straps, as well as a 90-degree hip belt was attempted to break up extensor tone in the hips

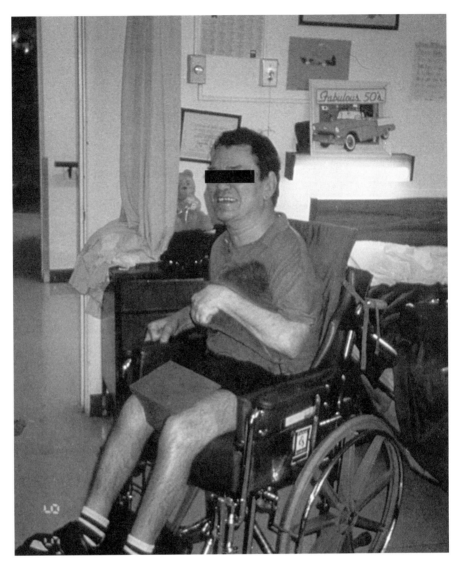

FIGURE 27.20 *Note the significant change of positioning with the antithrust cushion and drop back to inhibit the patient's severe extensor tone.*

and knees. These interventions made no impact on the knee extension. The equipment was also painful for the patient. Figure 27.21 shows a closer view of the knee extension contractures. Therapy achieved a 20-degree maximum knee flexion measurement on assessment, despite trials with tone-reducing position techniques. Therapists noted that they were physically not strong enough to stabilize the patient in side-lying or other positions that normally can assist in reducing extensor tone.

Figure 27.22 shows the available knee flexion after placement of the patient on the antithrust cushion with drop back configuration. An immediate 25-degree increase in knee flexion occurred. The antithrust cushion rose from back to front, from 3 in. to 5 in. in thickness. Cutout under the

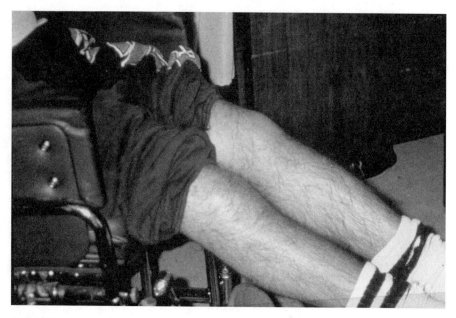

FIGURE 27.21   *A closer view of the knee extension contractures.*

coccyx was unnecessary, as the pressure was off-loaded from the coccyx and ischial tuberosities over the posterior thighs. With the utilization of the antithrust cushion and drop back, the extensor tone was reduced enough to allow footrests to be used comfortably by the patient. Gravity

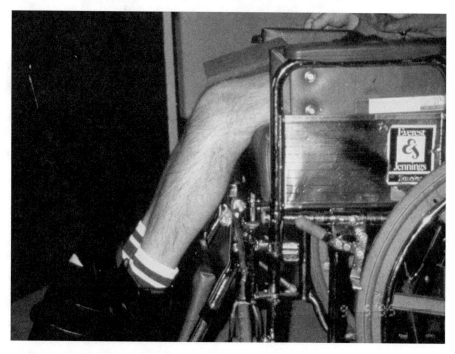

FIGURE 27.22   *The available knee flexion after placement of the patient on the antithrust cushion and drop back configuration.*

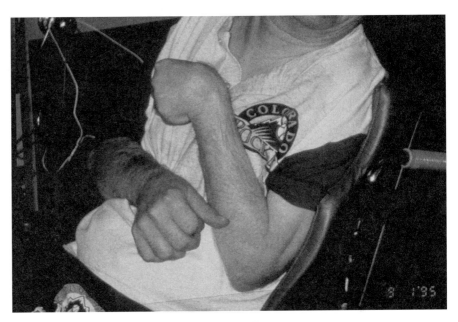

FIGURE 27.23   *Habitual positioning of the left arm.*

would further assist in the lengthening of the knee flexors and soft tissue to allow for a gentle increase in available range over time.

The left upper extremity had a history of skin breakdown at the elbow crease. Factors affecting skin integrity included friction, perspiration, and strong adduction and internal rotation against the ribcage. Figure 27.23 illustrates the habitual positioning of the left arm. The nursing staff could not keep the elbow extended long enough to complete hygiene or efficient dressing, and these activities were very painful for the patient. He was also at risk for skin problems along the rib cage. Trials to increase range were employed using both a Dynasplint and a JAS (Joint Active Systems) splint but the patient found these interventions very painful and eventually refused them altogether.

Figure 27.24 shows the patient accepting a 65-degree arm wedge. The shoulder adduction and internal rotation are adequate to keep the support in place without further strapping. The side closest to the thorax can be further customized to conform to the body shape, increasing comfort, wearing time, and stability in wearing. This support is softer than the orthotics but has adequate foam density to provide a firm static stretch over time, and the patient was able to tolerate wearing-times of 2 hours or more. Eventually this patient progressed to be able to tolerate a 90-degree arm wedge for further static stretching during wearing times.

The patient achieved a near symmetric sitting posture without neck, trunk, or pelvic rotation (Figure 27.25). Without these interventions, the patient could clearly have been risking a coccygeal pressure ulcer, skin breakdown in the left elbow crease, and very likely scoliosis in the spine in response to all the forces of pull in asymmetric sitting. The patient was also able to resume his leisure and limited self-feeding abilities. Extensive

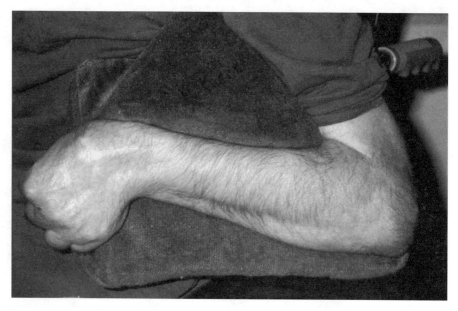

FIGURE 27.24   *The 65-degree arm wedge. (Courtesy of Positioning Solutions.)*

education was provided to direct care staff. Pictures of the chair with all the equipment placed in it were attached to the wheelchair as well as placed in the nursing chart. Consultation regarding protective skin barriers to ameliorate the effects of bladder incontinence was also completed. Most of the positioning pieces could be securely attached to the chair, with removal required only for cleaning, to assist with staff follow-through and ease of application.

Further improvements were expected over time, particularly in knee flexion and elbow extension. This patient needs to be periodically assessed for positioning needs the rest of his life due to the influence of abnormal tone.

This patient's history is an excellent example of the need for thorough assessment. Without identifying the lack of true hip flexion, none of the other interventions would have been successful. Also, this patient demonstrated the need to carefully grade therapeutic sitting. When the influence of strong extensor tone is lessened, a patient very often exhibits extremely weak postural support musculature both in flexors and extensors. These must be gradually strengthened in the absence of the overwhelming extensor tone. The patient very often "looks worse" after intervention if this important factor is not considered.

Conclusion

Therapeutic positioning falls in the no man's land of health care territorial issues—no one discipline sees itself having sole responsibility or proprietary knowledge for appropriate positioning in the bed and chair. As the case studies illustrate, the attention of the entire team is

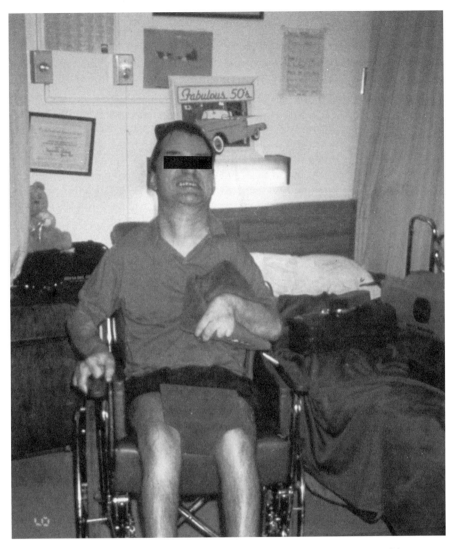

FIGURE 27.25 *The patient achieved a near symmetric sitting posture without neck, trunk, or pelvic rotation.*

commonly aroused only when the positioning problem has become acute and far less treatable. Excuses such as "If restorative had really done the range of motion . . ." and "the patient just wouldn't follow through with weight shifts" serve only to assuage guilt and place blame unfairly. Much like treatment for communication deficits, positioning intervention must take place in an integrated manner, not isolated in treatment rooms or disciplines.

One answer to the dilemma of "who does what" is to adopt the principle of team responsibility and individual accountability. In this principle, all team members are responsible for noting problems with positioning, skin integrity, restraint reduction, contracture management, and safety issues. All team members bear group responsibility for the outcome, but individual team members are accountable for specific interventions in the overall plan. Positioning is so complex and far reaching that no single discipline can assume all the responsibility in any case. Setting up systems to address positioning in a health care facility is the safest way to ensure that all patients who would benefit from intervention are identified and treated before problems become more difficult. Use of predictive measures such as the Braden scale can assist in the classification of clinical biographies of patients into mild, moderate, and high risk for development of pressure ulcers.[18] Through the systematic use of such a tool, the entire health care team can increase its awareness of facility-wide problems as well as problems with individual patients. Examples include an automatic referral to dietary for any patients identified as eating an average of one-half of the meal offered or less than three servings of meat or dairy products per day, or instituting the use of safe perineal cleanser (acidic rather than alkaline) and a moisture barrier with all incontinent patients to reduce effects of prolonged and damaging moisture on skin.

Information provided in this chapter is intended as both a resource and a stimulus to further expand the knowledge and skills in positioning in each group of consumers and health care providers. A suggested reading list is provided for further information.

References

1. Olshansky K. Essay on knowledge, caring, and psychological factors in the prevention and treatment of pressure ulcers. Adv Wound Care 1994;7(3):64.
2. Bergstrom N, Allman R, Alvarez O, et al. Treatment of Pressure Ulcers: Clinical Practice Guideline No. 15. Rockville, MD: Agency for Health Care Policy and Research, US Department of Health and Human Services. AHCPR Publication No. 95-0652, 1994.
3. Reimbursable Geriatric Service Delivery, Suppl 2, Pittsburgh, PA: Glickstein Neustadt, 1994;13:1–2.
4. Hoeman SP. Rehabilitation Nursing: Process and Application (2d ed). St. Louis: Mosby, 1996;241–244, 479–572.
5. Moody BL, Fanale JE, Thompson M, et al. Impact of staff education on pressure sore development in elderly hospitalized patients. Arch Intern Med 1988;148:224.
6. National Pressure Ulcer Advisory Panel (NPUAP). Pressure ulcers: prevalence, cost and risk assessment: consensus development conference statement. Decubitus 1989;2(2):24.
7. Chernoff R. Geriatric Nutrition (Vol. 15). Gaithersburg, MD: Aspen, 1991.
8. Russ GH, Motta GJ. Eliminating pressure: is less than 32 mm Hg enough for wound healing? Ostomy Wound Manage 1991;34:60.
9. Sussman C. Assessment of the Skin and Wound. In C Sussman, BM Bates-Jensen (eds), Wound Care: A Collaborative Practice Manual for Physical Therapists and Nurses. Gaithersburg, MD: Aspen, 1998;49.

10. Rappl LM. Management of Pressure by Therapeutic Positioning. In C Sussman, BM Bates-Jensen (eds), Wound Care: A Collaborative Practice Manual for Physical Therapists and Nurses. Gaithersburg, MD: Aspen, 1998;284.
11. Davies PM. Steps to Follow: A Guide to the Treatment of Adult Hemiplegia. Berlin: Heidelberg, 1985;24–28.
12. Davies PM. Steps to Follow: A Guide to the Treatment of Adult Hemiplegia. Berlin: Heidelberg, 1985;77–98.
13. Meehan M. Multisite pressure ulcer prevalence survey. Decubitus 1990;3(4):14.
14. Reprinted with permission from Positioning Solutions, Cheyenne Mountain Alliance, Colorado Springs, CO 80906.
15. McLean J. Pressure reduction or pressure relief: making the right choice. J ET Nurs 1993;20(5):211.
16. Levin ME, O'Neal LW, Bowker JH (eds). The Diabetic Foot (5th ed). St. Louis: Mosby, 1993;483–484.
17. Greenberg D. Geriatric seating and positioning: definitely a therapy task. A special interest section. Gerontology 1996;19(3):1.
18. Braden BJ, Bergstrom N. A conceptual schema for the study of etiology of pressure sores. Rehabil Nurs 1987;12(1):8.

Further Reading

Hasty JH, Krasner D, Kennedy KL. A new tool for evaluating patient support surfaces, part I: a guideline for making practice decisions. Ostomy Wound Manage 1991;36:51.

Hedrick-Thompson JK. A review of pressure reduction device studies. J Vasc Nurs 1992;10:3.

Jay ER. How different support surfaces address pressure and shear forces. Durable Med Equip Rev 1995;(2);60.

Kemp M, Krouskop T. Pressure ulcers—reducing incidence and severity by managing pressure. J Geriatr Nurs 1994;20(9):27.

Lubin BS, Powell T. Pressure sores and specialty beds: cost containment and ensurance of quality care. J ET Nurs 1991;18:190.

Plautz R. Positioning can make the difference. Nurs Homes Long-term Care Manage 1992;(41):30.

TABLE 27A.1 Bilateral Total Hips (Seated Position)

Medical diagnoses	Examination/evaluation	Functional diagnoses	Prognoses	Interventions	Outcomes
Osteoarthritis of femoral head and acetabulum, with recent, bilateral, total hips	Hip flexion measures 75 degrees, bilaterally, and wheelchair seat-to-back angle is 90 degrees, causing patient to slide forward on seat. Knee flexion is limited to 65 degrees, bilaterally, causing increased pain and inability to support feet on footrests of standard, removable footrest. Because of lack of adequate seat cushion and patient's position on seat, interface pressure over the sacrum and coccyx is >100 mm Hg. This is considered unsafe due to patient's immobility, incontinence, nutritional status, and impaired cognitive status, which is either due to pain medications or a reaction to the surgical anesthetic. Braden scale is 12, indicating high risk for pressure ulceration.	• Inability to sit at optimal 90 degrees seat-to-back angle and knee flexion angle in wheelchair, for maximal independence in ADLs and wheelchair mobility • Undue susceptibility to hip dislocation • Undue susceptibility to pressure ulceration over the sacrum and coccyx • Inability to perform position changes and transfers	• Patient will maintain upright positioning in wheelchair, with hips on back of seat for 4 hours, twice per day, in 1 week. • Patient will remain free of hip dislocation during this admission.	• Fit with positioning and pressure reducing foam seat cushion, at least 3 in. thick, with anti-sling insert, to eliminate upholstery sling, stabilize pelvis, and distribute interface pressure away from the weight-bearing bony prominences and onto the femurs • Carve out cushion anteriorly, under the thighs, to accommodate for the lack of hip flexion and to assist in avoiding hip flexion beyond 90 degrees • Equip with reclining backrest to further accommodate for range-of-motion limitations at the hips and to keep safe from dislocation • Equip with elevating leg rests to accommodate for the lack of knee flexion, initially, and adjust them to facilitate increasing knee flexion, as the patient increases knee flexion • Replace the elevating leg rests with standard footrests when sitting knee flexion is at least 90 degrees • Fit with back cushion that supports the spinal curves	• Patient has maintained upright sitting, as close to 90 degrees of hip and knee flexion as is allowed by range-of-motion and hip precaution limitations. • Patient has remained free of hip dislocation during this admission. • Patient has remained free of pressure ulcers during this admission. • Patient is independent in all position changes and transfers.

ADLs = activities of daily living.

TABLE 27A.2   Thoracic Kyphosis (Seated Position)

Medical diagnoses	Examination/evaluation	Functional diagnoses	Prognoses	Interventions	Outcomes
Thoracic kyphosis	Patient has a fixed thoracic kyphosis, weak cervical extensor muscles, and 80 degrees of hip flexion. She is sitting in a wheelchair with a 90-degree seat-to-back angle and slides forward on the seat due to the limited hip flexion and fixed thoracic kyphosis. Chin is resting on chest due to weak cervical extensor muscles and the fixed kyphosis. The thoracic kyphosis and limited hip flexion must be accommodated by opening up the seat-to-back angle >90 degrees. The seat-to-back angle will be determined by: the specific angle it takes to accommodate for the 80 degrees of hip flexion and the fixed kyphosis and to bring the head to midline, with a slight chin-tuck position for safe deglutition and swallowing. Due to inability to lift her head and see or access her food, the patient cannot interact with her environment or feed herself. Interface pressure measurements are 80 mm Hg over the sacrum, coccyx, and the thoracic spinous processes at the apex of the curve. These readings are considered unsafe due to the Braden score of 12, which suggests high risk for pressure ulceration.	• Inability to maintain 90 degrees hip flexion and keep face vertical, sitting in wheelchair • Undue susceptibility to pressure ulceration over the chin, chest, sacrum, coccyx, and the spinous processes on the apex of the thoracic curve • Susceptibility to wheelchair tipping posteriorly • Inability to self-feed	• Patient will sit for 2 hrs, three times per day, with hips back on seat, with face vertical, in 2 wks. • Patient will be free of pressure ulceration during this admission. • Patient will self-propel wheelchair throughout the facility without tipping wheelchair posteriorly. • Patient will self-feed with supervision of caregiver in 1 mo.	• Fit with reclining back-rest to accommodate for the fixed thoracic kyphosis and limited hip flexion. Modify, as necessary, to accommodate for prominent spinous processes. • Fit with stabilizing and pressure reducing seat cushion, modify to eliminate pressure over the sacrum and coccyx • Or, fit with a cushion that eliminates ischial, sacral, and coccyx pressure • Equip wheelchair with rear antitippers to prevent wheelchair from tipping posteriorly • Refer to occupational therapist for work on self-feeding • Refer to speech/language pathologist for determination of the appropriate position of the head and neck for safe deglutition and swallowing	• Patient is able to sit with face vertical and hips in the appropriate position on the seat with safe interface pressures. • Patient tolerates sitting 2 hrs, three times per day, coordinated with meal times. • Patient has had no evidence of irritation, friction, shearing, excessive moisture, or excessive interface pressure during this admission. • Patient can self-propel wheelchair and has not tipped wheelchair posteriorly. • Patient is able to feed self independently.

TABLE 27A.3   Above-the-Knee Amputation (Seated Position)

Medical diagnoses	Examination/evaluation	Functional diagnoses	Prognoses	Interventions	Outcomes
Left, above-the-knee amputation, secondary to peripheral vascular disease Peripheral vascular disease in right lower extremity	Patient has interface pressures over the ischial tuberosities, measuring 100 mm Hg on the left and 80 mm Hg on the right. The interface pressure on the left is higher than the right due to the inability to distribute the tissue load along the length of the femur. The interface pressures are considered unsafe, as patient is immobile and has a spiky bony skeletal structure without adequate muscle mass. Braden score is 12, indicating patient is at high risk for pressure ulceration. Patient has no shoe or protection for right foot and foot is resting on metal footrest and is in danger of developing trauma-related wounds.	• Undue susceptibility to pressure ulceration over ischial tuberosities • Undue susceptibility to ulceration of right foot	• Patient will sit erect in wheelchair with back and seat cushion that provides for postural support and pressure elimination over the ischial tuberosities and coccyx, by tomorrow. • Patient will have protection of right foot when up in wheelchair by 5 PM today.	• Fit with appropriate back cushion to support spinal curves • Fit with custom-modified, 4-in. foam seat cushion (a combination of a 2-in. layer of high density/high resiliency foam on the top and a layer of 2-in. medium density/medium resiliency foam on the bottom) to achieve pressure elimination for each ischial tuberosity, the sacrum, coccyx, and the perineum • Consider utilizing a reclining back to redistribute some of the pressure off the sitting surface and onto the back • Equip with antitippers (posterior), amputee adapters, or amputee wheelchair to move the wheels posteriorly to compensate for the loss of the weight of the left leg to avoid tipping posteriorly • Fit with foot pedal cover for foot pedal and Plastazote shoe with extra toe depth and width to protect the remaining foot	• Patient sits with postural alignment and positioning close to ideal, for 3 hrs, three times per day. • Patient has remained free of pressure ulceration during this admission. • Right limb has remained free of trauma-related ulcers.

TABLE 27A.4 Bilateral Above-the-Knee Amputations (Seated Position)

Medical diagnoses	Examination/evaluation	Functional diagnoses	Prognoses	Interventions	Outcomes
Bilateral, above-the-knee amputations, secondary to peripheral vascular disease	Patient is sitting in a wheelchair with a 90-degree seat-to-back angle, slung seat upholstery, and a soft foam seat cushion. Consequently, posture is characterized by: hips forward on the seat, hips adducted and internally rotated, and thoracic kyphosis. Sitting balance is poor, requiring constant manual support in maintain upright sitting. Nurses report that the patient tipped the wheelchair posteriorly and fell on the floor this morning. Wheelchair accommodation is necessary to compensate for the loss of the weight of the lower extremities, to prevent posterior tipping. This patient is in imminent danger of further injury from the chair tipping over posteriorly and from falling forward. Patient reports that sitting is painful and that he has pain over the ischial tuberosities. Interface pressures over the ischial tuberosities are >100 mm Hg and considered unsafe. This is caused by inability to off-load the ischial tuberosities onto the posterior thighs with the present seat cushion. The Braden score is 10, placing this patient at high risk for pressure ulcer development. For this patient to sit safely, the support surface must be changed to one that can support postural alignment and distribute the pressure away from the ischial tuberosities.	• Undue susceptibility to falls due to: inadequate weight distribution anteriorly and poor sitting balance • Undue susceptibility to pressure ulceration over ischial tuberosities • Inability to maintain an upright posture and neutral hip alignment due to poor sitting balance, ischial pain, and an inadequate seat and back cushion • Inability to tolerate sitting for more than 30 mins at one time • Inability to self-propel wheelchair	• Patient will be safe from falls from wheelchair by 5 PM today. • Patient will have safe interface pressures over the ischial tuberosities by 5 PM today. • Patient will have postural alignment close to ideal in the wheelchair. • Patient will tolerate sitting for 2 hrs, three times per day, in 2 wks. • Patient will self-propel wheelchair for functional distance throughout the facility in 1 mo.	• Equip wheelchair with amputee adapters, rear antitippers, and padded chest strap • Utilize same intervention as single above-the-knee amputee • Utilize back cushion to support the spinal curves • Consider using a reclining back to redistribute some of the pressure off the sitting surface and onto the back • Consider fitting with a 90-degree padded hip belt across the remaining limbs, to assist in off-loading the ischial tuberosities and transferring the tissue load to the remaining posterior thighs	• Patient has had no falls from the wheelchair since the second day of his admission. • Patient has interface pressure readings over the ischial tuberosities of 20 mm Hg, bilaterally, and has had no pressure ulceration over the sitting surface. • Patient is sitting upright, with proper alignment of head, neck, shoulders, and hips. • Patient tolerates sitting in the wheelchair for 6 hrs, twice per day, with no reported pain over sitting surface. • Patient can self-propel the wheelchair independently throughout the facility, including to the dining room and to activities.

TABLE 27A.5 Hip and Knee Flexion Contractures (Seated Position)

Medical diagnoses	Examination/evaluation	Functional diagnoses	Prognoses	Interventions	Outcomes
Hip and knee flexion contractures, fixed	Hip extension measures –45 degrees, bilaterally, and left knee extension measures –75 degrees, and right knee extension measures –90 degrees. Patient is immobile and dependent in all position changes, transfers, and ADLs. Patient is sitting in a recliner geriatric chair with hips forward, hips and knees flexed toward chest, and feet resting between the footrest and the seat. Her hips are forward on the seat secondary to the hip and knee flexion contractures, and the recliner geriatric chair that prohibits the accommodation of the contractures. Braden score is 12, indicating high risk for pressure ulceration. Interface pressure measures >100 mm Hg on the sacrum, coccyx, and heels, which is considered unsafe due to risk factors of immobility, cognitive impairment, nutritional status and incontinence. Patient is dependent in self-feeding and personal hygiene activities due to proximal instability that prohibits use of the upper extremities.	• Inability to achieve ideal upright position with hips and knees at 90 degrees and face vertical due to less than full hip and knee extension, secondary to joint integrity impairments at the hips and knees • Undue susceptibility to increasing the severity of the existing hip and knee joint integrity impairments, secondary to flexor spasticity • Undue susceptibility to pressure ulcer development over the sacrum, coccyx, and heels • Inability to perform self-feeding and personal hygiene activities	• Patient will achieve ideal upright sitting in a wheelchair with a 90-degree seat-to-back angle and 90 degrees of hip and knee flexion and face vertical in 2 wks. • Patient will maintain the existing hip and knee extension over the next 90 days. • Patient will remain free of pressure ulcers over the next 90 days. • Patient will self-feed and perform personal hygiene activities with supervision and verbal cues in 1 mo.	• Fit with appropriate size wheelchair with 90-degree seat-to-back angle and standard removable footrests • Fit with seat cushion that eliminates ischial tuberosity and coccygeal pressure, stabilizes the pelvis, and eliminates the sling in the seat upholstery • Fit with back cushion that supports the spinal curves and eliminates the sling in the back upholstery • Fit with appropriately sized footwear and an adjustable calf rest/foot support combo device that provides stabilization of the knee and ankle joints and protects and supports the feet • Fit with padded positioning hip belt over the thighs to stabilize the hips on the seat and to place a gentle stretch on the hip flexors • Consider fitting with a padded lap tray for trunk and upper extremity support, especially during the early phases of treatment intervention • Refer to occupational therapist for evaluation and instruction in self-feeding and personal hygiene activities	• Patient sits with erect posture in wheelchair with hips and knees at 90-degree and face vertical. • Patient tolerates sitting in the wheelchair for 2 hrs, three times per day, coordinated with meal times. • Patient has maintained hip and knee extension range of motion during the last 90 days. • Patient's skin has shown no signs of excessive pressure, shearing, moisture, or friction during the last 90 days. • Patient has been referred to occupational therapist and is working on self-feeding and personal hygiene activities.

ADLs = activities of daily living.

TABLE 27A.6 Bilateral Total Hips (Recumbent Position)

Medical diagnoses	Examination/ evaluation	Functional diagnoses	Prognoses	Interventions	Outcomes
Osteoarthritis of femoral head and acetabulum with bilateral total hips	Patient is unable to reposition self in bed due to pain, range-of-motion limitations at the hips and knees, and postanesthetic cognitive impairments. Patient is spending 20 hrs per day in bed and eating two meals per day in bed. Head and neck positioning are not safe for swallowing; Patient is choking on each bite of food. Interface pressure measurements are >100 mm Hg over sacrum and heels in supine on hospital mattress and are considered unsafe due to risk factors of impaired cognition and immobility. Braden score is 12, which indicates high risk for pressure ulcer development. Patient cannot tolerate full side-lying and prefers supine.	• Undue susceptibility to pressure ulceration over the sacrum and heels, secondary to risk factors of immobility, unsafe interface pressures over the sacrum and heels, and cognitive impairments • Undue susceptibility to hip dislocation due to recent bilateral total hip surgical procedures • Undue susceptibility to aspiration and subsequent aspiration pneumonia due to poor head and neck positioning in bed	• Patient will be able to reposition self and will have safe interface pressure measurements over all bony prominences in all positions by 5 PM today. • Patient will be safe from pressure ulceration for the duration of this admission. • Patient will be free from hip dislocation during this admission. • Patient will be safe from aspiration and aspiration pneumonia during this admission.	• Equip with pressure-reducing and firmly supportive mattress overlay and a 30-degree positioning wedge and to use under one side of the buttocks to relieve pressure over the sacrum in supine • Utilize the same wedge to achieve 30-degree and 150-degree side-lying to reduce interface pressure on the lateral trochanters and to enable patient to tolerate the side-lying position. Use the wedge to support the hips and trunk in side-lying. • Provide with an abduction wedge or knee extension splints to prevent the hips from flexing beyond 90 degrees • Fit with heel boots that reduce or eliminate the interface pressure over the posterior heels • Examine carefully the effectiveness of the heel boots and verify that the interface pressures are safe by placing the pressure sensor inside the boot, over the posterior heel, and then measure the interface pressure. Interface pressure should be 0–20 mm Hg. Verify interface pressures are safe by inspecting the skin after 2 hrs in one position with the boot in place. • Assess the interface pressure measurements over all bony prominences in all positions. Interface pressure readings should be 20–30 mm Hg. • Examine skin over bony prominences over time to verify that the support surface and positioning techniques are working effectively • Position patient's head and neck in a chin-tuck position for safe deglutition and swallowing • Consult with a speech/language pathologist to verify safe position for feeding and swallowing	• Patient has been safe from pressure ulceration and is able to reposition self. • Patient tolerates 30-degree and 150-degree side-lying for 2-hr periods. • Patient's hips did not dislocate during this admission. • Patient did not aspirate or develop aspiration pneumonia during this admission.

TABLE 27A.7 Thoracic Kyphosis (Recumbent Position)

Medical diagnoses	Examination/evaluation	Functional diagnoses	Prognoses	Interventions	Outcomes
Thoracic kyphosis, fixed	Patient has a fixed thoracic kyphosis. Preferred position is side-lying due to stated pain in back when supine. Patient has standard hospital mattress. Interface pressure is 100 mm Hg over lateral trochanters in full side-lying and considered unsafe, as patient is immobile and has a Braden score of 12.	• Undue susceptibility to pressure ulceration due to risk factors of immobility, unsafe interface pressures, and limited positions • Undue susceptibility to increasing the severity of the thoracic curve due to poor positioning in bed	• Patient will have safe interface pressures over all bony prominences in all positions in bed by 5 PM tomorrow. • Patient will tolerate 30-degree and 150-degree side-lying and supine positioning for 2-hr intervals in 2 wks.	• Replace the hospital mattress with a dynamic, nonpowered, air/foam combination mattress replacement that will accommodate for the kyphosis and provide for safe interface pressures • Assess the interface pressure measurements over all bony prominences in all positions. Interface pressures should be 20–30 mm Hg • Fit with a 30-degree positioning wedge to support the trunk and hips in 30-degree and 150-degree side-lying • Support the hips and knees with the wedge in supine to reduce the stress on the spine and give support to the lower extremities • Gradually increase the time spent in supine, as tolerance increases	• Patient has remained free from pressure ulcer development. • Patient tolerates 30-degree and 150-degree side-lying and supine positioning in bed for 2-hr intervals with no stated pain.

TABLE 27A.8   Above-the-Knee Amputation (Recumbent Position)

Medical diagnoses	Examination/evaluation	Functional diagnoses	Prognoses	Interventions	Outcomes
Left, above-the-knee amputation, secondary to peripheral vascular disease	Patient is unable to move and change positions due to fear and the instability of the water mattress overlay. Patient requires maximal assistance of one to sit on the edge of the bed and transfer to the wheelchair, due to the instability of the water and the patient's fear of falling. Interface pressure measurements over the lateral trochanters in full side-lying and over the sacrum in supine are 125 mm Hg and 80 mm Hg, respectively, and are considered unsafe due to Braden score of 12. Interface pressure measurement of the right posterior heel is 75 mm Hg and is considered unsafe due to the peripheral vascular disease present and the other risk factors.	• Undue susceptibility to pressure ulcer development on the sacrum, lateral trochanters, and right posterior heel due to Braden score of 12 and peripheral vascular disease • Inability to perform position changes and transfers due to instability of the mattress overlay and patient's fear of falling	• Interface pressure will be either eliminated or under 20 mm Hg over all bony prominences in all positions by 5 PM today. • Patient will be independent in all position changes and transfers in 1 mo.	• Replace the mattress with a dynamic, non-powered air/foam mattress replacement that will not only provide a more stable surface for position changes and transfers, but will provide interface pressures lower than 20 mm Hg over all bony prominences in all positions • Fit with heel boot that will eliminate interface pressure over the posterior heel • Utilize a 30-degree wedge to assist in achieving and maintaining the 30-degree and 150-degree side-lying positions; utilize same wedge to position under one buttock to achieve pressure elimination over the sacrum in supine	• Patient has remained free from pressure ulceration during this admission. • Patient is independent in all position changes and transfers. • Braden score has improved by 4 points, which changes the risk status from high to low.

TABLE 27A.9 Bilateral, Above-the-Knee Amputations (Recumbent Position)

Medical diagnoses	Examination/evaluation	Functional diagnoses	Prognoses	Interventions	Outcomes
Bilateral, above-the-knee amputations, secondary to peripheral vascular disease	Patient is dependent in all position changes and transfers due to instability of existing alternating air mattress overlay, poor sitting balance, and trunk muscle weakness. Patient cannot sit on the edge of the bed, without maximal assistance, due to the instability of the mattress overlay, poor sitting balance and trunk musculature weakness. Patient has been on existing alternating air mattress overlay for 1 mo and has no history of skin breakdown. Patient is spending 22 hrs per day in bed. Braden score is 10, which is considered high risk for pressure ulceration. Patient has a spiky-bony skeletal structure. Interface pressures over all bony prominences in all positions range from 20 to 30 mm Hg. Facility is renting current mattress overlay and now wishes to purchase the appropriate support surface for this patient. Considerations for the selection of a new bed support surface include the need for maximum pressure distribution away from the bony prominences due to the high-risk status and the spiky-bony skeletal structure, as well as the need for increased bed surface stability to facilitate mobility in position changes and transfers in bed. Preferred position is right side-lying to view the television.	• Inability to reposition self and perform bed-to-chair transfers due to the instability of the mattress, poor sitting balance and trunk muscle weakness • Undue susceptibility to pressure ulceration due to Braden score of 10, as well as preferred position and time spent in bed	• Patient will be independent in all position changes and transfers in 2 mos. • Patient will remain free of pressure ulcers for the next 90 days. • Patient will decrease time spent in bed from 22 hrs to 14 hrs in 2 mos.	• Fit patient with a non-powered, dynamic mattress replacement that is a combination air cylinder with a foam topper mattress. This mattress replacement will provide the stability for position changes and transfers and also will provide the safe interface pressures over all bony prominences in all positions. • Instruct and work with the patient on position changes and transfers, with the new mattress replacement • Equip patient with wedge cushion to facilitate 30-degree and 150-degree side-lying positions • Assess interface pressure measurements over all bony prominences in all positions. Interface pressure should be 20–30 mm Hg. • Examine and evaluate patient's skin condition after weight bearing on bony prominences, just after off-loading to assess for any signs of excessive interface pressure, shearing, friction, or moisture • Provide therapeutic positioning for the wheelchair; increase time out of bed	• Patient is independent in all position changes and transfers. • Braden score has improved by 4 points, which changes the risk status from high to low. • Interface pressure over all bony prominences in all positions is less than 30 mm Hg and is considered safe. • Patient has remained free from pressure ulcer development over the last 90 days. • Patient utilizes the following positions in bed: supine and left and right, 30-degree and 150-degree side-lying.

TABLE 27A.10 Hip and Knee Flexion Contractures (Recumbent Position)

Medical diagnoses	Examination/evaluation	Functional diagnoses	Prognoses	Interventions	Outcomes
Hip and knee flexion contractures	Due to hip and knee flexion contractures, the patient's preferred position is right side-lying, with hips and knees flexed past 90 degrees, with heels touching the buttocks. The Braden score is 11, indicating high risk for pressure ulceration. The patient is on a standard hospital mattress, and interface pressures over the right trochanter, shoulder, malleolus, and fifth metatarsal range from 75 to 110 mm Hg. This indicates that the mattress is ineffective in pressure distribution. The medial femoral condyles and the medial malleoli and first metatarsal heads are in contact and interface pressure ranges from 50 to 80 mm Hg, which is considered unsafe, due to high-risk status. Patient cannot be positioned supine; therefore, cannot be positioned safely for accessing food on the over-the-bed table. The head and neck are in an unsafe position for deglutition and swallowing, and the patient chokes with each bite of food or drink of liquid. The patient is immobile and unable to change positions or assist in transfers.	• Inability to achieve functional hip and knee extension, in supine and side-lying in bed, due to impairment in hip and knee joint integrity • Undue susceptibility to increasing the severity of the hip and knee flexion contractures • Undue susceptibility to necrosis of the lower leg secondary to vascular occlusion subsequent to severe hip and knee flexion contractures • Undue susceptibility to pressure ulceration, due to risk factors, inadequate positioning, and an ineffective bed support surface • Inability to self-feed • Undue susceptibility to aspiration and the development of aspiration pneumonia • Inability to change positions or assist in transfers	• Patient will be positioned in supine and 30-degree side-lying and achieve maximal hip and knee extension, within the joint impairment limitations, in 2 wks. • Patient will maintain hip and knee extension range-of-motion measurements for the next 90 days. • Patient will remain free of pressure ulcers for the next 90 days. • Patient will self-feed with supervision and verbal cues in 2 wks. • Patient will be free from aspiration and aspiration pneumonia for the next 90 days. • Patient will assist in position changes and transfers in 1 mo.	• Measure and fit with a custom-fitted, foam, contoured bed/leg cushion that facilitates the extension available in each hip and knee; eliminates interface pressure over the posterior heels; and protects the medial condyles, medial malleoli, and feet from any contact or weight bearing in supine and side-lying • Fit with a mattress replacement that provides for interface pressures of under 30 mm Hg over all bony prominences in all positions • Use 30-degree wedge to achieve 30-degree side-lying position and to achieve interface pressure elimination over the sacrum in supine • Refer to occupational therapist for work on self-feeding • Equip with a head cushion to achieve a head and neck position conducive to safe deglutition and swallowing; consult a speech/language pathologist • Instruct and practice in position changes and transfers	• Patient tolerates positioning in supine and side-lying, with maximal hip and knee extension available within the range-of-motion limitations, for 2 hrs each position. • Hip and knee extension remained unchanged for the past 90 days. • Patient has been free of pressure ulcers for the past 90 days. • Patient has been referred to occupational therapy for work on self-feeding. • Patient has been referred to speech/language pathology and is scheduled for a video swallow evaluation. • Patient is assisting in rolling side-to-side and in wheelchair-to-bed transfers.

TABLE 27A.11 Medically Complex Patient Example and Cost Study (Seated Position)

Medical diagnoses	Examination/evaluation	Functional diagnoses	Prognoses	Interventions/cost of equipment	Outcomes
CVA, old hip fracture, incontinence, depression, dysphagia, tube-fed, chronic GERD, CHF, HTN, CAD, aspiration pneumonia, low back pain, seizures	Patient presents as a recent admission to the nursing facility, with a right CVA, onset 3 wks ago, with left hemiplegia and severe left neglect syndrome. Since the CVA, patient had two seizures in the hospital, but has been controlled with medications and has had no seizures for the past 2 wks. Patient has no awareness of the left side of her body and has left visual field impairment. Patient is dependent in all position changes, transfers, and ADLs. Sitting balance is poor, and she is unable to sit unsupported. No righting or equilibrium reactions are present. She cannot stand without maximal assistance of two. Urge and functional urinary incontinence is present, and she is constantly wet.	• Undue susceptibility to injury of left extremities due to lack of awareness, lack of sensory and kinesthetic sensation on the left side, and visual field deficit • Impaired mobility and inability to perform ADLs • Inability to perform position changes and transfers • Inability to control urine output due to functional limitations and urge incontinence • Inability to control fecal output due to functional limitations and impaired sensation • Undue susceptibility of aspiration due to impaired sensation and function of the swallowing musculature, as well as unsafe positioning in the wheelchair and bed	• Patient will be free from injury for the next 30 days. • In 1 mo, patient will self-propel wheelchair for functional distances, with right extremities, requiring only verbal cues to compensate for visual field impairment. • Patient will be able to perform upper-body dressing and personal hygiene activities with moderate verbal and manual cueing in 1 wk. • Patient will perform position changes and transfers, requiring verbal and manual cues and moderate assistance of one person, in 2 wks. • Patient will be dry at night in 1 wk. • Patient will be dry during the day, 50% of the time, in 2 wks. • Patient will be continent of bowel in 1 wk.	• Refer to physical therapy to determine appropriate size wheelchair. Utilize the following accessories: extended brake handles, removable foot-rests, and a seat height that is 2 in. less than the patient's back-of-the-knee to-the-floor measurement (Hemi or Super Hemi wheelchair), with seat cushion in place, to facilitate wheelchair propulsion with right extremities. • Secure rental wheelchair (cost: $125/mo, rental; 2 mos rental while on part A is $250) • Fit with left slide-away lap tray to support and protect the left upper extremity (cost: $190) • Fit with reclining back, with head support to accommodate for the hip flexion impairment and to support the head and neck in a safe position for deglutition and swallowing (cost: $550)	• Patient has been free of injury of left extremities for the past 30 days. • Patient can self-propel wheelchair independently throughout the facility, utilizing right extremities. • Patient is able to perform upperbody dressing and personal hygiene activities with supervision and verbal cues. • Patient can perform position changes and transfers, requiring only supervision and verbal cues. • Patient is dry at night 90% of the time.

continued

She is also incontinent of bowel. Patient has a history of dysphagia, aspiration pneumonia, and GERD and is currently being tube-fed. Braden score is 9, indicating high risk for pressure ulceration. She has a history of old left hip fracture with internal fixation. Hip flexion range of motion is limited to 75 degrees, indicating a need to accommodate for this fixed deformity with the seat cushion and a reclined back for the wheelchair. Interface pressures were examined over all bony prominences, in all positions, and are as follows: 120 mm Hg over the right ischial tuberosity, 40 mm Hg over the left ischial tuberosity, and 65 mm Hg over the sacrum and coccyx.

- Inability to feed self secondary to poor positioning in the wheelchair, related to lack of stabilization of the pelvis and trunk
- Undue susceptibility to pressure ulceration related to sensory impairment, incontinence, immobility, nutritional status, and unsafe interface pressures over the right ischial tuberosity, sacrum, and coccyx
- Undue susceptibility to injuries related to falls from wheelchair
- Inability to maintain upright position in wheelchair due to joint integrity impairment of right hip and impaired balance and kinesthetic sense
- Impaired sitting tolerance related to poor positioning and back pain

- Patient will be free of aspiration pneumonia for the next 30 days.
- Patient will be referred in 1 wk to speech/language pathologist for a video swallow evaluation at the hospital and intervention in deglutition and swallowing.
- Patient will be positioned in the wheelchair so that the head and neck are in a safe position for deglutition and swallowing by today at 5 PM.
- Patient will be positioned in the wheelchair so that accessing the dining table and food are possible by tomorrow at 5 PM.
- Patient will self-feed finger foods in 2 wks.
- Patient will be free of pressure ulceration for the next 30 days.
- Braden score will improve from a score of 9 to a score of 15 in 30 days, which shifts the pressure ulcer risk from high to low.

- Consult with speech/language pathologist for the appropriate food and liquid consistencies and the appropriate position of the head and neck for safe deglutition and swallowing
- Coordinate with dietary, nursing, occupational therapy, and physical therapy to establish and eliminate the bladder irritants and the functional barriers to urinary and fecal continence and to discover urge suppression techniques (supply cost: $100)
- Use appropriate incontinence containment devices (cost: $100 per mo, 2-mo supply = $200)
- Protect the patient's skin from urine and feces with a perineal cleanser, moisturizer, and skin barrier after each incontinent episode (cost: $60 per mo, 2-mo supply = $120)
- Secure a video swallow evaluation at the hospital in coordination with speech/language pathologist
- Fit with seat cushion that eliminates the pressure on the ischial tuberosities and stabilizes the pelvis (cost: $300)

- Patient is continent of urine 75% of the time, during the day, and has improved from using eight pads per day to using two pads per day.
- Patient is continent of bowel.
- Patient has had no episodes of aspiration pneumonia during the last 30 days.

Medical diagnoses	Examination/evaluation	Functional diagnoses	Prognoses	Interventions/cost of equipment	Outcomes
	These readings are considered unsafe because of the Braden score. The high interface readings over the coccyx and right ischial tuberosity are the result of her sliding forward and to the right to self-accommodate for the limited hip flexion. Because this has not been accommodated for in the past, she has developed back pain that has made her sitting tolerance very limited. She is currently sitting for 30 mins, twice per day, and in bed 23 hrs of the day. Her positioning in the wheelchair is characterized by a hips-forward position with a severe lean to the right and a constant gaze to the right. The nursing assistants must constantly reposition her in the wheelchair to keep her from falling on the floor. Her endurance is poor, and she has situational depression.		• Patient will be safe from injuries related to falls from the wheelchair for the next 30 days. • Patient will maintain a position in the wheelchair characterized by the following: hips back on the seat, face vertical, hip flexion impairment accommodated, and left extremities protected from injury by 5 PM tomorrow. • Sitting tolerance will improve from 30 mins twice per day to 2 hrs, three times per day, coordinated with meal times, within 30 days.	• Fit with a padded positioning hip belt that assists in maintaining the hips back on the seat, while the patient self-propels the wheelchair (cost: $40) • Refer to occupational therapist for instruction and practice in self-feeding and ADLs • Instruct patient, caregivers, and family in the techniques to utilize in position changes, transfers, self-care activities, and in care and utilization of the equipment • Increase the sitting time gradually, as the patient's endurance, strength, and tolerance increases • Total cost (seated): $1,900	

ADLs = activities of daily living; CAD = coronary artery disease; CHF = congestive heart failure; CVA = cardiovascular accident; GERD = gastric esophageal reflux disease; HTN = hypertension.

TABLE 27A.12   Medically Complex Patient Example and Cost Study (Recumbent Position)

Medical diagnoses	Examination/evaluation	Functional diagnoses	Prognoses	Interventions/cost of equipment	Outcomes
CVA, old hip fracture, incontinence, depression, dysphagia, tube-fed, chronic GERD, CHF, HTN, CAD, aspiration pneumonia, low back pain, seizures	The patient has no awareness of the left side of her body and has left visual field impairment. There is a risk of injury to the left extremities due to total lack of awareness. This danger is especially high when she is being repositioned or when she begins to be more mobile. She is immobile and dependent in all position changes. The supine position facilitates extensor tone in the cervical and trunk extensor musculature, as well as in the hip extensor and adductor musculature. Extensor tone dominates in the Fowler's position as well, causing the head and neck to be in an unsafe position for deglutition and swallowing. The head of the bed should be elevated 45 degrees due to tube feeding and GERD. A slight flex in the hips and knees and a firm head cushion inhibits the extensor tone. Braden score is 9, placing patient at high risk for pressure ulceration.	•Undue susceptibility to injury related to impaired sensation, proprioception, kinesthetic sense, and visual field impairment •Inability to position change and reposition self due to impaired volitional movement of left side of body, presence of abnormal muscle tone, and lack of sensation, kinesthesia, and proprioception •Undue susceptibility to aspiration due to poor head and neck positioning and known dysphagia •Inability to achieve ideal supine position due to extensor tone domination •Undue susceptibility to pressure ulcer development •Inability to tolerate full side-lying	•Patient will be free of injury related to trauma to left extremities for the next 30 days. •Patient will reposition self in bed, independently, in 60 days. •Patient will have an effective mattress replacement and interface pressures of less than 30 mm Hg over all bony prominences in all positions, by 5 PM today. •Patient will tolerate the Fowler's position and 30-degree and 150-degree side-lying in 1 wk. •Patient will be positioned in bed with the head and neck in a slight chin-tuck position by 5 PM today. •Patient will be free of aspiration pneumonia for the next 60 days.	•Fit with side rail covers, bolsters, or pillows to support and protect the left extremities (cost: $75) •Utilize pillow between the lower extremities in side-lying to support and prevent one extremity from weight bearing on the other •Instruct and practice in position changes and transfers •Refer to speech/language pathologist to determine safe position of the head and neck for safe swallowing; fit with a firm head cushion to inhibit extensor tone and to facilitate a safe swallow (cost: $55) •Fit with heel boots that eliminate interface pressure over posterior heels; the Lunax boot is appropriate when the patient must use the boots for ambulation; Heellift boots are appropriate for use in bed or the wheelchair; examine and evaluate the interface pressures on the posterior heel or any other bony prominence inside the boot to assure effectiveness; interface pressure should be 0–20 mm Hg (cost: $106 and $95, per pair, respectively) •Fit with 30-degree wedge cushion to utilize in supine to place under the knees to inhibit extensor tone and to utilize in 30-degree and 150-degree side-lying (cost: $68)	•Patient has been free from injury for 60 days. •Patient has been free from pressure ulceration. •Patient is independent in position changes, in bed, using the side rails. •Patient is positioned safely in bed with a slight chin-tuck position for the head and neck. •She has had no reported instances of aspiration pneumonia. •Patient is positioned in bed in the Fowler's position with ideal body alignment.

continued

Medical diagnoses	Examination/evaluation	Functional diagnoses	Prognoses	Interventions/cost of equipment	Outcomes
	She is currently on a 2-in. soft foam mattress overlay. The interface pressures, in supine, over the sacrum, coccyx, and posterior heels range from 80 to 100 mm Hg, which are considered unsafe due to Braden score. She has a spiky-bony skeletal structure. In full side-lying the interface pressures over the lateral trochanters and shoulders range from 100 mm Hg to 150 mm Hg, which are considered unsafe. Due to the high-risk status for pressure ulceration and the high interface pressures, this patient is in eminent danger of pressure ulcer development.	• Inability to access available visual field due to the placement of the bed in the room • Undue susceptibility to agitation, anger, fear, and combative behavior due to patient's inability to appropriately interact with her environment	• Patient will be supine-positioned with the head of the bed elevated 45 degrees, head and neck slightly flexed and in midline, trunk in midline, and hips and knees slightly flexed. • Patient will be free of pressure ulceration for the next 60 days. • Patient's bed will be repositioned so that she can access her available visual field by 5 PM today. • Patient will be less fearful and more interactive and cooperative with family and caregivers.	• Fit with a mattress replacement that is nonpowered but dynamic, has air cylinders and foam topper for stability, has a firm foam edge for sitting stability, and adjusts to the patient's movement (cost: $1,080) • Reposition patient's bed so that she can access her available visual field • Refer to occupational therapist to begin work on assisting patient in learning to compensate for the visual field deficit • Gradually increase time out of bed after wheelchair is adapted for patient • Total cost (recumbent position): $1,384	• Patient has an effective mattress replacement for both safe pressure distribution and facilitation of independence in bed mobility. • She tolerates supine, 30-degree and 150-degree side-lying for 2-hr intervals with no signs of excessive interface pressure or discomfort. • She can now access visual field and interact with her environment in her room, since the repositioning of her bed in the room.

An effective support must be secured today. Because part of her intervention is working on position changes and transfers, a support surface is needed that not only decreases interface pressure, but also provides sufficient stability to facilitate independence in position will also provide a firm edge for sitting balance for performing ADLs and for sit-to-stand position changes. Because of the visual field impairments and the position of the bed in the room, the patient's visual field is limited to the wall. She is in bed 23 hrs per day due to a very limited sitting tolerance due to back pain, weakness, and poor endurance.

• Patient's behavior has improved from being characterized as combative and uncooperative to being characterized as cheerful, cooperative, and fully participatory in her care and therapy program.

ADLs = activities of daily living; CAD = coronary artery disease; CHF = congestive heart failure; CVA = cardiovascular accident; GERD = gastric esophageal reflux disease; HTN = hypertension.

APPENDIX 27.2 Therapeutic Positioning Suppliers

- Heellift® suspension boot to eliminate pressure over the posterior heel (DM Systems, Inc., ground floor, 1316 Sherman Avenue, Evanston, IL 60201; 800-254-5438)
- Lunax Boot™ eliminates pressure over the posterior heel and is safe for ambulation (Lunax Boot, PO Box 214725, Auburn Hills, MI 48304; 800-355-8629)
- Body Aligner to assist with three-quarter side-lying and to eliminate pressure over the sacrum in supine by placing under one side of the buttocks (Positioning Solutions™, 660 Southpointe Court, Suite 100, Colorado Springs, CO 80906; 800-701-9173)
- Geo-Matt® 30° Body Wedge to assist with three-quarters side-lying and to eliminate pressure over the sacrum in supine by placing under one side of the buttocks (Span-America Medical Systems, Inc., PO Box 5231, Greenville, SC 29606; 800-888-6752)
- Cradle Boot to eliminate pressure over the posterior heel (Span-America Medical Systems, Inc., PO Box 5231, Greenville, SC 29606; 800-888-6752)
- Foot Drop Stop (Span-America Medical Systems, Inc., PO Box 5231, Greenville, SC 29606; 800-888-6752)
- BedLeg™ Positioning Cushion for use when knee flexion contractures are present to accommodate for the contractures, make supine positioning possible, inhibit flexor tone, prevent further contracture development, and eliminate pressure over the posterior heels (Positioning Solutions™, 660 Southpointe Court, Suite 100, Colorado Springs, CO 80906; 800-701-9173)
- Foot pedal covers that cover and pad the foot pedals to protect the feet and lower leg from trauma (Positioning Solutions™, 660 Southpointe Court, Suite 100, Colorado Springs, CO 80906; 800-701-9173)
- Hinge covers that cover and pad the elevating footrest hinge to protect the head of the fibula from pressure and trauma (Positioning Solutions™, 660 Southpointe Court, Suite 100, Colorado Springs, CO 80906; 800-701-9173)
- Pressore™ Monitor is a hand-held, single-pad sensor, interface pressure evaluator to objectively measure interface pressure over any bony prominence in any position; with choice of large or small sensor to correlate with size of bony prominence to be measured (Cleveland Medical Devices, Inc., 11000 Cedar Avenue, Suite 130, Cleveland, OH 44106, 877-253-8363)
- Pressure elimination seat cushion, Isch-Dish™ (Span-America Medical Systems, Inc., PO Box 5231, Greenville, SC 29606; 800-888-6752)
- Wheelchair and bed positioning supplies (Positioning Solutions™, 660 Southpointe Court, Suite 100, Colorado Springs, CO 80906; 800-701-9173)
- Pressure elimination back cushion, Sacral Dish™ (Span-America Medical Systems, Inc., PO Box 5231, Greenville, SC 29606; 800-888-6752)
- Positioning Hip Belts to keep the hips from sliding forward on the seat cushion (Positioning Solutions™, 660 Southpointe Court, Suite 100, Colorado Springs, CO 80906; 800-701-9173)

- Mattress overlay, Geo-Matt® Overlay (Span-America Medical Systems, Inc., PO Box 5231, Greenville, SC 29606; 800-888-6752)
- Static therapeutic mattress replacement, PressureGuard® Renew™ (Span-America Medical Systems, Inc., PO Box 5231, Greenville, SC 29606; 800-888-6752)
- Dynamic, powered mattress replacement, PressureGuard® APM (Span-America Medical Systems, Inc., PO Box 5231, Greenville, SC 29606; 800-888-6752)
- Dynamic, nonpowered mattress replacement, PressureGuard® CFT™ (Span-America Medical Systems, Inc., PO Box 5231, Greenville, SC 29606; 800-888-6752)
- Rotational surface to be utilized when a patient cannot turn due to pain or other medical conditions, PressureGuard® Turn Select™ (Span-America Medical Systems, Inc., PO Box 5231, Greenville, SC 29606; 800-888-6752)
- Drop Back to accommodate for inadequate hip flexion, trunk weakness, or fixed thoracic kyphosis (Positioning Solutions™, 660 Southpointe Court, Suite 100, Colorado Springs, CO 80906; 800-701-9173)
- Adjustable calf and footrest support to accommodate for knee flexion contractures, inhibit knee flexor tone, and to support and protect the posterior lower legs and feet, Foot Rest/Calf Support Combo (Positioning Solutions™, 660 Southpointe Court, Suite 100, Colorado Springs, CO 80906; 800-701-9173)
- Slide-Away Lap Tray™ to support one upper extremity and easily slide away to the side for ease in transfers, (Positioning Solutions™, 660 Southpointe Court, Suite 100, Colorado Springs, CO 80906; 800-701-9173)
- Drop Back with Adjustable Head Support to accommodate for inadequate hip flexion, trunk weakness, or fixed thoracic kyphosis and support the head and neck at the appropriate angle for safe swallowing and deglutition (Positioning Solutions™, 660 Southpointe Court, Suite 100, Colorado Springs, CO 80906; 800-701-9173)
- Drop Seat to decrease the distance from the seat to the floor (Positioning Solutions™, 660 Southpointe Court, Suite 100, Colorado Springs, CO 80906; 800-701-9173)
- Transparent liquid cyanoacrylate film skin protectant to protect wounds that are in the maturation phase of healing and to protect skin from friction and moisture, Liquishield™ (Medlogic Global Corporation, 4815 List Drive, Colorado Springs, CO 80919, 800-475-0173)
- Wheelchair and bed positioning supplies (Smith & Nephew, Inc., Rehabilitation Division, One Quality Drive, PO Box 1005, Germantown WI 53022-8205; www.easy-living.com)
- Wheelchair and bed positioning supplies (North Coast Medical, 18305 Sutter Boulevard, Morgan Hill, CA 95037; 800-821-9319, Fax: 877-213-9300; www.ncmedical.com)
- Wheelchair and bed positioning supplies (Sammons® Preston, PO Box 5071, Bolingbrook, IL 60440; 800-323-5547, Fax: 800-547-4333, www.sammonspreston.com)

- Wheelchair and bed positioning supplies (AliMed® Inc., 297 High Street, Dedham, MA 02026; 800-225-2610, Fax: 800-437-2966; www.alimed.com)
- Wheelchair and bed positioning supplies (Skil-Care™, 29 Wells Avenue, Yonkers, NY 10701; 800-431-2972, Fax: 914-963-2567)
- Braden scale (for predicting pressure ulcer risk) and other health care forms and products (Briggs Corporation, PO Box 1698, Des Moines, IA 50306; 800-247-2343, Fax: 800-222-1996; www.BriggsCorp.com)
- Wheelchairs, wheelchair accessories, and positioning supplies (Otto Bock™ Rehab, 3000 Xenium Lane North, Minneapolis, MN 55441; 800-328-4058, Fax: 800-962-2549)
- Roho wheelchair cushions and other positioning supplies (Crown Therapeutics, Inc., 100 Florida Avenue, Belleville, IL 62221; 800-851-3449, Fax: 618-277-6518)
- Wheelchair cushions and other positioning supplies and equipment (Jay Medical, Ltd., Jay a Division of Sunrise Medical, PO Box 18656, Boulder, CO 80308; 800-648-8282)
- Custom molded seating systems (Signature 2000, 489 W. Exchange Street, Akron, OH 44302; 800-227-2152, Fax: 330-376-9723)
- Custom molded seating systems (PinDot, Invacare, 800-333-6900)

Index

Note: page numbers followed by *f* indicate figures; page numbers followed by *t* indicate tables.

Bethanechol chloride, for overflow incontinence due to impaired detrusor contractility, 275, 275t

Bilateral above-the-knee amputation, therapeutic positioning for, seated, examples of, 471t

Bilateral total hips, therapeutic positioning for recumbent, examples of, 473t
    seated position, examples of, 468t

Bilirubin, urine, in urinalysis, 164t, 168

Bimanual examination, in examination of female genitalia in incontinence assessment, 78–79

Biofeedback therapy
    in involuntary detrusor contractions, 264–265
    in wound care pain management, 394–395

Bladder
    function of, 27
    neurologic modulation of, 29–34, 30f, 32f, 33f
        afferent sensory pathways in, 29–31, 30f
        sensation in, pathologic changes in, 132
        uninhibited, 262
    urinary, anatomy of, 18–20, 19f, 20f

Bladder accommodation, pathologic changes in, 132–133

Bladder augmentation, for instability incontinence, 252t, 255, 256f–258f

Bladder body, 19, 19f

Bladder capacity, pathologic changes in, 131–132, 132t

Bladder contractility, pathologic changes in, 133, 134f, 134t

Bladder function, evaluation of, CMG in, 126, 128–131, 129f–131f

Bladder instability
    idiopathic, involuntary detrusor contractions caused by, 262
    pathologic changes in, 133, 134f, 134t

Bladder irritants, elimination of, in involuntary detrusor contractions, 264

Bladder outlet obstruction, 220
    benign prostatic hypertrophy and, 277
    features of, 278
    gender predilection for, 269
    involuntary detrusor contractions caused by, 261–262

Bladder stability, pathologic changes in, 133, 134f, 134t

Bladder voiding patterns, in incontinence assessment, 47–48

Bladder wall, inflammation of, involuntary detrusor contractions caused by, 262

Blood, urine, in urinalysis, 164t, 167

Blood glucose, serum fasting, in genitourinary disorders, 187

Blood supply, to kidney, 5–6, 7f, 8f

Blood urea nitrogen (BUN), in genitourinary disorders, 187–188

Blood vessels, 327

Body loading, types of, 343–344

Body temperature, as factor in skin wounds, 345

Bone pain, prostate cancer–related, 313–316, 316t

Braden scale, in pressure ulcer assessment, 356, 357f

Brain, base of, arterial arrangement at, 52, 53f

Brain tumors, dysfunction due to, 54–55

Burn(s), pain associated with, 412

Calcium
    serum, in genitourinary disorders, 188
    urine, 24-hour, 178–179

Calcium stones, 197–199, 197t–199t
    diagnosis of, 197
    metabolic and clinical disorders with, 197, 198f
    treatment of, 197–198

Calculus(i), urine, laboratory assessment of, 201–202, 202t

Cancer, prostate, See Prostate cancer

Candidal rashes, in extraurethral incontinence, treatment of, 293

Capacity, defined, 130–131

Capillary(ies), glomerular, endothelium of, 9–10

Carbamazepine (Tegretol), in wound care pain management, 397–398

Caregiver education, pressure ulcer–related, 366–367

Carotid circulation ischemia, symptoms of, 54t

Catheter(s), indwelling
    in benign prostatic hypertrophy, 285
    in incontinence assessment, 49
    in stability incontinence, 255

Catheterization
    in benign prostatic hypertrophy, 280
    indwelling catheters in, for instability incontinence, 255
    intermittent. See Intermittent catheterization

Cauda equina syndrome
    patient history in, 271
    physical examination in, 272
CBC count. *See* Complete blood cell
        (CBC) count
Cerebral arteries, regions supplied by,
        52, 54f
Cerebral cortex, in voiding control,
        262
Cerebrovascular accident (CVA), void-
        ing dysfunction due to,
        52–53, 53f, 54f, 54t
Chemotaxis, defined, 181, 339
Chemotherapy, for prostate cancer,
        315–316, 316t
Chemstrip, in genitourinary disorders,
        160t, 162–164
Chloride
    in genitourinary disorders, 185
    urine, in 24-hour urine collection, 176
Chronic benign pain, opioids for, 399–
        407, 402t–404t
Chronic nonmalignant pain, opioids for,
        399–407, 402t–404t
Chronic renal failure (CRF), 210t,
        210–214, 213f
    amyloidosis and, 211
    causes of, 211
    course of, 211
    laboratory diagnosis of, 212–214, 213f
    management of, 214
    pathophysiology of, 211–212, 212t
Chronic urinary retention, defined, 220
Chronic wound pain experience,
        defined, 382
Clearance, defined, 177
Clonazepam (Klonopin), in wound care
        pain management, 398
Clonidine (Catapres), in wound care
        pain management, 399
CMG. *See* Cystometrogram (CMG)
Codeine, 402t
Cognition
    deficits in, functional incontinence
        due to, 297
        treatment of, 303–304
    evaluation of, in patient history and
        physical examination, 65
Colic, acute, presentation of, 195–196
Collagen, dermal, 325–326
Collecting system, anatomy of, 11–13, 13f
Color flow duplex imaging, in venous
        ulcer diagnosis, 376
Comparative tourniquet test, in venous
        ulcer diagnosis, 376
Complete blood cell (CBC) count
    defined, 179
    in genitourinary disorders, 179–184,
        179t, 180t, 181f

differential WBC count, 179t,
        180–182, 180t, 181f
    hematocrit, 179t, 183
    hemoglobin, 179t, 183–184
    mean corpuscular volume,
        179t, 184
    red blood cell count, 182–183
    white blood cell count, 179t, 180
Computed tomography (CT)
    in incontinence assessment, 104–105,
        105f, 106f
        clinical implications of, 105, 106f
        introduction to, 104, 105f
        procedure for, 104–105
    in overflow incontinence due to
        impaired detrusor contrac-
        tility, 274
Condom drainage, for instability incon-
        tinence, 252t, 253
    device for, 254–255
Constipation, opioid-related, 405
Containment devices, in incontinence
        assessment, 48–49
Continence
    drug effects on, 61, 62t
    management of, 1–317. *See also spe-
        cific problem and type of
        incontinence*
    urinary. *See* Urinary continence; Uri-
        nary incontinence
Continuous incontinence, 50–51
Contractility, detrusor, drug effects on,
        61
Contraction(s)
    detrusor
        impaired, overflow incontinence
            due to, 221–222
        involuntary
            incontinence due to, 219–220
            storage problems caused by,
                261–267
        uninhibited. *See* Involuntary detru-
            sor contractions
    wound, 342
Contracture(s), hip and knee flexion,
        therapeutic positioning for
    recumbent, examples of, 477t
    seated, examples of, 472t
Contrast agents, in radiography of uri-
        nary tract in incontinence
        assessment, 86
Controlled attention, in wound care
        pain management, 394
Corticosteroid(s), wound healing
        effects of, 349
Creatinine
    clearance, in 24-hour urine collec-
        tion, 177, 177t
    serum, in genitourinary disorders, 188

Genitalia—*continued*
    bimanual examination, 78–79
    pelvic examination, 79–80
    rectal examination, 79
    speculum examination, 77–78, 78f
    technique of examination, 74–77, 76f, 77f
  male
    anatomy of, 72–73
    physical examination of, in incontinence assessment
    anal and rectum examination, 72–73
    general examination, 71–73, 71f
    palpation, 72
Genitourinary disorders, urinary function in, laboratory assessment of, 159–191
Genitourinary infections, 193. *See also* Urinary tract infections
Genitourinary system, physical examination of, in incontinence assessment, 65–83
  abdominal examination, 66–69, 67f, 68f, 70f. *See also* Abdominal examination, in incontinence assessment
  female genitalia, 73–80, 74f–78f. *See also* Genitalia, female
  male genitalia, 71–73, 71f. *See also* Genitalia, male
  neurologic examination, 80–83
Gittes procedure, for stress incontinence with pelvic descent, 234
Glomerular capillaries, endothelium of, 9–10
Glomerular filtrate, 8, 10
Glomerulus
  anatomy of, 6, 8–10, 9f, 10f
  defined, 8
Glucose
  blood, serum fasting, in genitourinary disorders, 187
  urine
    in 24-hour urine collection, 175–176
    in urinalysis, 164t, 168
    urine dipstick in determination of, 160t, 163
Glucose tolerance test, in genitourinary disorders, 188–189
Glycosaminoglycan(s), 327
Grip strength, physical examination of, 81
Ground substance, 327

Hair follicles, 328–329
Head position instability, causes and treatment of, 444t

Health care team, role in therapeutic positioning, 425–429
Heels(s), pressure on, causes and treatment of, 445t
Hematocrit, in genitourinary disorders, 179t, 183
Hematuria, 209–210, 210t
  approach to patient with, 210
  causes of, 209, 210t
  diagnostic tests in, 209–210, 210t
  prevalence of, 209
  symptoms of, 209
Hemidesmosome(s), 324
Hemiparesis, spastic, gait abnormality due to, 81
Hemoglobin
  in genitourinary disorders, 179t, 183–184
  urine, in urinalysis, 164t, 167
  urine dipstick in determination of, 160t, 163
Hesitancy, urinary, 48
Hilum, renal, 3, 5f
Hip(s)
  adduction of, causes and treatment of, 444t
  bilateral total, therapeutic positioning for
    recumbent, examples of, 473t
    seated, examples of, 468t
  external rotation of, causes and treatment of, 444t
Hip and knee flexion contractures, therapeutic positioning for
  recumbent, examples of, 477t
  seated, examples of, 472t
Hip flexion, less than 90-degree, causes and treatment of, 444t
Hormonal therapy
  for benign prostatic hypertrophy, 286
  for prostate cancer, 315, 316t
Hyalin casts, urine, microscopic examination of, 169t, 170–171
Hydrocodone bitartrate, 402t
Hydromorphone hydrochloride, 403t
Hydronephrosis, 11, 13
Hydrotherapy, for pressure ulcers, 363
Hyperbaric oxygen therapy, for pressure ulcers, 363
Hypercalcemia, 197–199, 197t–199t
  causes of, 197–198, 198t
  diseases associated with, 178
  hypercalciuria not associated with, causes of, 197, 197t
  signs and symptoms of, 198, 199t
Hypercalciuria, 197–199, 197t–199t
  not associated with hypercalcemia, causes of, 197, 197t

Hyperextension, neck, causes and treatment of, 444t
Hyperkalemia, 186
Hyperparathyroidism, results of, 178
Hyperpigmentation, venous ulcer–related, 374
Hypnosis, distraction, in wound care pain management, 394
Hypodermis, 329
Hypokalemia, 186

Ice therapy, for pressure ulcers, 364
Imaging of urinary tract, in incontinence assessment, 85–115. *See also specific modality and* Urinary tract, imaging of, in incontinence assessment
Imipramine (Tofranil), for involuntary detrusor contractions, 266
Immune system
    effect on inflammatory response, 348
    in epidermal regulation, 331
Impaired detrusor contractility
    chronic, causes of, 269–270
    overflow incontinence due to, 269–276. *See also* Overflow incontinence, impaired detrusor contractility and
    transient, causes of, 269
Incontinence
    assessment of, 47–64, 63t. *See also specific assessment techniques;* Patient history, in incontinence assessment
        abdominal examination, 66–69, 67f, 68f, 70f
        cognition in, 65
        dexterity in, 66
        gait in, 66
        general survey, 65–66
        mobility in, 66
        patient history in, 47–64, 63t
        physical examination of genitourinary system, 65–83
        pudendal nerve conduction studies, 147–149, 148f
        skin in, 66
        transfer skills in, 66
        urinary tract imaging, 85–115
        urodynamic studies, 117–145
        vital signs in, 65–66
    continuous, 50–51
    defined, 217
    diagnosis for, 218
    extraurethral. *See also* Extraurethral incontinence, 221–222, 291–293

functional. *See* Functional incontinence
    instability, 50, 153t, 219, 247–260. *See also* Instability (reflex) incontinence
    involuntary detrusor contractions and, 219–220
    obstructive uropathy and, 220–221
    overflow. *See* Overflow incontinence
    patterns of, 49–52. *See also specific types*
    pudendal nerve conduction velocity studies in relation to, clinical use of, 149
    reflex, 50, 153t, 219, 247–260. *See also* Instability (reflex) incontinence
    sphincteric, 219
        causes of, 237
        defined, 237
        stress incontinence and, 237–246. *See also* Stress incontinence, sphincter incontinence and
        stress incontinence due to, 237–246
    stress. *See* Stress incontinence
    stress-urge, 232
    types of, 217–233. *See also specific types*
    uninhibited bladder, 50
        urodynamic and electrophysiologic features in, 153t
    urge, 50
        defined, 218
        in diabetes mellitus, 202–203
Indwelling catheter
    in benign prostatic hypertrophy, 285
    in incontinence assessment, 49
    in instability incontinence, 255
Infection(s), skin wounds due to, 344
Inflammation
    of bladder wall, involuntary detrusor contractions caused by, 262
    in inflammatory-exudative phase of wound healing, 337–338, 338f
Inspection, in abdominal examination in incontinence assessment, 67
Instability (reflex) incontinence, 50, 219, 247–260
    autonomic dysreflexia, associated with, 248–248
    causes of, 219
    complications of, 247–248
        prevention and management of, 252t, 253–254
    defined, 218
    diagnostic studies in, 249–252, 250f, 251f

Negative pressure with external application of vacuum, for pressure ulcers, 363–364
Neospinothalamic tract, 386
Nephron, anatomy of, 11, 12f
Nephropathy
    diabetic, 203
    obstructive, 221
Nephroscopy, in incontinence assessment, 112
Neurologic disorders, in incontinence assessment, 52–59, 53f, 54f, 54t, 57f
Neurologic examination
    in incontinence assessment, 80–83
        mental status, 80
        motor system, 80–82
        sensory system, 82
        speech, 80
        reflexes, 82–83
Neurologic lesions
    effect on micturition, 44
    involuntary detrusor contractions caused by, 262
Neuron(s), motor, lower, 34
Neuropathy(ies)
    autonomic, in incontinence assessment, 59
    peripheral
        electrodiagnostic studies in, 273
        in incontinence assessment, 59
        physical examination in, 271–272
Neuropsychological screening, in functional incontinence, 301
Neutropenia, 182
Neutrophil(s), 180–182, 180t, 181f
    function of, 181
    size of, 180, 181f
Neutrophil precursor cell, myeloblast, 180, 181f
Neutrophilia, defined, 181–182
Nicotine patches, skin wounds due to, 348
Nitrate, urine, urine dipstick in determination of, 160t, 163
Nonkeratinocyte cells, of epidermis, 323–327, 325f, 326f
Nonopioid analgesics, in wound care pain management, 396, 396t
Normal flow pattern, 119f, 120
Normal-pressure hydrocephalus, dysfunction due to, 55
Norton scale, in pressure ulcer assessment, 357, 357f
Nuclear imaging, in incontinence assessment, 108, 110–111, 110f
Nuclear magnetic resonance (NMR) imaging, defined, 106

Nursing professionals, role in therapeutic positioning, 428

Obstructive nephropathy, 221
Obstructive uropathy
    causes of, 220
    defined, 278
    incontinence due to, 220–221
Obtrusive flow pattern, 121–123, 123f
Occupational therapist, role in therapeutic positioning, 426–427
Occupational therapy, in wound care pain management, 392–393
Open prostatectomy, for benign prostatic hypertrophy, 288–290
Opioid(s), in wound care pain management, 399–407, 402t–404t
    addiction to, 400
    constipation due to, 405
    controversies related to, 399–400
    forms of, 400
    gastrointestinal effects of, 45, 406t
    mechanism of action of, 404
    morphine, 401
    nausea and vomiting due to, 405
    pharmacologic effects of, 401
    risks associated with, 400
    side effects of, 404–407, 406t
    types of, 402t–404t
Oral glucose tolerance test (OGTT)
    in diabetes mellitus, 203, 204t
    in genitourinary disorders, 188–189
Orchiectomy, for prostate cancer, 315, 316t
Osmolality, urine, in 24-hour urine collection, 174–175
Overflow incontinence, 51–52
    defined, 218
    gender predilection for, 269
    impaired detrusor contractility and, 269–276
        back imaging workup in, 274
        CT in, 274
        electrodiagnostic studies in, 273–274
        laboratory data in, 274
        MRI in, 274
        myelography in, 274
        patient history in, 270–271
        physical examination in, 271–272
        radiography in, 274
        treatment of, 274–276, 275t
            catheterization in, 276
            conservative, 274–275, 275t
            drugs in, 275–276, 275t
        urodynamic and electrophysiologic features in, 153t
        urodynamics in, 272–273